Metabolism and Nutrition

First and second edition authors:
Sarah Benyon
Jason O'Neale Roach

Third edition author:
Ming Yeong Lim

Fourth edition authors:
Amber Appleton
Olivia Vanbergen

5th Edition

CRASH COURSE

SERIES EDITORS

Philip Xiu
MA MB BChir MRCP
GP Registrar
Yorkshire Deanery
Leeds, UK

Shreelata Datta
MD MRCOG LLM BSc (Hons) MBBS
Honorary Senior Lecturer
Imperial College London,
Consultant Obstetrician and Gynaecologist
King's College Hospital
London, UK

FACULTY ADVISOR

Marek Dominiczak
dr hab med, FRCPATH
Hon. Professor of Clinical Biochemistry and Medical Humanities
University of Glasgow,
Consultant Biochemist
NHS Greater Glasgow and Clyde

Metabolism and Nutrition

Olivia Vanbergen
MA Oxon, MSc, MBBS (distinction)
Clinical fellow in anaesthesia at Hampshire hospitals,

Gareth Wintle
3rd year Biomedical science undergraduate
University of Reading
Berkshire, UK

For additional online content visit StudentConsult.com

ELSEVIER

ELSEVIER

Content Strategist: Jeremy Bowes
Content Development Specialist: Alexandra Mortimer
Project Manager: Andrew Riley
Design: Christian Bilbow
Illustration Manager: Karen Giacomucci
Illustrator: MPS North America LLC
Marketing Manager: Deborah Watkins

First edition 1998
Second edition 2003
Reprinted 2004
Third edition 2007
Fourth edition 2013
Updated Fourth edition 2015
Fifth edition 2019

ISBN: 978-0-7020-7341-0
eISBN: 978-0-7020-7342-7

your source for books,
journals and multimedia
in the health sciences

www.elsevierhealth.com

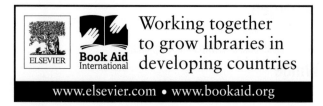

Working together
to grow libraries in
developing countries

www.elsevier.com • www.bookaid.org

The
publisher's
policy is to use
**paper manufactured
from sustainable forests**

Printed in Poland
Last digit is the print number: 9 8 7 6 5 4 3 2 1

Series Editors' foreword

The *Crash Course* series was conceived by Dr Dan Horton-Szar who as series editor presided over it for more than 15 years - from publication of the first edition in 1997, until publication of the fourth edition in 2011. His inspiration, knowledge and wisdom lives on in the pages of this book. As the new series editors, we are delighted to be able to continue developing each book for the twenty-first century undergraduate curriculum.

The flame of medicine never stands still, and keeping this all-new fifth series relevant for today's students is an ongoing process. Each title within this new fifth edition has been re-written to integrate basic medical science and clinical practice, after extensive deliberation and debate. We aim to build on the success of the previous titles by keeping the series up-to-date with current guidelines for best practice, and recent developments in medical research and pharmacology.

We always listen to feedback from our readers, through focus groups and student reviews of the *Crash Course* titles. For the fifth editions we have reviewed and re-written our self-assessment material to reflect today's 'single-best answer' and 'extended matching question' formats. The artwork and layout of the titles has also been largely re-worked and are now in colour, to make it easier on the eye during long sessions of revision. The new on-line materials supplement the learning process.

Despite fully revising the books with each edition, we hold fast to the principles on which we first developed the series. *Crash Course* will always bring you all the information you need to revise in compact, manageable volumes that still maintain the balance between clarity and conciseness, and provide sufficient depth for those aiming at distinction. The authors are junior doctors who have recent experience of the exams you are now facing, and the accuracy of the material is checked by a team of faculty editors from across the UK.

We wish you all the best for your future careers!

Philip Xiu and Shreelata Datta

Faculty advisor

The aim of this book, now in its 5th edition, remains unchanged: to help the readers pass their examination. It contains a large amount of basic and clinical knowledge in a remarkably concise form.

It covers what one would call the 'classic" biochemistry i.e. description of the main metabolic pathways, enzymes and key regulatory mechanisms, and then it links these to clinical topics, which cover clinical examination, history taking and interpretation of laboratory tests, all in relation to metabolic disease.

It highlights the topics important for a doctor, such as diabetes mellitus or thyroid disease. This edition contains more detailed account of the principal subjects related to nutrition, including biochemical mechanisms of appetite control and obesity. Many self-assessment questions are based on cases, which reflect the everyday clinical situations. As in previous editions, the Authors keep the exam in the reader's mind throughout, pointing out examiners' favorite topics.

This edition has again been extensively rewritten and updated. We carefully sought better ways of explaining complex subjects, and scrutinized clinical topics to ensure that they reflect current recommendations and practice.

It has been a great pleasure for me to work with Olivia Vanbergen and Gareth Wintle, and seeing the book take shape. The previous editions of the Crash Course have served students in the UK and beyond since 1998. I am convinced that the 5th edition will be even more sought after than the previous ones.

Marek Dominiczak

Acknowledgements

This book is dedicated to my son Jonathan, who is the light of my life. I hope it proves useful for those studying medicine, biology, nutrition or any discipline that demands a good understanding of the topics included. Professor Dominiczak has been a fantastic mentor as our faculty editor, and I'm also very grateful to Barbara and Alex for their professional expertise and support in writing this book. Please enjoy!

Olivia Vanbergen

I would like to thank Professor Dominiczak for his feedback and guidance during the writing of this book, as well as that from my co-author, Livvi. I am also extremely grateful to Dr's Renee Lee, Andrew Bicknell, and David Leake at the University of Reading for their support over the course of this project. It has been an incredible privilege to be involved in producing this book, and I truly hope that, wherever possible, it provides readers a suitable platform to help achieve academic success.

Gareth Wintle

Series Editors' acknowledgements

We would like to thank the support of our colleagues who have helped in the preparation of this edition, namely the junior doctor contributors who helped write the manuscript as well as the faculty editors who check the veracity of the information.

We are extremely grateful for the support of our publisher, Elsevier, whose staffs' insight and persistence has maintained the quality that Dr Horton-Szar has set-out since the first edition. Jeremy Bowes, our commissioning editor, have been a constant support. Alex Mortimer and Barbara Simmons our development editors have managed the day-to-day work on this edition with extreme patience and unflaggable determination to meet the ever looming deadlines, and we are ever grateful for Kim Benson's contribution to the online editions and additional online supplementary materials.

Philip Xiu and Shreelata Datta

Contents

Contents

Cellular biology

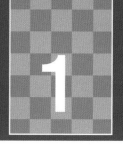

1

INTRODUCTION

This chapter is an overview of eukaryotic cells, addressing their intracellular organelles and structural components. A basic appreciation of cellular structure and function is important for an understanding of the following chapters' information concerning metabolism and nutrition. For further detailed information in this subject area, please refer to a reference textbook.

The eukaryotic cell

Humans are multicellular eukaryotic organisms. All eukaryotic organisms are composed of eukaryotic cells. Eukaryotic cells (Fig. 1.1) are defined by the following features:

- A membrane-limited nucleus (the key feature differentiating eukaryotic cells from prokaryotic cells) that contains the cell's genetic material.

- Specialized intracellular membrane-bound organelles (Fig. 1.2), such as mitochondria, Golgi apparatus, endoplasmic reticulum (ER).
- Large size (relative to prokaryotic cells).

EUKARYOTIC ORGANELLES

Nucleus

The nucleus is surrounded by a double membrane (nuclear envelope). The envelope has multiple pores to allow transit of material between the nucleus and the cytoplasm. The nucleus contains the cell's genetic material, DNA, organized into linear structures known as chromosomes. As well as chromosomes, irregular zones of densely staining material are also present. These are the nucleoli, which are

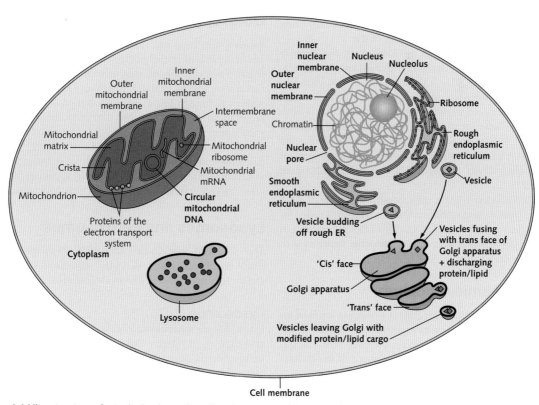

Fig. 1.1 Ultrastructure of a typical eukaryotic cell and structure of important intracellular organelles. *ER,* Endoplasmic reticulum.

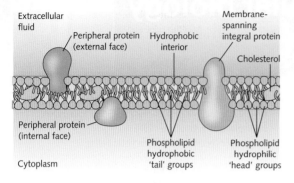

Extracellular fluid

Peripheral protein (external face)

Hydrophobic interior

Membrane-spanning integral protein

Cholesterol

Peripheral protein (internal face)

Cytoplasm

Phospholipid hydrophobic 'tail' groups

Phospholipid hydrophilic 'head' groups

Fig. 1.2 Cross-section of a typical cell membrane. Note the phospholipid bilayer membrane and integral and peripheral proteins.

responsible for ribosomal RNA (rRNA) synthesis and ribosome assembly. Messenger RNA (mRNA) synthesis (translation of genetic material; see Chapter 9) occurs within the nucleus. mRNA can then exit the nucleus via the nuclear pores into the cytoplasm.

Mitochondrion

The ultrastructure of a mitochondrion is illustrated in Fig. 1.2. Mitochondria are present in all human cells except mature red blood cells. Mitochondria are semiautonomous, self-replicating organelles. They are separated from the cytoplasm by a double membrane, the inner membrane being highly folded into inward-projecting 'cristae'.

The inner membrane is the location of the electron transport chain (see Chapter 4), where oxidative phosphorylation takes place. This is the main role of mitochondria; oxidative phosphorylation is responsible for the vast majority of adenosine triphosphate (ATP) production. ATP is the intracellular energy currency used to 'power' nearly all intracellular endergonic reactions. The tricarboxylic acid (TCA) cycle (see Chapter 3) is another extremely important metabolic pathway that occurs only in the mitochondrial matrix.

Mitochondria contain mitochondrial versions of RNA and ribosomes, and synthesize their own proteins coded for by distinct mitochondrial DNA. This DNA is arranged in circular form, rather than the chromosome structure seen in the nucleus.

Endoplasmic reticulum

The endoplasmic reticulum (ER) is a complex series of interconnected, flattened membranous sacs or 'cisternae'. The ER possesses a double membrane, the interior of which is contiguous with the intermembrane space of the double-membraned nucleus at distinct points. Intracellular ER is divided into two types: rough and smooth. Both smooth and rough ER are continuous with each other as well as with the intermembrane space of the nuclear membrane.

Rough ER

Rough ER is far more abundant than smooth ER. It is distinguished from smooth ER on electron microscopy by the presence of membrane-associated ribosomes (presenting a 'rough' appearance). The ribosomes intermittently attach/detach to the rough ER. Attachment occurs when ribosomes bind with mRNA strands (see Chapter 9) that encode proteins destined for secretion. The developing polypeptide is extruded into the rough ER interior, where it may remain to complete its development (see Chapter 9). Alternatively, nascent proteins may be transported via vesicles to the Golgi apparatus or another destination for further posttranslation modifications.

Smooth ER

Smooth ER differs from rough ER by the absence of membrane-bound ribosomes. The main function of smooth ER is lipid synthesis – assembling phospholipids, steroids and other lipids. It is therefore more abundant in cell types with secretory roles. The large surface area of the convoluted structure also presents a useful intracellular surface for enzyme attachment, for example, glucose-6-phosphatase, a key enzyme in gluconeogenesis (see Chapter 5). Smooth ER also plays an important role in attaching nascent receptors to membrane proteins prior to their membrane insertion.

Golgi apparatus

Because of its large size, the Golgi apparatus (Fig. 1.2) was one of the first identified intracellular organelles. It is a system of 5 to 8 cup-shaped interconnected membranous sacs that receive vesicles containing lipids and proteins from the smooth and rough ER, respectively. It modifies these molecules in various ways and then distributes them to appropriate areas within the cell, packaged within vesicles. The overall structure possesses a 'cis' and a 'trans' face. The cis face is the 'entry' portal to the Golgi apparatus, and modified molecules exit at the trans face. The Golgi apparatus has another important function – it manufactures lysosomes.

Lysosomes and peroxisomes

The cytoplasm contains two different types of specialized single-membrane-bound vesicular structures: lysosomes and peroxisomes. These differ by their enzyme contents.

Lysosomes

Lysosomes are spherical membrane-bound vesicles with an acidic (pH 4–5) interior. They are the intracellular spaces for enzyme-mediated degradation of obsolete intracellular molecules or imported extracellular material. They are derived from the trans face of the Golgi. Lysosomes are highly variable in size and contain multiple pH-sensitive hydrolases. These can degrade most biomolecules.

Peroxisomes

Peroxisomes are vesicular, ER-derived structures. They are smaller than lysosomes and contain different enzymes, primarily oxidative enzymes. They participate in the β-oxidation of fatty acids with very long chains (see Chapter 7) and in the pentose phosphate pathway (see Chapter 5). Peroxisomal catalase also detoxifies reactive oxygen species such as hydrogen peroxide.

Ribosomes

Eukaryotic cells contain 80S ribosomes, composed of a small 40S and a large 60S subunit. They are composed of rRNA and are manufactured in the nucleus. The two subunits unite immediately prior to beginning translation (see Chapter 9). Ribosomes translate information contained in the mRNA into polypeptides by assembling peptides from amino acids in the order dictated by the mRNA sequence. Ribosomes within the cytoplasm typically synthesize cytoplasmic proteins, whereas those producing proteins destined for the plasma membrane or vesicles associate with the rough ER.

THE CELL MEMBRANE

The cell membrane (Fig. 1.2) is a biological barrier that separates the cellular interior from the external environment. The main function of the cell membrane is to separate the cell from its surroundings and provide a distinct intracellular environment. However, the cell membrane also participates in many important cellular processes, for example:

- Maintenance of the resting membrane potential via regulation of ion entry/exit.
- Interaction with the intracellular cytoskeleton.
- Transport of ions, metabolites and nutrients.
- Cell adhesion to external structural elements within the surrounding tissue or to neighbouring cells.

Cell membranes are impermeable to most molecules, however specialized membrane-spanning transport proteins permit selective permeability to specific ions/molecules. Structural and functional modification of these proteins allows regulation of entry and exit of the relevant transported molecule.

Membrane components

Cell membranes are composed of a phospholipid bilayer studded with membrane proteins and cholesterol (Fig. 1.3).

Phospholipids

Phospholipids consist of a hydrophilic 'head', containing phosphate, and a hydrophobic fatty acid 'tail' of varying length and saturation. The amphiphilic nature of the molecule means that phospholipids spontaneously adopt a bilayer structure. The hydrophilic 'heads' form the surfaces of the membrane, and the hydrophobic 'tails' interact with each other, forming the interior of the bilayer. In this way, the hydrophilic components are in contact with the intracellular and extracellular environments.

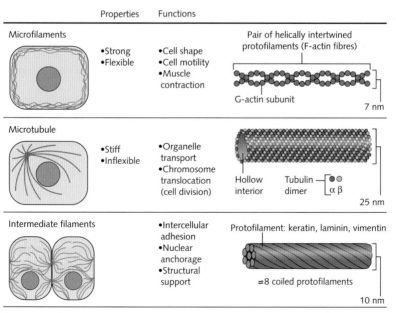

Fig. 1.3 Cytoskeletal components.

Cholesterol

Cholesterol is a sterol, which is an integral part of cell membranes. It intercalates between the phospholipids that make up the bilayer. The presence of cholesterol affects the membrane in different ways, depending on the temperature:

- At lower temperatures, cholesterol disrupts the interaction between phospholipids, increasing membrane viscosity.
- At higher temperatures, cholesterol increases membrane fluidity by raising the bilayer melting point.

The fluidity of the bilayer is significant because it affects the movement of membrane proteins within the bilayer and thus influences local membrane permeability. The role of cholesterol in metabolism is discussed further in Chapter 7.

Membrane proteins

Protein components of the cell membrane may span the membrane completely (integral proteins) or be associated with either the internal or external face of the membrane (peripheral proteins). These proteins may fulfil various roles including:

- Receptor function: allowing external messengers (e.g. hormones) to effect intracellular changes, usually via intracellular signalling cascades.
- Bidirectional transmembrane transport of a myriad of ions and molecules.
- Integral structural functions – acting as anchors for the internal cytoskeleton (integral or internal peripheral proteins).
- Adhesion to neighbouring cells – intercellular adhesion and adhesion to extracellular structural tissue components, stabilizing the cell location within a tissue (integral or external peripheral proteins).
- Some of these proteins are enzymes (integral, internal peripheral and external peripheral proteins).

Permeability and transmembrane transport

Passive (simple) diffusion

Simple diffusion describes the free movement of molecules across a membrane down their concentration gradient. Small nonpolar molecules (e.g. O_2 and CO_2) and uncharged polar molecules (e.g. urea) may diffuse directly through the lipid bilayer in this manner. No energy is required to drive the molecular movement, and diffusion continues until an equilibrium is attained between the intracellular and extracellular compartments.

Facilitated diffusion

Because charged molecules cannot diffuse directly through the lipid bilayer, they rely on specific proteins to traverse the membrane. Proteins mediating facilitated diffusion are typically ion channels or carrier proteins.

The rate of movement of ions through a membrane via channels depends on:

- The ion concentration gradient *and* the charge difference across the membrane relative to the ion's charge. The combination of these two features is known as the 'electrochemical gradient'.
- The number of open channels. Regardless of the electrochemical gradient, an ion cannot cross the membrane if the specific ion channels are closed. This permits an additional level of regulation; channels may be 'gated' such that traffic is possible only in certain situations.

Active transport

Active transport couples the movement of molecules *against* electrochemical gradient with a thermodynamically favourable reaction 'powering' the energetically unfavourable direction of travel. Active transport may be primary or secondary:

- Primary active transport is coupled directly to the hydrolysis of ATP.
- Secondary active transport is coupled indirectly to the hydrolysis of ATP.

Primary active transport

Primary active transport requires energy to transport molecules across a membrane against their electrochemical gradient. Sodium and potassium are examples of ions that are transported across the cell membrane against their electrochemical gradient by primary active transport. This transport is via the Na^+/K^+-dependent adenosine triphosphatase (ATPase). For every ATP hydrolysed, this transporter pumps three Na^+ ions outward and two K^+ ions inward.

Secondary active transport

Secondary active transport is not *directly* coupled to ATP hydrolysis, but exploits a concentration gradient that itself is maintained by primary active transport coupled directly to ATP hydrolysis.

The Na^+/K^+–ATPase establishes an Na^+ gradient across the membrane. This renders Na^+ influx into the cell thermodynamically favourable, because the ion is following its electrochemical gradient. This energetically favourable sodium influx can be coupled to the movement of another molecule against its gradient, for example, glucose (see Chapter 5).

THE CYTOSKELETON, CELL MOTILITY AND INTRACELLULAR TRANSPORT

The cytoskeleton (Figs 1.3 and 1.4) is a dynamic system of structural proteins that support the cell membrane. It

(A) microfilaments

(B) microtubules

(C) intermediate filaments

(D) a + b + c merge

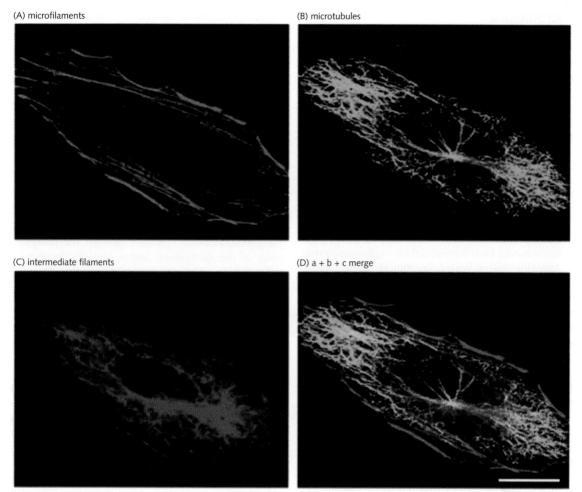

Fig. 1.4 Fluorescence microscopy of cytoskeletal elements. Each of the different types ((A) microfilaments; (B) microtubules and (C) intermediate filaments) is stained and assigned its own colour in this image (D). (From Omary MB, Ku NO, Tao GZ, Toivola DM, Liao J: "Heads and tails" of intermediate phosphorylation: multiple sites and functional insights, *Trends Biochem Sci* 31:383–394, 2006 Box 2, Fig. I.)

contributes significantly to determining cellular three-dimensional (3D) shape and cellular motility. Cytoskeletal components are also paramount for normal mitotic and meiotic cellular division. The major components of the cytoskeleton are:

- Microfilaments (actin polymers)
- Microtubules (tubulin polymers)
- Intermediate filaments (IFs)

Components of the cytoskeleton

Microfilaments

Microfilaments, composed of actin, form a parallel lamina closely associated with the internal face of the cell membrane. They also traverse the cytoplasm in multiple directions. Microfilaments are crucial for cell polarization and motility. Neutrophil chemotaxis, macrophage movement and muscle contraction are prime examples of the dynamism that microfilaments confer to the cytoskeleton.

Actin

Actin is the most abundant cellular protein. Actin filaments (F-actin) consist of linear polymerized globular subunits (G-actin). Bundles of actin filaments are able to form linear structures, as well as two-dimensional and 3D meshwork.

Actin polymerization is closely regulated by the cell and may be influenced by extracellular signalling by surface receptors.

Actin-binding proteins—Protein binding to actin causes changes to the 3D structure of the actin molecules. The most important example of this is myosin, found in contractile cells (e.g. muscle or cardiac myocytes). However, myosin is by no means the only one; actin participates in a large number of protein–protein interactions.

Microtubules

Microtubules, like microfilaments and intermediate filaments (IF) are cytoskeletal components that contribute to maintaining cellular structure. They are present in all cell types except red blood cells.

As well as structural support, microtubules also enable various types of intracellular movement to occur: intracellular transport and organelle movement during mitosis or meiosis.

Microtubules are formed from assembled linear protofilaments, arranged in parallel in a hollow cylindrical structure. Protofilaments consist of linearly polymerized tubulin heterodimers, with each heterodimer consisting of α- and β-tubulin. Microtubules extend from distinct origins or microtubule-organizing centres. These origins act as a focus for microtubule development; developing microtubules radiate outwards from the microtubule-organizing centres.

Like the microfilament constituent actin, tubulin interacts with specific proteins. These are known as 'microtubule-associated proteins'. ATP-reliant molecular motors such as dynein and kinesin exploit microtubules as intracellular roadmaps, allowing cargo such as secretory vesicles or organelles to travel along the microtubule to specific locations within the cell.

Intermediate filaments

Intermediate filaments (IFs) are the most abundant components of the cytoskeleton. They are extremely stable, more so than microfilaments and microtubules, as their subunits do not dissociate under physiological conditions. They therefore represent the more permanent structural components of the cytoskeleton, which is their main function.

IF subunits consist of a family of α-helical proteins. The particular components vary with cell type. These subunits wind together to form the rope-like structure that characterizes IF. IF are present in both the nucleus and the cytoplasm, where they form meshworks of laminae closely associated with the internal leaflet of the enclosing membranes in a similar manner to microfilaments. IF also form supportive internal frameworks for intracellular spatial organization, for example, by interconnecting the external nuclear membrane to the cellular membrane.

GENETICS

Deoxyribonucleotides

To understand the structure of *deoxyribonucleic acid*, or 'DNA', one must first appreciate the components of the basic units (deoxyribonucleotides). The basic 'unit' of DNA is the *deoxyribonucleotide* (Fig. 1.5). Each deoxyribonucleotide is composed of:

- a deoxyribose sugar
- a phosphate group
- a nitrogenous base (adenine, cytosine, guanine or thymine)

Polymerized deoxyribonucleotides form the strand of the *deoxyribonucleic acid*.

Nitrogenous bases

The nitrogenous bases of DNA are heterocyclic molecules derived from purines (adenine and guanine) or pyrimidines (cytosine and thymine). Note that RNA does not include thymine and instead contains uracil, a pyrimidine derivative. For details of purine and pyrimidine metabolism, please see Chapter 10.

Deoxyribonucleotide polymerization

Deoxyribonucleotides polymerize in linear fashion via phosphodiester bond formation between the phosphate group of one deoxyribonucleotide and the deoxyribose group of the neighbouring deoxyribonucleotide. These interactions underpin the assembly of consecutively linked deoxyribonucleotides. The macromolecule (or 'polymer') formed is a *nucleic acid*.

The double helix: paired strands of DNA

Discovered by Watson and Crick in 1953, the structure of DNA consists of two intertwined nucleotide strands, held together in a double helical structure by nitrogenous base pairing. Adenine and thymine pair via two hydrogen bonds between opposing strands, whereas guanine and cytosine pair via three hydrogen bonds. Base pairing results in two 'complementary' strands of nucleic acid, orientated antiparallel to each other (i.e. one runs in the 5′→3′ direction, and the other runs in the 3′→5′ direction). The structure is characterized by a 'core' of inwardly orientated nitrogenous bases and an outer 'shell' of externally protruding phosphate groups.

HINTS AND TIPS

DIRECTIONALITY OF NUCLEIC ACIDS

Nucleic acids have directionality. One end is the five-prime (5′) end, where the phosphate group is attached to carbon 5 of the deoxyribose ring. At the three-prime (3′) end, the phosphate group is attached to carbon 3 of the deoxyribose.

Complementary pairing of nucleic acids

Each strand is described as 'complementary' to its partner strand. Complementary polynucleotide strands interact with each other through hydrogen bonds between the nitrogenous base component of each deoxyribonucleotide as described earlier. Note that in DNA each single strand is partnered by another single strand. When the term 'DNA' is used, this refers to the *pair* of helically intertwined polynucleotide chains.

Strand terminology

Genetic information is only carried by *one* of the two nucleic acid strands making up a length of DNA. This strand is known as the 'coding' strand. The coding strand is the 5'→3' strand, whereas the noncoding template strand is the 3'→5' strand. Confusingly, the 'coding' strand is also known as the 'sense' strand and the 'nontemplate strand', and the noncoding (template) strand as the 'antisense' strand. Essentially:

- Coding strand=nontemplate strand (5'→3') = sense strand (contains codons). This is a strand with a nucleotide sequence **identical** to that which will appear in the mRNA transcribed from the template strand, with the exception that thymine (T)

deoxyribonucleotides in the DNA sequence will be substituted by uracil (U) ribonucleotides in the mRNA sequence.

- Noncoding strand = template strand (3'→5') = antisense strand (contains anticodons). A strand with the sequence of nucleotides **complementary** to what will be the transcribed mRNA. RNA polymerase (RNA pol II) binds to this strand, transcribing it into mRNA.

The gene

A gene is the basic functional unit of heredity responsible for the passage of genetic information from one generation to the next. Genes also play a vital role in protein synthesis, encoding the information needed to assemble the primary structure (see Chapter 9) of any particular protein. A gene (Fig. 1.5) is composed of a length of DNA.

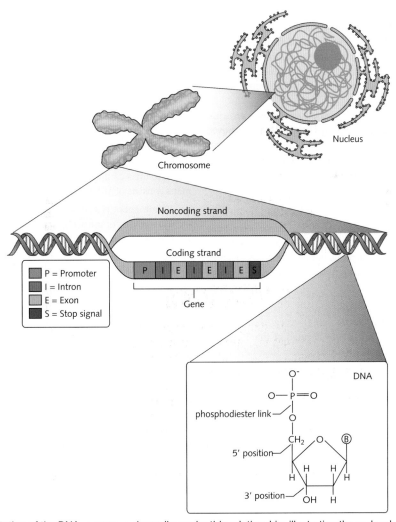

Fig. 1.5 Representation of the DNA → gene → deoxyribonucleotide relationship, illustrating the molecular structure of a deoxyribonucleotide.

Gene expression

Each gene encodes its specific polypeptide in the following way:

1. The gene acts as a blueprint determining the order of ribonucleotide assembly into mRNA, which occurs in the nucleus. This process is called 'transcription'.
2. The mRNA moves out of the nucleus and into the cytoplasm.
3. In the cytoplasm, mRNA attached to ribosomes functions as a physical blueprint for ribosomes, dictating the order of polypeptide assembly; the specific order of the amino acids represents the primary structure (see Chapter 9) of the new polypeptide.

The processes of transcription and translation are discussed in much greater detail in Chapter 9.

Gene components

Exons and introns

Each individual gene consists of exons, which are functional coding regions. The exons are separated from each other by noncoding introns. Together, the separate exons make up a coding sequence, which encodes the genetic information that ultimately dictates the primary sequence of the encoded protein.

Introns from the coding strand do *not* encode proteins, despite being on the coding strand. Their mRNA is removed or 'spliced' out of the developing mRNA during its synthesis (see Chapter 9). Introns do not therefore contribute to the genetic code for each polypeptide.

Noncoding deoxyribonucleotide sequences

Between different genes, there are large expanses of noncoding deoxyribonucleotide sequences. These were once thought to serve no function, but now are believed to undergo transcription, forming noncoding RNA strands. Noncoding RNAs play various roles in the regulation of gene expression.

Promoter sequences

A promoter sequence is typically located at the 5′ end of a gene (although promoter sequences can also be located at completely separate sites within the coding strand). Promoter sequences function as binding sites for RNA polymerase (see Chapter 9), an enzyme necessary for transcription of the gene.

The genetic code

The 'one gene, one polypeptide' hypothesis states that the base sequence of DNA determines the amino acid sequence in a single corresponding polypeptide. By convention, gene sequences are described in the 5′→3′ direction, because this is the direction of *in vivo* nucleic acid synthesis. Do not slip into the error of stating 'one gene, one *protein*;' the phrase is 'one gene, one *polypeptide*', because multiple polypeptides may contribute to a fully formed protein, that is, multiple genes would contribute to a single protein.

The process of translation (see Chapter 9) from mRNA to protein is directed by the ribonucleotide sequence, which itself is determined by the original gene sequence (minus the introns). Each of the amino acids is represented within the mRNA sequence by a codon. A codon consists of a triplet of consecutive ribonucleotides. As there are four different bases in DNA, there are 4^3 (64) possible codons. Of these 64 possible codons, the genetic code consists of 61 amino acid-encoding codons and three termination codons, which arrest translation.

Although there are 61 amino acid-coding codons, only 20 amino acids are commonly used in polypeptide synthesis – thus more than one codon may represent an amino acid. For example, the codons GGU, GGC, GGA and GGG all encode the amino acid glycine. This feature is described as 'degenerate'.

mRNA transcript codons correspond to (and form temporary base pair hydrogen bonds with) transfer RNA (tRNA) 'anticodons', which define which amino acid is transported by that particular tRNA. Three mRNA codons (UAA, UAG and UGA) are not recognized by tRNAs, and these are termed 'stop codons'. They mark the end of a polypeptide and signal to the ribosome to finish synthesis.

Mitochondrial DNA and the genetic code

Mitochondria contain their own unique DNA, which in humans consists of 16 kb of circular DNA coding for:

- 22 mitochondrial (mt) tRNAs
- two variants of mitochondrial rRNAs
- 13 separate mitochondrial proteins (e.g. subunits of the electron transfer system responsible for oxidative phosphorylation).

Chromosomes

The human genome (i.e. the entirety of human genes) is divided into DNA superstructures packaged around DNA-associated proteins such as histones. Each of these superstructures represents a chromosome. Each chromosome represents a segment of the individual's genome.

The combination of DNA with DNA-associated proteins is termed 'chromatin'. Chromatin allows the enormous lengths of DNA comprising the chromosome to occupy a relatively tiny volume within the nucleus.

Chromosomal inheritance

Every human cell (apart from gametes) contains 23 pairs of chromosomes stored within the nucleus. Each pair of an individual's chromosomes consists of one chromosome derived from the mother and one from the father.

EPIGENETICS

Epigenetics refers to heritable characteristics that are *not* related to the genetic code sequence of the parents. Environment-induced changes to parental DNA-binding proteins (such as histones) or covalent modifications (e.g. methylation of cytosine base in the DNA) may be inherited in their offspring.

The significance of this is that these changes can facilitate or impede expression of a gene. In an epigenetic change, the inherited gene itself is identical, but its ability to be expressed, or 'switched-on', may be different after the change.

● **Chapter Summary**

- Eukaryotic cells are defined by the presence of a membrane-bound nucleus, which contains the cell's genetic material, and several types of membrane-bound organelles, which are responsible for specific intracellular functions.
- Cell membranes are composed of phospholipid bilayers, studded with proteins responsible for specific functional roles, and cholesterol. Transport across membrane is governed by presence of transport proteins and electrochemical gradients or direct/indirect adenosine triphosphate hydrolysis when the direction of transfer is against an electrochemical gradient.
- Human DNA consists of a double helix of deoxyribonucleotide polymers. A deoxyribonucleotide consists of a nitrogenous base (purine or pyrimidine), a phosphate group and a deoxyribose sugar group.
- A gene consists of discontinuous lengths of DNA. Coding introns are interspersed by noncoding exons. Arrays of genes specific to the individual together comprise the genetic code. A chromosome represents a portion of the total DNA content of the nucleus; in humans there are 46 chromosomes (23 pairs). Each member of a pair is either paternally or maternally derived.
- Chromosomal inheritance underpins the transfer of genetic information between parents and offspring. Chromosomes consist of condensed DNA, complexed with specific proteins such as histones, which can also play a part in controlling expression of genes.

Introduction to metabolism

2

INTRODUCTORY CONCEPTS

Metabolism

The term 'metabolism' encompasses all the biochemical reactions occurring within a living organism. These reactions allow extraction of chemical energy from food and biosynthesis of all the molecules necessary to sustain life. Key points to appreciate are as follows:

- Reactions involve molecular conversion of substrates into products.
- In living organisms, reactions never occur in isolation. Products from one reaction go on to participate in other reactions as substrates.
- A set of consecutive reactions is described as a 'pathway'. Components of the pathway are known as 'intermediates' (Fig. 2.1).

In metabolism, pathways tend to be named according to their overall role. A pathway with the suffix '-lysis' is a reaction sequence devoted to degrading the molecule named in the prefix. For example, 'glycogenolysis' pathway is a glycogen degradation pathway.

Because most molecules participate in more than one reaction pathway, different pathways 'intersect' where they have a common participant. Therefore metabolism can be considered analogous to a route map – the 'roads' representing reaction pathways criss-crossing one another.

Instead of traffic lights and speed humps, reaction pathway 'traffic' is regulated by various biological mechanisms. These regulatory mechanisms govern the rate at which molecules enter and proceed through a pathway.

HINTS AND TIPS

The key to understanding metabolism is to appreciate that the particular details are less important than the overall picture. It is more important that you understand the metabolic role, location and regulatory mechanisms of a pathway than to have memorized every individual reaction.

ENZYMES

Enzymes are specialized, highly specific proteins. Each enzyme mediates a particular biochemical reaction by acting as a biological catalyst. Without enzymes, biological reactions would occur far too slowly for cell viability. Each enzyme temporarily binds a specific ligand (substrate) and imposes a particular molecular modification before releasing a product of the reaction. Enzymes are not altered or consumed by the reactions they catalyse, so they are effectively 'reusable'.

The efficiency of an enzyme at catalysing a reaction determines the rate at which the reaction proceeds. In this way, enzyme function is comparable to a tuning dial controlling the reaction's rate. Modulation of enzyme function (activity) is therefore a major biological regulation strategy. Several terms are frequently used in enzymology; these are given in Table 2.1.

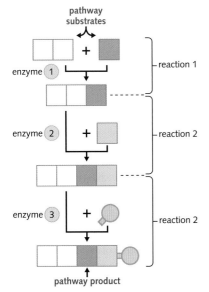

Fig. 2.1 Example of a short metabolic pathway. Circled numbers 1, 2 and 3 represent the enzymes responsible for catalysing each reaction.

HINTS AND TIPS

Recall that enzyme activity is analogous to a tuning dial controlling reaction rates. The rate-limiting enzyme may be thought of as a master dial that controls the pathway rate.

Table 2.1 Enzyme-related terms and definitions

Term	Definition
Active site	The structural region of an enzyme responsible for binding to its specific substrate
Conformation	This term describes the 3D structure of an enzyme or protein. A change in conformation results in a change to the enzyme's behaviour and function. Any molecule binding to an enzyme can potentially have an effect on the overall 3D structure (i.e. alter the conformation). Such changes in conformation may be subtle or dramatic and each specific conformational change may increase or decrease the enzyme's functional capacity (see 'Activity').
Activity	This term describes ability of an enzyme to convert its substrate into the reaction product. Activity is influenced by the environmental pH, temperature, enzyme conformation and the relative concentrations of enzyme and substrate. Presence of inhibitors or activators (see below) also affects enzyme activity.
Affinity	This term describes the avidity of the association between an enzyme and its substrate. An enzyme with low affinity binds its substrate weakly, and vice versa.
Inhibitor	An inhibitor binds the enzyme and reduces its activity for substrate→product conversion. This is usually by mediating a conformational change. The inhibitor may bind to the enzyme's active site (competitive inhibition) or at a site separate from the active site (noncompetitive inhibition). Both mechanisms decrease the enzyme's maximum rate of activity and thus the substrate→product conversion.
Activator	The opposite of inhibitors, activators bind to an enzyme, increasing enzyme activity and thus the rate of substrate→product conversion.
Coenzyme	A specific 'companion molecule' required by some enzymes to allow them to perform their function. They can be thought of as mandatory activators – without the coenzyme the enzyme is unable to function.
Cofactor	Similar to a coenzyme, in that a cofactor is required by some enzymes (apoenzymes) to allow them to perform their function; however, a cofactor is **not** part of an enzyme. Often cofactors are metal ions or vitamin derivatives.
Apoenzyme	An apoenzyme is an inactive enzyme which is activated by binding and association with its specific cofactor.
Holoenzyme	A holo enzyme consists of an apoenzyme and a cofactor. Essentially, an activated apoenzyme.
Proenzyme	A biologically inactive enzyme precursor, which requires further modification or processing (e.g. proteolytic cleavage) to render it active and competent to perform its catalytic function.
Isoenzyme	A subtly different version of enzyme that catalyses an identical reaction. Isoenzymes catalyse the same reaction but are not identical.

Enzyme nomenclature

Enzymes are named according to the reaction they catalyse, so their reaction can often be inferred from the name. Table 2.2 provides common examples.

BIOENERGETICS

Reactions are described as exergonic (energy releasing) or endergonic (energy requiring). Reactions will occur only if they are energetically favourable. Energetic favourability is quantified by a change in the Gibbs free energy (ΔG) of a reaction. Exergonic reactions have negative ΔG values (they release energy), whereas endergonic reactions have positive ΔG values (they require energy input). A reaction with a positive ΔG value cannot occur spontaneously; it occurs only when coupled with a separate exergonic reaction,

for example, adenosine triphosphate (ATP) hydrolysis (Fig. 2.2).

Activation energy

A reaction can only proceed spontaneously if it is energetically favourable, that is, the total free energy of the reaction product(s) is lower than the total free energy of the substrate(s). The Gibbs free energy defines the free energy change.

However, there is an additional consideration – the activation energy (E_a) of the reaction. Even in a reaction where the overall ΔG is negative, some activation energy may be required for the reaction to occur. The requirement for activation energy is due to the temporary formation of transient, unstable, high-energy intermediates.

Enzymes catalyse their reactions by reducing the activation energy of the reaction. In the presence of the enzyme, the high-energy intermediates are stabilized by interactions

Table 2.2 Enzyme nomenclature

Enzyme	Molecular reaction catalysed
Kinase	Addition of a phosphate group to the substrate (phosphorylation).
Phosphatase	Removal of a phosphate group from the substrate (dephosphorylation).
Synthase	Synthesis of a molecule (the molecule's name precedes the 'synthase', e.g. glycogen synthase – synthesis of glycogen).
Carboxylase	Incorporation of a carbon atom and two oxygen molecules into the substrate.
Decarboxylase	Removal of a carbon atom and two oxygen atoms from the substrate. These interact to form carbon dioxide.
Dehydrogenase	Oxidation of the substrate by virtue of transfer of (one or more) hydride (H^-) ions to an electron acceptor such as NAD^+ or FAD.
Isomerase	Rearrangement of the molecular structure of the substrate molecule. The product will have the same chemical formula.
Mutase	Transfer of a functional group to a new location within the substrate molecule. The product and substrate have the same chemical formula. Mutases are technically also isomerases.
Transferase	Transfer of a functional group between different molecules, for example, aminotransferase.

FAD, Flavin adenine dinucleotide; NAD^+, nicotinamide adenine dinucleotide.

with the enzyme, thus the energy required to drive the reaction (E_a) is significantly reduced (Fig. 2.3).

Enzyme kinetics

Enzyme kinetics refers to the study of enzymatic reactions. Appreciating these concepts is quite challenging, but often examined.

Plotting the product against time allows reaction velocity to be quantified (Fig. 2.4). Reaction velocity is represented by the gradient of the graph.

The reaction velocity (identified from the graph relating product accumulation to time) can then be plotted against substrate, illustrating that substrate availability also influences the maximum rate of reaction (Fig. 2.5). It is assumed for the purposes of this graph that the enzyme is fixed.

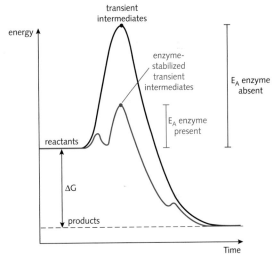

Fig. 2.3 Reaction profile for uncatalysed *(black)* and catalysed *(red)* reactions. E_a, Activation energy.

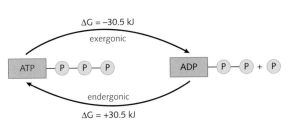

Fig. 2.2 Adenosine triphosphate (ATP) hydrolysis. Energy released by the highly exergonic forward hydrolytic release of a phosphate group may be used to 'power' simultaneous endergonic reactions where products have higher free energy than the reactions (+ve ΔG) that would otherwise not proceed. *ADP*, Adenosine diphosphate.

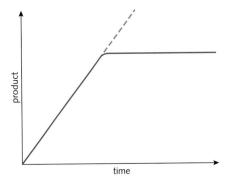

Fig. 2.4 Reaction product formation against time. Note that the graph plateaus once no further product formation occurs. This scenario develops due to both substrate exhaustion and product-mediated enzyme inhibition.

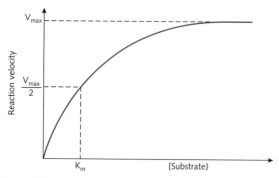

Fig. 2.5 Reaction velocity against substrate concentration. Note that the graph plateaus at a maximum velocity, regardless of increasing the substrate concentration. The reaction cannot proceed at a higher velocity without addition of additional enzyme, that is, beyond a given substrate, the enzyme limits reaction velocity.

The initial velocity will increase with increasing substrate concentration until it closely approaches the maximum velocity. If the concentration increases further, the graph flattens out (the gradient approaches zero); further increase in reaction rate is negligible.

The type of graph is called a 'Michaelis–Menten graph', and the shape of the curve is described as a 'rectangular hyperbola'.

First-order kinetics

At low substrate, the graph is approximately linear – the reaction velocity is proportional to the substrate. This relationship is described as 'first-order kinetics'.

Zero-order kinetics

At high substrate, the graph flattens and above a certain substrate is completely flat – no matter how much additional substrate is available, the reaction rate increase will be minimal due to the enzyme operating at maximal capacity. This relationship is described as 'zero-order kinetics'.

The Michaelis–Menten equation

The Michaelis–Menten equation relates the reaction rate to the substrate concentration:
where K_1, K_2, K_3 and K_4 are the individual rate constants. K_4 is insignificant in this context and can be ignored.

The Michaelis constant (K_m) quantifies the rate of dissociation of the enzyme–substrate complex:

$$E + S \underset{K_2}{\overset{K_1}{\rightleftarrows}} ES \underset{K_4}{\overset{K_3}{\rightleftarrows}} E + P$$

$$K_m = \frac{K_2 + K_3}{K_1}$$

The maximum velocity (V_{max}) is reached under enzyme-saturation conditions, at high substrate concentration:

$$V_{max} = K_3 \big[ES \big]$$

where K_3 is rate of enzyme and product formation and [ES] is enzyme–substrate complex concentration.

The velocity (V) of the reaction at a given substrate for any enzyme can be calculated using the Michaelis–Menten equation (if the V_{max} and K_m are known):

$$V = \frac{V_{max} \big[S \big]}{K_m + \big[S \big]}$$

Note that both V_{max} and K_m can be derived from the graph of substrate against reaction velocity (Fig. 2.5). These parameters are specific to each individual enzyme. The equation of the line in Fig. 2.5 is given by the Michaelis–Menten equation.

K_m (the Michaelis constant) corresponds to a substrate concentration at which the reaction rate is half of the maximum ($V_{max}/2$). The primary feature influencing a particular enzyme's K_m value is the affinity of the enzyme for its specific substrate. A low K_m value would be expected when there is a low rate of enzyme–substrate dissociation due to a high affinity (i.e. strong binding interaction between enzyme and substrate).

Because of the shape of the rectangular hyperbola, accurately determining the V_{max} and K_m from the Michaelis–Menten graph is challenging. Mathematically converting the graph to a straight line allows easier derivation of these values (Fig. 2.6).

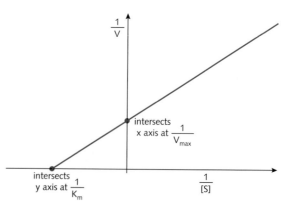

Fig. 2.6 Graph illustrating the reciprocal of the reaction velocity (1/[V]) against the reciprocal of the substrate concentration (1/[S]). The y-axis intersection occurs at $1/V_{max}$, and the x-axis intersection at $1/K_m$. This representation of the velocity–substrate concentration relationship is called a 'Lineweaver–Burk' plot.

ANABOLISM AND CATABOLISM

Metabolic pathways are either anabolic or catabolic. Anabolic pathways generate complex molecules from simpler substrates, whereas catabolic pathways break down complex molecules into simpler products (Fig. 2.7). 'Metabolism' describes all reactions occurring in the living organism: both the anabolic and catabolic processes. The balance between the two reflects the energy status of a cell or organism.

Anabolic pathways consume energy and are typically synthetic processes. The suffix of a synthetic pathway is '-genesis', for example, lipogenesis (lipid synthesis). Anabolism is analogous to 'construction'; construction requires raw materials (substrates) and energy.

Catabolic pathways liberate intrinsic chemical energy from biological molecules, usually via ATP generation. They involve sequential molecular degradation. Catabolic pathways are suffixed with '-lysis', for example, glycolysis (glucose degradation).

PATHWAY REGULATION

Different pathways have different maximum rates of activity. Note that a pathway cannot proceed at a rate independent of the activity of the coexisting pathways. Coordination and regulation of pathways are therefore vital aspects of metabolism.

There are three main control mechanisms in cells that regulate metabolic pathways in an integrated fashion. These include:

- Substrate availability
- Hormonal regulation
- Enzyme modification

Pathway regulation: substrate availability

Pathway progression or 'activity' is limited by availability of the initial pathway substrate. An important mechanism cells exploit to regulate the quantity of substrate available for participation in a pathway is by regulating membrane traffic of substrate molecules. This refers to traffic across organelle membranes and the cell membrane itself.

Membranes are not freely permeable to the majority of substrates, so varying the supply of substrate by regulating import/export across the membranes adds an additional level of potential regulation (see Chapter 1). Essentially, sequestering enzymes in different compartments away from their substrates limits their ability to participate in metabolic pathways.

Pathway regulation: hormonal regulation

Hormones are molecular messengers, released from endocrine glands into the bloodstream. At responsive (target) cells, hormones exert their effects by:

- Binding to external surface receptors (Fig. 2.8)
- Binding to intracellular receptors (Fig. 2.9)

To bind to intracellular receptors, a hormone must first traverse the cell membrane. This is usually via passive diffusion; such hormones are typically lipid soluble (e.g. steroid hormones).

Hormones ultimately impose their influence via alteration of the activity of the key enzymes in specific intracellular pathways (Fig. 2.11). Altering the activity of either phosphorylating enzymes (kinases) or dephosphorylating enzymes (phosphatases) is a common mechanism.

Some hormones (e.g. steroid hormones) bind to DNA within the cell nucleus at target DNA sequence (hormone-response elements), directly influencing the rate of synthesis of enzymes. Increased or decreased enzyme synthesis (enzyme induction and repression, respectively) influences the pathway in which the enzyme participates.

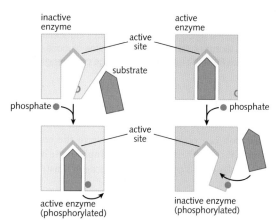

Fig. 2.8 In the scenario on the left, phosphorylation activates the enzyme by imposing a conformational change that exposes the active site *(bold)*. On the right, the converse scenario is shown; phosphorylation inhibits the enzyme by imposing a conformational change that impedes substrate access to the active site.

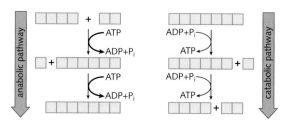

Fig. 2.7 Schematic of a catabolic *(right)* and anabolic *(left)* pathway. Enzymes omitted for simplicity. *ADP,* Adenosine diphosphate; *ATP,* adenosine triphosphate; *Pᵢ,* inorganic phosphate.

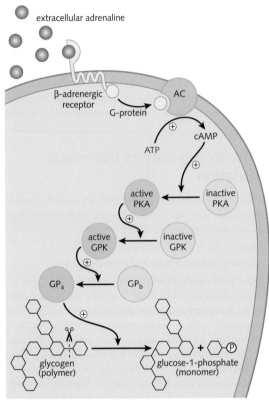

Fig. 2.9 Hormonal regulation: cell-membrane receptor binding. Extracellular adrenaline (epinephrine) binds to the receptor, activating important signal transduction molecules known as 'G proteins'. In this example, the G proteins, in turn, activate the membrane-embedded adenylate cyclase enzyme (AC), which synthesizes cyclic adenosine monophosphate (cAMP) from adenosine triphosphate (ATP). cAMP activates protein kinase A (PKA), which in turn activates (via phosphorylation) glycogen phosphorylase kinase (GPK). This activates glycogen phosphorylase (GP), which releases glucose-1-phosphate from branched glycogen polymer. Via this intracellular cascade, extracellular adrenaline liberates glucose-1-phosphate from the intracellular storage polymer glycogen.

In human metabolism, hormonal control is a mechanism by which intracellular catabolism and energy production can respond appropriately to the energy requirements of the organism. The example of the opposing intracellular effects of insulin and glucagon illustrates this principle.

Insulin

Insulin is produced by the pancreas in response to a rise in blood glucose following a meal (i.e. in the 'fed' state). Insulin released into the bloodstream binds to cell membrane surface receptors. This activates an array of intracellular pathways, including synthesis of storage macromolecules such as glycogen and lipids. This is energetically appropriate in the context of the glucose abundance in the fed state. At the same time, energy-demanding pathways such as gluconeogenesis and catabolic pathways such as glycogenolysis and lipolysis (which were necessary during the fasting state to maintain circulating glucose and fatty acid levels) are suppressed.

Glucagon

Glucagon, conversely, is released into the bloodstream in response to a fall in blood glucose, which occurs in the fasting state. Glucagon activates various intracellular pathways, for example, catabolism of storage molecules such as lipids and glycogen, and promotes gluconeogenesis. The overall effect is to supply tissues with substrates for cellular catabolism and ATP generation. These substrates are derived from endogenous stores (e.g. fatty acids from triacylglycerols and glucose from glycogen). These actions are necessary during fasting, because in this context these molecules are no longer being assimilated from ingested food. Insulin and glucagon are discussed further in Chapter 6.

Pathway regulation: enzyme modification

Within a metabolic pathway, the slowest individual reaction is known as the 'rate-limiting reaction'. The enzyme responsible for this reaction is the rate-limiting enzyme. The pathway cannot proceed at a rate exceeding the rate of this reaction. Thus the activity of the rate-limiting enzyme ultimately dictates the rate of the entire pathway.

- An increase in the rate-limiting enzyme's activity permits the entire pathway to proceed at an increased rate.
- A decrease in the rate-limiting enzyme's activity slows the entire pathway. The activity of the rate-limiting enzyme can be considered as one of three main 'speed dials' which together govern the rate of progression of the pathway. Hormonal regulation and substrate availability are the other two 'speed dials'. However, the effects of enzyme modification are by far the most rapid mechanism of altering the activity of the pathway.

The greatest impact on pathway progression is achieved by altering the activity of the rate-limiting enzyme. Activity can be altered by:

- Structural modification (covalent and/or noncovalent) of the enzyme molecule (may ↑ or ↓ activity).
- Increasing the enzyme concentration by increased gene expression (↑ activity).
- Decreasing the enzyme concentration by increased degradation of the enzyme (↓ activity).

Allosteric regulation

Allosteric modification describes binding of a small regulatory molecule(s) to an enzyme, to a site different from its active site. This interaction imposes a conformational change that alters the enzyme's catalytic function. This may increase or decrease the enzyme's activity. Allosteric modulators act as enzyme inhibitors or activators. A very common example of allosteric regulations is 'negative feedback' (Fig. 2.10). This is where a downstream pathway intermediate imposes allosteric inhibition to an upstream enzyme.

Presence of enzyme inhibitors

Competitive inhibitors (in contrast to allosteric modulators) bind to enzymes at the active site, that is, they 'compete' with the enzyme's usual substrate for binding to the active site. Noncompetitive inhibitors bind to enzymes at a site other than the active site, imposing a conformational change which usually impedes access of the usual substrate to the enzyme's active site.

In terms of enzyme kinetics, the presence of a competitive inhibitor increases the K_m value of the enzyme (for its normal substrate) without altering the V_{max}. A noncompetitive inhibitor reduces the V_{max} but does not affect the K_m value.

Phosphorylation

Phosphorylation is an extremely important enzyme modification. Phosphorylation is the covalent addition of a phosphate moiety (PO_3^{2-}) to a molecule. This moiety is (relatively) large and strongly charged. It therefore has a major impact on the structure (and the activity) of the enzyme. Phosphorylation is mediated by kinase enzymes. Removal of the phosphate moiety, 'dephosphorylation', is mediated by phosphatases.

Influencing a molecule's ability to traverse membranes

Phosphorylation is also important for molecules other than enzymes. In the case of glucose, the presence of the phosphate moiety determines whether the glucose molecule can cross the cell membrane. Phosphorylated glucose (glucose phosphate) is unrecognizable to the glucose-specific membrane transport systems that allow unphosphorylated glucose to pass across the membrane. This essentially 'traps' the glucose inside the cell.

Influencing the molecule's function

In enzyme molecules, the phosphate moiety typically associates with amino acids serine and threonine. Depending on where exactly in the three-dimensional structure of the enzyme these amino acid residues are situated, phosphorylation may influence an enzyme's activity positively or negatively (Fig. 2.9).

This ability of phosphorylation to result in activation or inhibition of enzymes is vital to appreciate, because phosphorylation is a ubiquitous intracellular mechanism that influences enzyme activity. Whether (or not!) a phosphorylation leads to an increase or decrease in an enzyme's activity depends on the precise structural modification it imposes.

REDOX REACTIONS

Reduction and oxidation

In biochemistry, oxidation of a molecule (Fig. 2.12) means the loss of electron(s).

This is often associated with:

• losing a hydrogen atom or
• gaining an oxygen atom.

The molecule undergoing oxidation is termed the 'reductant'.

Reduction of a molecule (Fig. 2.12) means the gain of electron(s).

This is often associated with:

• gaining a hydrogen atom or
• losing an oxygen atom.

The molecule undergoing reduction is termed the 'oxidant'.

The word 'redox' is a combination of 'reduction' and 'oxidation'. It highlights that neither process can occur

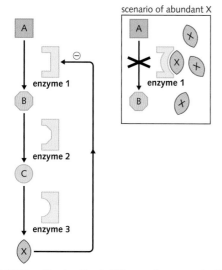

scenario of abundant X

Fig. 2.10 Negative feedback. When pathway product X is abundant (inset), it inhibits the activity of upstream enzyme 1 by binding and distorting its structure. If enzyme 1 is rate limiting, this will slow the rate of the entire pathway. Abundant X implies that sustained high activity of the X-generating pathway would be superfluous to cellular requirements.

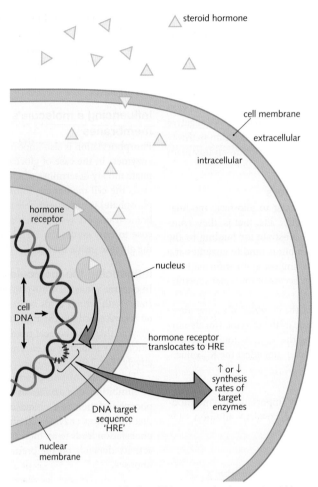

Fig. 2.11 Hormonal regulation: intracellular receptor binding. This example shows steroid hormone diffusing into a cell, accessing the nucleus and binding to its receptor. The activated receptor binds the relevant hormone-response element (HRE) in the DNA sequence, leading to altered synthesis rates of target enzymes.

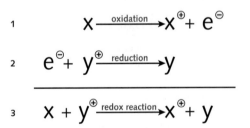

Fig. 2.12 Example redox reaction. X loses an electron, that is, it is oxidized; X is the 'reductant' (1). Y gains an electron, that is, it is reduced; Y is the 'oxidant' (2). These reactions are each 'half-reactions' because together they comprise a complete redox reaction (3).

without the other. Whenever a reduction occurs, an oxidation must also occur. X and Y in Fig. 2.12 are redox partners. Note that in Fig. 2.12 the division into 'half-reactions' is to aid comprehension – electrons never 'float' around freely on their own.

Free radicals

Free radicals are molecules or atoms containing an unpaired electron (see Box 2.3). Because of this unpaired electron, they are extremely reactive and indiscriminately enter undesirable redox reactions with other biological molecules such as DNA or proteins. This is known as 'oxidative damage', as the free radicals, acting as oxidants, are reduced during the process whilst the target molecule is oxidized.

HINTS AND TIPS

When referring to atoms/molecules of oxygen with an unpaired electron, one uses the term 'reactive oxygen species'. These include the superoxide anion O_2^-, peroxide (H_2O_2) and hydroxyl, OH^-. All are highly reactive.

Free radical damage is thought to contribute to cell damage associated with ageing, inflammation and the complications of diabetes.

Numerous exogenous factors such as radiation, smoking and various chemicals all promote free radical formation. Surprisingly, free radicals are also produced in the course of normal cellular metabolism. However, excessive oxidative damage is prevented by antioxidant compounds such as vitamins C and E and glutathione. These 'scavenge' (mop-up) free radicals, limiting the potential damage. Specific enzymes also inactivate free radicals (e.g. catalase).

KEY MOLECULES IN METABOLISM

Adenosine triphosphate: cellular 'energy currency'

ATP is a molecule composed of an adenine ring attached to C1 of a ribose sugar. A 'tail' of three phosphate groups is attached to the C5 of the ribose (Fig. 2.13).

The two phosphoanhydride bonds illustrated in Fig. 2.13 are responsible for the high chemical energy content of the molecule. These bonds require a large amount of energy to form, and release a large amount of energy on hydrolysis (Fig. 2.2). ATP is never 'stored' intracellularly; it is continuously utilized (yielding adenosine diphosphate (ADP) or adenosine monophosphate (AMP)) and resynthesized.

Roles of ATP

ATP hydrolysis provides energy (indirectly or directly) to drive the vast majority of endergonic cellular reactions. ATP also participates in numerous reactions as a vital phosphate donor as well as an energy source. It also has important roles in intracellular signalling. It is required for synthesis of adenine nucleotides necessary for RNA and DNA synthesis. ATP is responsible for an enormous amount of membrane traffic; all transport systems involving adenosine triphosphatases (ATPases) require an uninterrupted supply of ATP to maintain active transport of the various ions and molecules necessary to sustain the cell. All secondary active transport systems indirectly rely on concentration gradients maintained by ATP-driven primary transport as described earlier (see Chapter 1: Primary active transport).

Sources of ATP

ATP is generated by two principal mechanisms; oxidative phosphorylation and substrate-level phosphorylation. The 'phosphorylation' refers to the phosphorylation of ADP. 'Oxidative' refers to ATP synthesis coupled to oxidation of the reduced intermediates NADH+H$^+$ (reduced nicotinamide adenine dinucleotide) and FADH$_2$ reduced flavin adeninine dinucleotide in the electron transport chain (ETC) (see Chapter 4: The electron transport chain (ETC)). 'Substrate-level phosphorylation' refers to ADP phosphorylation occurring *away* from the ETC, for example, during the glycolysis reactions (see Chapter 5: Glycolysis) and the tricarboxylic acid (TCA) cycle (see Chapter 3) reactions.

Nicotinamide adenine dinucleotide and flavin adenine dinucleotide

Nicotinamide adenine dinucleotide (NAD$^+$) and flavin adenine dinucleotide (FAD) are two crucial team players in cellular metabolism. Their structures are given in Fig. 2.14. They usually function as redox partners in oxidation reactions, and act as cofactors for the enzymes mediating these reactions.

Both NAD$^+$ and FAD function as electron carriers, because they readily accept and donate electrons during interaction with other molecules. They participate in catabolic oxidation reactions (as the oxidant, where they are reduced). Once reduced, they each transfer an electron pair to ETC complexes (at the mitochondria inner membrane). This is fundamental to the process of oxidative phosphorylation, in which they act as reductants and are reoxidized, reforming NAD$^+$ and FAD. Their redox behaviour is illustrated in Fig. 2.15, where 'X' represents a substrate molecule undergoing oxidation in any catabolic pathway.

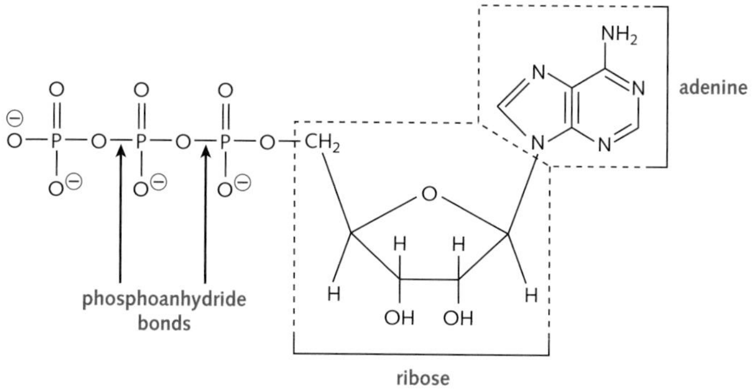

Fig. 2.13 Molecular structure of adenosine triphosphate (ATP).

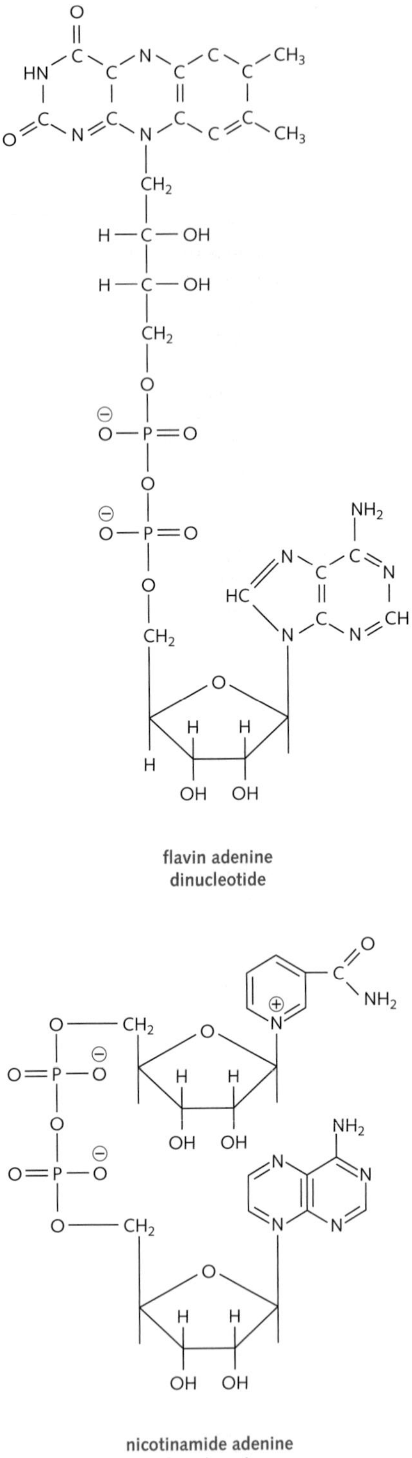

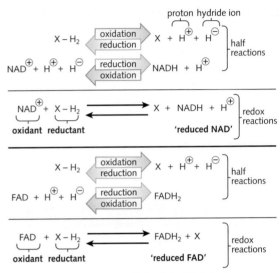

Fig. 2.14 Structures of flavin adenine dinucleotide and nicotinamide adenine dinucleotide.

Fig. 2.15 Redox reactions of nicotinamide adenine dinucleotide (NAD$^+$) and flavin adenine dinucleotide (FAD). Note in both reactions that X is oxidized, whereas NAD$^+$ or FAD is reduced, as seen in the half-equations. The two H atoms are removed from X–H$_2$ in the form of a hydride ion (H$^-$) and a proton (H$^+$ ion).

Conventional notation

Some scientists prefer to write 'NADH', rather than 'NADH+H$^+$' for simplicity. The former causes confusion as it implies that the second hydrogen atom is covalently associated with NADH. The second 'atom' is in fact a hydrogen ion, and because it 'disappears' into solution, some scientists prefer to completely omit the H$^+$ ion from equations. This also causes confusion as the equation then appears unbalanced. Understand that whenever you see 'NADH' written alone, the writer has assumed you appreciate that a free H$^+$ ion was also produced. In addition, note that 'NADH$_2$' is sometimes used interchangeably with 'NADH+H$^+$'.

Role of NAD$^+$ and FAD in ATP generation

NAD$^+$ and FAD integrate catabolism of all the major energy substrates (carbohydrates, lipids and proteins). Energy released from oxidation of these molecules is used to reduce NAD$^+$ and FAD by addition of a hydrogen ion (H$^+$) and a hydride ion (H$^-$). This reaction generates the reduced intermediates NADH+H$^+$ and FADH$_2$. NADH+H$^+$ and FADH$_2$ are then reoxidized when they transfer their two hydrogen atoms (and associated electrons) to the complexes of the ETC (see Chapter 4: The electron transport chain).

Nicotinamide adenine dinucleotide phosphate

Nicotinamide adenine dinucleotide phosphate (NADP$^+$) shares a structure with NAD$^+$ but has an additional phosphate group at C2 of the ribose moiety. The structure is shown in Fig. 2.16. The reduced form of NADP$^+$ is NADPH+H$^+$. NADPH+H$^+$ functions as a redox partner in numerous reductive biosynthetic reactions, including nucleotide (see Chapter 10), fatty acid and cholesterol synthesis (see Chapter 7; Table 2.3). The redox behaviour of NADP$^+$ is shown in Fig. 2.17.

Acetyl coenzyme A

The structure of acetyl coenzyme A (acetyl CoA) consists of an acetyl group (CH$_3$COO$^-$) covalently linked to CoA. The functional group of CoA is a thiol group (–SH), and to highlight this CoA is sometimes written as CoA–SH. The structure is shown in Fig. 2.18.

This molecule is central to metabolism (Fig. 2.19). Most cellular catabolic pathways (including carbohydrate, fat and protein metabolism) eventually lead to acetyl CoA. Oxidation of the acetyl residue of acetyl CoA in the TCA cycle (see Chapter 3, Fig. 3.1) generates ATP directly (substrate-level phosphorylation) and indirectly (via oxidative phosphorylation of TCA cycle-generated FADH$_2$ and NADH+H$^+$). It is also a substrate for several synthetic pathways, including fats, steroids and ketones.

Pyruvate

Pyruvate is another pivotal molecule with multiple roles in various anabolic and catabolic pathways. These are summarized in Fig. 2.20.

Table 2.3 Metabolic pathways requiring NAD$^+$/NADH+H$^+$ and FAD$^+$/FADH$_2$

Pathway	Requisite electron carrier
Glycolysis, TCA cycle, ethanol catabolism, ketone oxidation, β-oxidation of fatty acids, mitochondrial phase of citrate shuttle, mitochondrial phase of malate–aspartate shuttle, oxidative deamination of glutamate, serine synthesis, glycine synthesis	NAD$^+$
Oxidative phosphorylation (Chapter 4) cytoplasmic phase of the citrate shuttle, cytoplasmic phase of the glycerol-3-phosphate shuttle, glycerol synthesis, ketone synthesis	NADH+H$^+$
TCA cycle, β-oxidation of fatty acids, mitochondrial component of the carnitine shuttle, mitochondrial component of the glycerol-3-phosphate shuttle	FAD
Oxidative phosphorylation (Chapter 4)	FADH$_2$
Oxidative deamination of glutamate, pentose phosphate pathway, cytoplasmic phase of the citrate shuttle	NADP$^+$
Fatty acid synthesis, cholesterol synthesis, reductive amination, folate reduction, glutathione reduction, mitochondrial phase of the citrate shuttle	NADPH+H$^+$

FAD, Flavin adenine dinucleotide; NAD+, nicotinamide adenine dinucleotide; TCA, tricarboxylic acid.

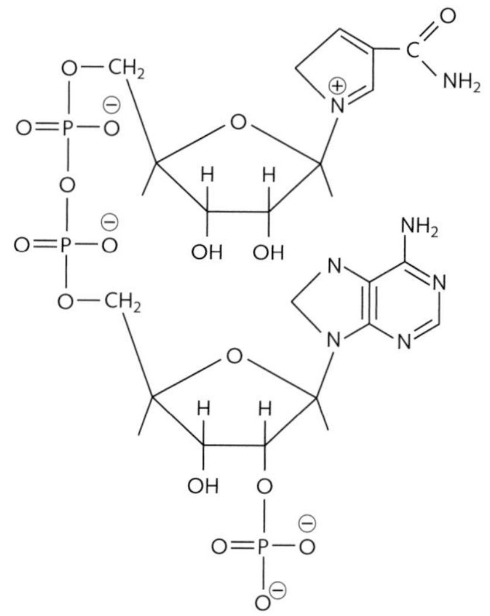

Fig. 2.16 Structure of nicotinamide adenine dinucleotide phosphate.

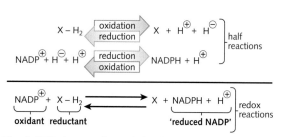

Fig. 2.17 Redox reactions of nicotinamide adenine dinucleotide phosphate (NADP$^+$.). Note in this reaction that X is oxidized, and NADP+ reduced. The two H atoms are removed from X–H$_2$ in the form of a hydride ion (H$^-$) and a proton (H$^+$ ion).

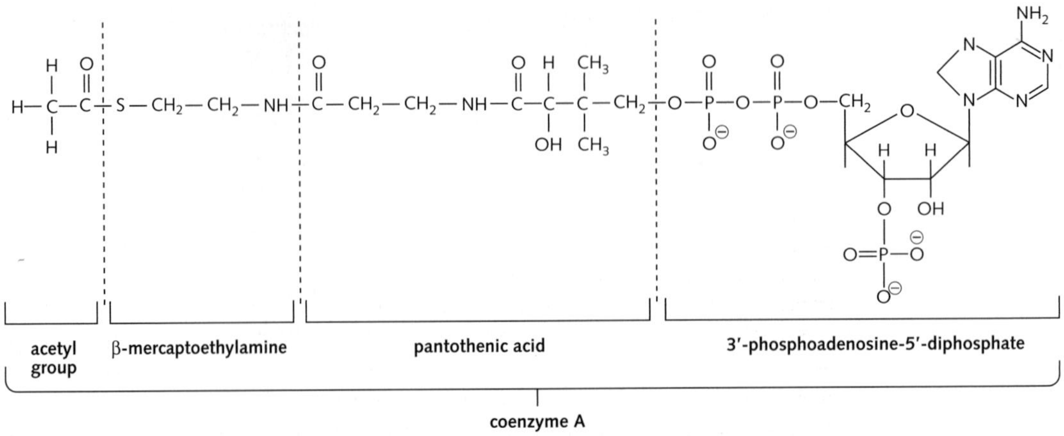

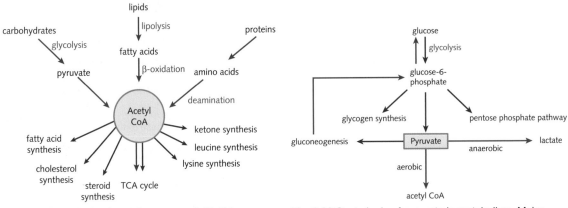

Fig. 2.18 Structure of acetyl-coenzyme A. Note the three components of coenzyme A.

Fig. 2.19 Central role of acetyl-coenzyme A (CoA) in metabolism. Major catabolic pathways are shown in *red* and major anabolic pathways in *blue*. *TCA*, Tricarboxylic acid.

Fig. 2.20 Central role of pyruvate in metabolism. Major catabolic pathways are shown in *red* and major anabolic pathways in *blue*. *CoA*, coenzyme A.

● Chapter Summary

- Catabolic pathways typically degrade biological molecules releasing energy, whereas anabolic pathways are usually synthetic, energy-consuming pathways.
- Enzymes play a pivotal role in metabolism by catalysing the biochemical reactions underpinning metabolic pathways.
- Pathway regulation is usually mediated by enzyme regulation, which may occur by a variety of mechanisms including substrate availability, allosteric regulation and hormonal regulation.
- Nicotinamide adenine dinucleotide (NAD^+), flavin adenine dinucleotide (FAD), nicotinamide adenine dinucleotide phosphate ($NADP^+$) are electron carriers which allow chemical potential energy to be transferred between different metabolic pathways. They readily participate in biological redox reactions.
- Adenosine triphosphate (ATP), acetyl coenzyme A and pyruvate are all key molecules in metabolism.

The tricarboxylic acid (TCA) cycle

3

INTRODUCTION

The tricarboxylic acid (TCA) cycle (also called the 'Krebs cycle' or the 'citric acid' cycle) is a cyclical reaction sequence (illustrated in Fig. 3.1) of oxidation reactions (Table 3.1) generating metabolic energy.

KEY POINTS

Key points regarding the TCA cycle include:

- It consists of eight individual reactions.
- The cycle can only function in the presence of oxygen (it is aerobic).
- It occurs in the mitochondrial matrix (and is thus limited to mitochondria-containing cells).
- The cycle initiates by accepting an acetyl-coenzyme A (acetyl-CoA), which combines with an oxaloacetate (generated by a previous 'turn' of the cycle) to form citrate (Fig. 3.1).
- Reactions 1, 3 and 4 are irreversible and represent the main regulation points for the cycle.
- Adenosine triphosphate (ATP) is generated *indirectly* via production of $FADH_2$ (reduced flavin

adenine dinucleotide) and $NADH+H^+$ (reduced nicotinamide adenine dinucleotide) in reactions 3, 4, 6 and 8 (see Fig. 3.1 and Table 3.1 for responsible enzymes).
- One molecule of guanosine triphosphate (GTP) is generated by substrate-level phosphorylation during reaction 5.

ROLE IN METABOLISM: INTEGRATING MACRONUTRIENT CATABOLISM

Because acetyl-CoA is produced from catabolism of carbohydrates, fatty acids and amino acids (the three macronutrients), the TCA cycle is pivotal in metabolism. It functions as a common pathway for (indirect) ATP generation from multiple different macronutrient molecules.

Cycle intermediates also function as substrates (raw materials) for numerous anabolic (synthetic) pathways. As the TCA cycle possesses both catabolic (breakdown of energy-rich molecules to release energy) and anabolic (synthetic) features, it is known as an 'amphibolic' pathway.

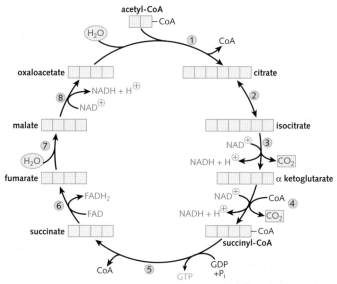

Fig. 3.1 The tricarboxylic acid cycle intermediates, enzymes and reaction participants. This takes place in the mitochondrial matrix. Enzymes are shown by letters: *1*, citrate synthase; *2*, aconitase; *3*, isocitrate dehydrogenase; *4*, α-ketoglutarate dehydrogenase; *5*, succinyl-CoA synthetase; *6*, succinate dehydrogenase; *7*, fumarase; *8*, malate dehydrogenase. Note each square represents a carbon atom. *CoA*, Coenzyme A; *FAD*, flavin adenine dinucleotide; *GDP*, guanosine diphosphate; *GTP*, guanosine triphosphate; *NAD*, nicotinamide adenine dinucleotide; *P*$_i$, inorganic phosphate.

Table 3.1 Details of each reaction of the tricarboxylic acid cycle

Reaction number (see Fig. 3.1)	Responsible enzyme	Reactants	Products	Notes
1	Citrate synthase	Acetyl-coenzyme A (acetyl-CoA) Oxaloacetate H_2O	Citrate CoA	Irreversible reaction Rate-limiting reaction Acetyl group from acetyl-CoA incorporated into oxaloacetate generated by a previous 'turn' of the cycle
2	Aconitase	Citrate	Isocitrate	
3	Isocitrate dehydrogenase	Isocitrate NAD^+	α-Ketoglutarate $NADH+H^+$ CO_2	Irreversible reaction Rate-limiting reaction
4	α-Ketoglutarate dehydrogenase	α-Ketoglutarate-CoA NAD^+	Succinyl-CoA $NADH+H^+$ CO_2	Irreversible reaction Rate-limiting reaction
5	Succinyl-CoA synthetase	Succinyl-CoA Guanosine diphosphate (GDP) Inorganic phosphate (P_i)	Succinate Guanosine triphosphate (GTP) CoA	One GTP molecule generated by substrate-level phosphorylation
6	Succinate dehydrogenase	Succinate FAD	Fumarate $FADH_2$	
7	Fumarase	Fumarate H_2O	Malate	
8	Malate dehydrogenase	Malate NAD^+	Oxaloacetate $NADH+H^+$	

ENERGY YIELD OF THE TCA CYCLE

GTP is directly generated by substrate-level phosphorylation (reaction 5, Fig. 3.1). ATP, however, is generated indirectly, via production of the reducing equivalents $FADH_2$ and $NADH+H^+$.

One complete cycle generates one molecule of $FADH_2$ and three molecules of $NADH+H^+$. $FADH_2$ and $NADH+H^+$ equate to approximately 1.5 and 2.5 ATP, respectively (see Chapter 4). The single GTP generated in reaction 5 is energetically equivalent to 1 ATP. Therefore, in total, 10 [1.5 + 3(2.5) + 1 = 10] ATP molecules are generated per molecule of acetyl-CoA oxidized by one complete revolution of the TCA cycle:

$$Acetyl\text{-}CoA + 2H_2O + 3NAD^+ + FAD + GDP + P_i \rightarrow 2CO_2$$
$$+3\left(NADH+H^+\right) + FADH_2 + GTP + CoA$$

REGULATION OF THE TCA CYCLE

Allosteric regulation

The three irreversible reactions (1, 3 and 4) are catalysed by the enzymes citrate synthase, isocitrate dehydrogenase

and α-ketoglutarate dehydrogenase. Because these reactions are rate limiting, modulating the activity of these enzymes controls cycle activity (see Chapter 2).

These three enzymes are allosterically activated by calcium ions. Intracellular Ca^{++} is elevated when energy-demanding processes (such as muscle contraction) are highly active. In this setting, TCA cycle activity is enhanced, allowing greater ATP production potential when the demand is greater (Fig. 3.2).

HINTS AND TIPS

High intracellular Ca^{2+} correlates with adenosine triphosphate (ATP)-demanding cellular activities. This is because Ca^{2+} ions represent chemical 'signals' initiating a vast number of key biochemical processes. Examples include muscle contraction, cell division and neurotransmitter release (exocytosis). This explains why Ca^{2+} has such a powerful influence on cellular energy homeostasis.

Cycle products $NADH+H^+$ and ATP (though note ATP production is indirect) allosterically inhibit the three rate-limiting enzymes. Abundance of these molecules

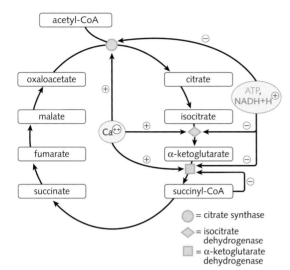

Fig. 3.2 Tricarboxylic acid cycle regulation. Note that the figure only illustrates the key regulatory enzymes. *ATP,* adenosine triphosphate; *CoA,* coenzyme A.

reflects high cellular ATP availability. TCA cycle activity is thus depressed when the demand for ATP is low.

Respiratory control (substrate provision)

TCA cycle activity, in common with all metabolic pathways, is limited by substrate availability. An available pool of nicotinamide adenine dinucleotide (NAD^+) and flavin adenine dinucleotide (FAD) is required. Thus NAD^+ and FAD renewal (from $NADH+H^+$ and $FADH_2$) contributes to TCA cycle activity. These molecules are regenerated during oxidative phosphorylation, meaning that an increased rate of oxidative phosphorylation (respiration) permits greater TCA cycle activity. Acetyl-CoA availability also influences TCA rate.

TCA CYCLE INTERMEDIATES AS METABOLIC PRECURSORS

Many important synthetic pathways use TCA cycle intermediates as substrates (raw materials). This is the synthetic (anabolic) aspect of the cycle, and is illustrated in Fig. 3.3. Key examples include:

- Gluconeogenesis, which utilizes oxaloacetate as a substrate (see Chapter 5).
- Oxaloacetate may also be diverted to aspartate synthesis, which in turn may be diverted towards purine and pyrimidine synthesis (see Chapter 10) or the synthesis of asparagine, lysine, methionine, threonine and isoleucine (see Chapter 9).
- Several pathways of amino acid synthesis use α-ketoglutarate as a substrate: glutamate, glutamine, arginine, proline and histidine (see Chapter 9).
- Porphyrin synthesis (e.g. haem) requires succinyl-CoA as a substrate (see Chapter 10).
- Fatty acids, ketone and cholesterol synthesis use acetyl-CoA as a substrate (see Chapter 7). Excessive carbohydrate intake is ultimately diverted towards fatty acid synthesis, because acetyl-CoA may be generated from citrate conversion. This in part explains the fattening tendency of diets excessively high in carbohydrates.

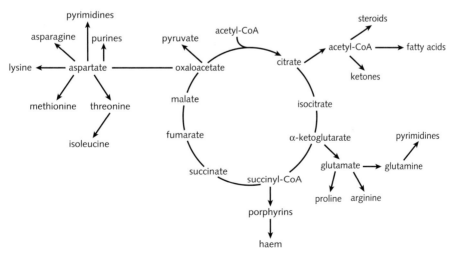

Fig. 3.3 Biosynthetic pathways that use tricarboxylic acid cycle intermediates as substrates. Note that reducing intermediates, additional reaction participants and enzymes are not shown for clarity. Also appreciate that each amino acid may be incorporated into proteins, but this is not shown on the diagram due to space limitation. *CoA,* Coenzyme A.

ANAPLEROTIC REACTIONS

When TCA cycle intermediates are recruited for use in other synthetic pathways, to sustain ongoing activity of the cycle, they must be replenished so the cycle can continue operating (Fig. 3.4). Pathways and reactions that replenish pathway molecules are known as 'anaplerotic' (Table 3.2). Try not to fall into the trap of assuming that simple reversal of the synthetic reactions always accounts for all TCA cycle anaplerosis.

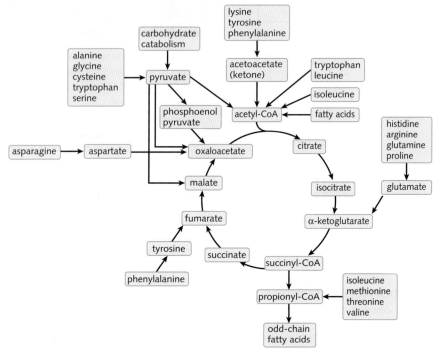

Fig. 3.4 Anaplerotic reactions of the tricarboxylic acid cycle. Note that reducing intermediates, additional reaction participants and enzymes are not shown for clarity. Also appreciate that each amino acid may be derived from protein hydrolysis, but this is not shown on the diagram due to space limitation.

Table 3.2 Example anaplerotic reactions of the tricarboxylic acid (TCA) cycle

Intermediate replenished	Substrate(s)	Reaction notes
Oxaloacetate	Pyruvate	Carboxylation
Oxaloacetate	Phosphoenolpyruvate	Carboxylation by pyruvate carboxylase (which is activated by acetyl-coenzyme A (acetyl-CoA), which accumulates when the downstream TCA cycle intermediate deficiency is holding up cycle progression)
Oxaloacetate	Aspartate	Transamination by aspartate transaminase
Succinyl-CoA	Propionyl-CoA (valine, methionine, threonine, isoleucine metabolism)	Propionyl-CoA is derived from catabolism of odd-numbered carbon chain fatty acids (see Chapter 7). It is converted to succinyl-CoA via a series of reactions including a reaction catalysed by the vitamin B12-dependent methylmalonyl-CoA mutase. Amino acids in brackets are first converted to propionyl-CoA.
α-Ketoglutarate	Glutamate (histidine, arginine, proline, glutamine)	Glutamate dehydrogenase catalyses the glutamate → α-ketoglutarate reaction. Amino acids in brackets first convert to glutamate
Fumarate	Tyrosine (phenylalanine)	Phenylalanine → tyrosine is catalysed by phenylalanine hydroxylase. Tyrosine is converted to fumarate, forming acetoacetate (a ketone (see Chapter 7) in the process.

INDIRECT ATP GENERATION BY THE TCA CYCLE

The principal role of the TCA cycle is generation of reducing equivalents ($FADH_2$ and $NADH+H^+$), which can then participate in oxidative phosphorylation. Oxidative phosphorylation (rather than substrate-level phosphorylation) is responsible for the vast majority of intracellular ATP generation. Oxidative phosphorylation is discussed in the following chapter.

Chapter Summary

- There are several tricarboxylic acid (TCA) cycle intermediates. It is unnecessary to memorize these; it is more advisable to focus on the key features such as the main substrate for the pathway (i.e. acetyl-coenzyme A (acetyl-CoA)), the main role of the cycle as an integration point for products of macronutrient (lipid, carbohydrate and protein) catabolism and the regulatory points within the cycle (the irreversible reactions: 1, 3 and 4).
- The direct energy yield of one 'turn' of the cycle is 10 adenosine triphosphate (ATP) molecules per incoming molecule of acetyl-CoA.
- The ATP yield is from both substrate-level phosphorylation (i.e. guanosine triphosphate generation) and also indirectly via the generation of reduced intermediates ($NADH+H^+$ and $FADH_2$), which subsequently enter the electron transport chain.
- The TCA cycle plays an important anaplerotic role. Cycle intermediates may be withdrawn from the pathway and directed towards other synthetic pathways, including amino acid synthetic substrates, purines, pyrimidines, porphyrins, fatty acids and ketones.

Oxidative phosphorylation

4

ADENOSINE TRIPHOSPHATE GENERATION

Adenosine triphosphate (ATP) molecules are all generated by phosphorylation of adenosine diphosphate (ADP). This can occur by either 'substrate-level' phosphorylation or 'oxidative' phosphorylation.

SUBSTRATE-LEVEL PHOSPHORYLATION

Substrate-level phosphorylation describes where ADP (or guanosine diphosphate) is modified by addition of a phosphoryl group (PO_3^{2-}), forming ATP (or guanosine triphosphate) independently of the mitochondrial electron transport chain (ETC). The phosphoryl group is derived from metabolic intermediate (substrate; Fig. 4.1). Substrate-level phosphorylation is an endergonic reaction, and therefore must be accompanied by an exergonic reaction to provide the energy required to drive the reaction forward.

Substrate-level phosphorylation does not require oxygen, and thus is vital for energy generation in anaerobic environments, such as rapidly contracting skeletal muscle. This form of ATP generation is also seen during glycolysis (reactions 7 and 10; see Chapter 5: Table 5.2), the tricarboxylic acid (TCA) cycle (reaction 5; see Chapter 3: Fig. 3.1 and Table 3.1) and creatine kinase-mediated hydrolysis of phosphocreatine in muscle cells.

PHOSPHOCREATINE (ALSO CALLED CREATINE PHOSPHATE)

Creatine is either absorbed from the diet or synthesized in the liver from glycine and arginine. It is then transported in the circulation to skeletal muscle. Once intracellular, it is phosphorylated, forming phosphocreatine (also called 'creatine phosphate'), effectively trapping the molecule inside the cell.

The phosphocreatine pool functions as a supply of immediately available phosphate. This allows ATP generation by substrate-level phosphorylation of ADP to take place during the first few seconds after initiations of high-intensity, energy-demanding activities such as muscle contraction (Fig. 4.2). As ATP is highly reactive and inherently unstable, it is energetically unfeasible to have a large available ATP pool intracellularly. In the absence of phosphocreatine, available intracellular ATP would be rapidly exhausted and muscle contraction would cease.

Phosphocreatine allows muscle contraction to be sustained after the initial (extremely small) amount of

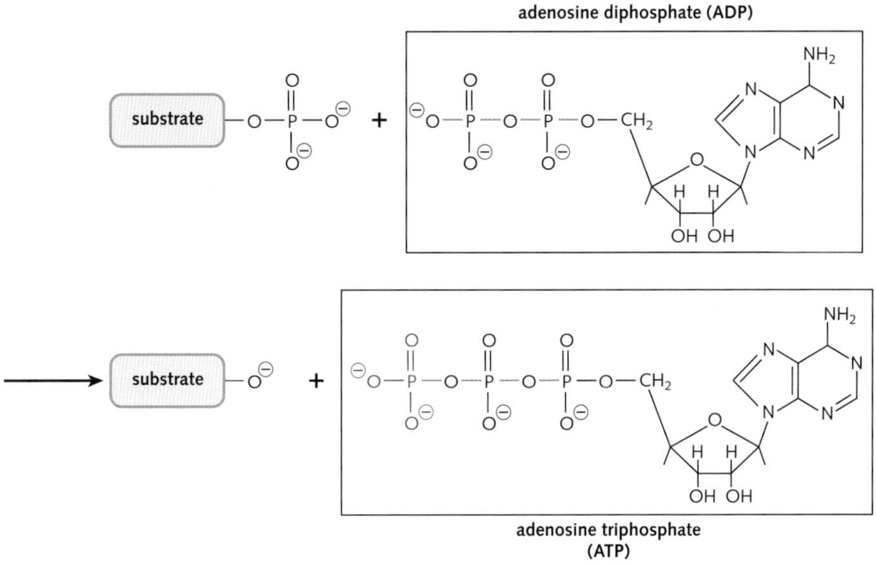

Fig. 4.1 Substrate-level phosphorylation. No oxygen is involved in this reaction. Note the two high-energy phosphoanhydride bonds in adenosine triphosphate (ATP), shown in *red*.

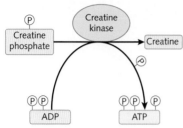

Fig. 4.2 Creatine phosphate: donation of phosphate group to adenosine diphosphate (ADP). *ATP,* Adenosine triphosphate.

available ATP is consumed, but before upregulation of glycolysis is sufficient to satisfy any increased demand for ATP (see Chapter 6).

OXIDATIVE PHOSPHORYLATION

This type of ATP production does require oxygen and occurs only at the *inner mitochondrial membrane* (IMM). This highly productive form of ATP generation is thus limited to cells containing mitochondria.

The energy required to perform the phosphorylation reaction is derived from the electron pairs associated with NADH+H$^+$ (reduced nicotinamide adenine dinucleotide) and FADH$_2$ (reduced flavin adenine dinucleotide). Recall that NADH+H$^+$ and FADH$_2$ are generated by catabolism of high-energy macronutrient molecules such as carbohydrates, fatty acids and amino acids.

The electron pairs are transferred from NADH+H$^+$ and FADH$_2$ (along with hydride and hydrogen ions) to the acceptor complexes of the ETC, also known as the electron transport system or respiratory chain. The electrons pairs are then sequentially transferred between the ETC complexes. The sequential oxidation of ETC complexes forms the 'oxidative' component of oxidative phosphorylation.

Every electron pair transfer between ETC complexes results in:

- The protein complex that donates the electrons being oxidized.
- The protein complex that receives the electrons being reduced.

Electron movement in an electronegative direction releases energy. This energy is used to import H$^+$ ions into the intermembranal space, generating a chemical gradient of hydrogen ions (protons) across the IMM.

Discharge of protons down their concentration gradient, back into the mitochondrial matrix, through the ATP synthase protein pore is highly exergonic. It provides the energy required for formation of the phosphoanhydride bond between inorganic phosphate (P$_i$) and ADP, forming ATP. This is the 'phosphorylation' stage of the oxidative phosphorylation.

The electron transport chain

The ETC consists of four protein structures embedded in the IMM. Each contains structural features (Table 4.1) that allow complexes to readily accept and release electrons. Each structure or 'complex' is numbered in order of increasing electron affinity and redox potential.

Two mobile transfer proteins (Fig. 4.3) also participate in oxidative phosphorylation:

- Coenzyme Q (also called 'ubiquinone'), which ferries two e$^-$ and two H$^+$ ions between complexes I and III, and between complexes II and III.
- Cytochrome c, which transfers the electron and proton pair from complex III to complex IV.

Electron pairs: where do they come from?

Electron pairs arrive at the ETC incorporated in NADH+H$^+$ and FADH$_2$ molecules.

- NADH+H$^+$ transfers two e$^-$ to complex I, forming nicotinamide adenine dinucleotide (NAD$^+$).
- FADH$_2$ transfers an e$^-$ pair to complex II, re-forming flavin adenine dinucleotide (FAD).

In receiving the e$^-$ pairs, each embedded protein complex is itself reduced.

Electron pair transfer between ETC complexes

After accepting an e$^-$ pair (and an H$^+$ pair, in the case of complexes I, II and IV), a complex then switches function, from e$^-$ pair recipient to donor. The e$^-$ pair is donated to the next unit of the ETC. Complexes I, II and IV pump protons into the intermembranal space.

Table 4.1 Structural features of proteins that confer the ability to accept and donate electrons

Feature	Description
Iron–sulphur centres	Iron ions are complexed with cysteine residue, sulphur atoms or inorganic sulphide groups. Iron in this configuration can undergo oxidation and reduction by cycling between the ferric and ferrous states.
Haem groups	These also contain an iron ion associated with four nitrogen atoms. The iron ion likewise can undergo oxidation and reduction by cycling between the ferric and ferrous states.

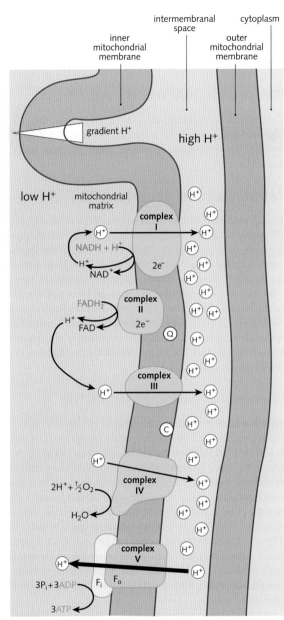

Fig. 4.3 Schematic of oxidative phosphorylation. Note the direction of the proton concentration gradient. *ADP*, Adenosine diphosphate; *ATP*, adenosine triphosphate; *C*, cytochrome C; *FAD*, flavin adenine dinucleotide; *NAD*, nicotinamide adenine dinucleotide; *Q*, coenzyme Q.

Complex III receives electron pairs from either complex I or II via coenzyme Q, and complex IV receives electron pairs from complex III via cytochrome c.

The final transfer occurs when complex IV transfers the electron pair to molecular oxygen (O_2), forming H_2O. This requirement for oxygen as the terminal electron (and hydrogen ion) pair acceptor explains why the process of oxidative phosphorylation requires oxygen (Fig. 4.4).

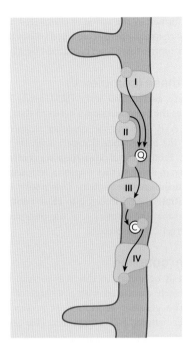

Fig. 4.4 Pathway of electron transfer. *Yellow circle* represents the transferred electron pair. *C*, cytochrome C; *Q*, coenzyme Q.

Generation of the proton gradient

The significance of electron transfer between complexes of the ETC is that it is highly exergonic. Electron transfer releases energy. This energy is harnessed by complexes I, III and IV and coupled to pumping of protons (originally delivered from NADH+H$^+$ and FADH$_2$) from the mitochondrial matrix compartment into the intermembranal space (across the IMM). This transfer is endergonic (requires energy), as this movement is against the H$^+$ gradient. In this way, receipt of the e$^-$ pairs is like an 'energy delivery', providing the complexes with the energy needed to transport protons across the IMM against their concentration gradient.

Differential ATP generation capacity of NADH+H$^+$ and FADH$_2$

Note that electron pairs originating from FADH$_2$ bypass complex I and arrive at complex II. Thus oxidation of FADH$_2$ leads to proton pumping only at complexes III and IV. NADH+H$^+$ oxidation, by contrast, leads to proton pumping at complexes I, III and IV. This explains why oxidation of FADH$_2$ leads to generation of less ATP per molecule than NADH+H$^+$ (approximately 1.5 ATP and approximately 2.5 ATP, respectively).

ATP synthesis

Formation of the second phosphoanhydride bond of ATP (from ADP and P$_i$) is highly endergonic. Once a proton gradient is formed by the action of complexes I, III and IV, the intrinsic chemical energy contained within the gradient (the 'proton-motive force') can be utilized by ATP synthase.

ATP synthase (complex V)

ATP synthase, also located at the IMM, binds ADP and P_i and catalyses the bond formation between the two species, generating ATP. The enzyme contains an intrinsic pore, connecting the mitochondrial matrix with the intermembrane space. Protons travel down their concentration gradient; however, in doing so they impose a transient structural alteration in the enzyme protein. This results in the ADP and P_i substrates being forced into close contact by ATP synthase, so that the formation of the phosphoanhydride bond is energetically favourable.

The term 'coupling'

ATP synthesis occurring in this manner can only occur when intimately associated with discharge of the proton gradient. The gradient generation is powered by electron transfer between ETC complexes. This association is termed 'coupling' or 'chemiosmotic coupling' and refers to ATP synthesis coupled with proton gradient discharge.

HINTS AND TIPS

Exploiting a chemical gradient as a source of chemical energy to power an energy-demanding biological process is conceptually similar to secondary active transport (see Chapter 1).

Uncoupling

Recall that 'coupling' describes the simultaneous discharging of the H^+ gradient with ATP synthesis. 'Uncoupling' describes the scenario where the permeability of the IMM to H^+ ions is significantly increased. H^+ ions are then able to discharge back into the matrix without travelling through the ATP synthase pore. This route of return cannot generate ATP; instead, the energy of the gradient discharge is dissipated as heat. ATP synthesis is thus uncoupled from discharge of the H^+ gradient. Any molecule that increases permeability of the IMM to H^+ ions is capable of uncoupling. 2,4-Dinitrophenol and carbonyl cyanide p-(trifluoromethoxy)-phenyl hydrazone uncouple mitochondria, short-circuiting the H^+ gradient accumulated by the ETC and blockading the main source of ATP production.

Uncoupling is only physiologically advantageous if heat is required, for example, in hairless newborn mammals. Newborn babies possess specialized heat-generating cells, termed 'brown fat' cells. These contain large numbers of uncoupled mitochondria, which are devoted to heat

production. The mitochondria are uncoupled by the presence of proteins in the IMM that contain a proton pore, allowing the accumulated H^+ gradient to discharge. These proteins are known as 'uncoupling proteins (UCPs)'.

Sources of NADH+H$^+$ and FADH$_2$

Catabolism of carbohydrates, fatty acids and the carbon skeletons of amino acids all produce NADH+H$^+$ and FADH$_2$ from their respective redox partners NAD$^+$ and FAD.

Mitochondrial access: NADH+H$^+$

Both β-oxidation of fatty acids and the TCA cycle occur in the mitochondrial matrix. NADH+H$^+$ and FADH$_2$ produced by these pathways are therefore already in the appropriate location for accessing the ETC and for participation in oxidative phosphorylation. However, NADH+H$^+$ generated in the cytoplasm by glycolysis or other pathways is in the 'wrong' place. The mitochondria are impermeable to NADH+H$^+$. So how does NADH+H$^+$ gain access to the mitochondrial interior to participate in oxidative phosphorylation? Two distinct 'shuttle mechanisms' exist, discussed in the following section.

Glycerol-3-phosphate shuttle

This mechanism recruits cytoplasmic NADH+H$^+$ into a redox reaction with dihydroxyacetone phosphate (DHAP): NADH+H$^+$ is oxidized to NAD$^+$, whereas DHAP is reduced to glycerol-3-phosphate (G3P). G3P *can* diffuse across the outer mitochondrial membrane and into the intermembrane space. Here, the G3P is reoxidized back to DHAP by glycerol-3-phosphate dehydrogenase, which spans the IMM and is thus appropriately spatially located. The redox partner for the second oxidation is FAD, located in the mitochondrial matrix, on the other side of the IMM. Reduced FAD (FADH$_2$) is then able to participate in oxidative phosphorylation by donating the electron pair to complex II of the ETC.

Although this is not a scenario identical to an NADH+H$^+$ itself travelling into the matrix, the results are similar: there is no longer an NADH+H$^+$ in the cytoplasm and there is a reduced equivalent (FADH$_2$) in a site where it may participate in oxidative phosphorylation.

Malate–aspartate shuttle

This system uses cytoplasmic NADH+H$^+$ as the redox partner in the reduction of oxaloacetate to malate. This shuttle exploits the fact that malate *can* cross mitochondrial membranes. It is illustrated in Fig. 4.5 and described here:

- Cytoplasmic malate dehydrogenase catalyses the reduction of malate to oxaloacetate, coupled with the simultaneous oxidation of NADH+H$^+$ to NAD$^+$.

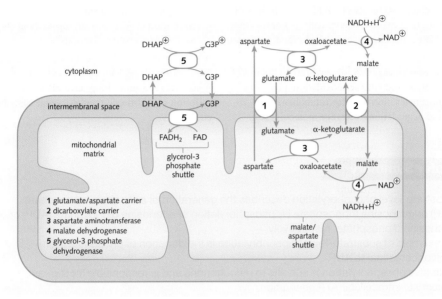

Fig. 4.5 The glycerol-3-phosphate and malate–aspartate shuttles. Note that there are both mitochondrial and cytoplasmic isoforms of the enzymes aspartate aminotransferase (3) and glycerol-3-phosphate dehydrogenase (5). *DHAP*, dihydroxyacetone phosphate.

- The cytoplasm-located malate then travels across both mitochondrial membranes into the matrix (via an antiport in the IMM; in exchange, α-ketoglutarate from the matrix is extruded into the cytoplasm).
- Once in the matrix, the reaction reverses. Matrix oxaloacetate is oxidized to malate, and matrix NAD$^+$ is reduced, forming NADH+H$^+$. Thus the reducing equivalent (NADH+H$^+$) 'appears' in the matrix to participate in oxidative phosphorylation.
- Matrix oxaloacetate is then converted to aspartate, which is extruded from the mitochondria by an antiport in exchange for glutamate.
- Once in the cytoplasm, the aspartate is converted to oxaloacetate.
- The matrix glutamate is converted to α-ketoglutarate, completing the cycle.

NAD$^+$ regeneration

Activity of the malate–aspartate or G3P shuttles ensures that cytoplasmic NAD$^+$ is continuously available. Shuttle activity is driven by oxidative phosphorylation, because this is the process that consumes the reducing equivalents in the mitochondrial matrix. Thus sustained oxidative phosphorylation ensures the maintenance of an available pool of NAD$^+$ in the cytoplasm.

Under anaerobic conditions, when oxidative phosphorylation cannot occur due to lack of molecular oxygen, NAD$^+$ is regenerated from NADH+H$^+$ by the reduction reaction pyruvate → lactate by lactate dehydrogenase.

FREE RADICAL PRODUCTION DURING OXIDATIVE PHOSPHORYLATION

Oxidative phosphorylation is the major intracellular generator of free radicals (see Chapter 2). Recall that the ultimate destination for sequentially transferred electron–hydrogen pairs is molecular oxygen (forming a water molecule). In a very small (<2%) proportion of reactions, oxygen is incompletely reduced, forming a superoxide radical (O_2^-) instead. This contains an unpaired electron, which reacts indiscriminately with biological molecules, causing oxidative damage.

ADENOSINE MONOPHOSPHATE-ACTIVATED PROTEIN KINASE

This enzyme is the major component maintaining the balance between intracellular ATP generation and utilization, that is, regulating cellular energy status. Adenosine monophosphate (AMP)-activated protein kinase (AMPK) activity approximates to the rate of intracellular ATP consumption, that is, AMPK can be considered as an integrated energy 'sensor' reflecting endergonic intracellular activities, such as muscle contraction.

The enzyme is named for its principal activator: AMP. AMP is generated by ATP hydrolysis, and is therefore present at high levels when ATP consumption is high.

Factors that deplete intracellular ATP (e.g. ischaemia, hypoxia or muscle contraction) typically generate AMP, activating AMPK. Its effects can be divided into two groups:

- Stimulation of pathways that increase intracellular ATP, such as glycolysis and fatty acid oxidation, processes which import macronutrients for catabolism (e.g. glucose) and degradation of storage molecules (e.g. lipolysis) for catabolism.
- Inhibition of ATP-consuming anabolic pathways such as lipid and protein synthesis.

AMPK primarily achieves these effects rapidly, via phosphorylation of regulatory enzymes in the relevant pathways. It also exerts a more long-term effect by influencing transcription of additional regulators that contribute to its own effects.

● Chapter Summary

- Substrate-level phosphorylation describes the generation of adenosine triphosphate (ATP) or guanosine triphosphate by phosphorylation of adenosine diphosphate (ADP) or guanosine diphosphate, respectively.
- An example of substrate-level phosphorylation is the donation of phosphate (from phosphocreatine) to ADP.
- Oxidative phosphorylation is specific to mitochondria and is responsible for the vast majority of intracellular ATP generation.
- Reduced intermediates (NADH+H$^+$ and FADH$_2$) generated by macronutrient catabolism function as the primary electron donors to the electron transfer chain (ETC).
- The electron transport chain is a series of proteins embedded in the inner mitochondrial membrane (IMM).
  Sequential oxidation and reduction of the ETC proteins (terminating with reduction of molecular oxygen) produce the energy required to generate a proton gradient between the intermembranal space and the mitochondrial matrix (i.e. across the IMM).
- Discharge of this proton gradient provides energy for ATP synthesis (ATP synthesis is 'coupled' to the discharge of the proton gradient).
- Import of reducing equivalents to the site of oxidative phosphorylation is mediated by the glycerol-3-phosphate and the malate–aspartate shuttles.
- Adenosine monophosphate-activated protein kinase functions as a molecular 'sensor' of intracellular energy status.

Carbohydrate metabolism

5

CARBOHYDRATES: A DEFINITION

A carbohydrate (also called 'saccharide') is a molecule containing only carbon, hydrogen and oxygen. The ratio of these atoms is always C:H:O = 1:2:1. The basic examples of a carbohydrate 'unit' are the 6-carbon 'monosaccharides' such as glucose, fructose or galactose. Disaccharides comprise two linked monosaccharides. Sucrose (glucose + fructose) and lactose (glucose + galactose) are shown in Fig. 5.1. The more complex 'polysaccharides' consist of numerous monosaccharide units linked by glycosidic bonds. A physiological example is glycogen (Fig. 5.2).

In biochemistry, carbohydrate metabolism encompasses glycolysis, glycogen synthesis and degradation, gluconeogenesis and the pentose phosphate pathway (PPP). These will be discussed in turn.

> ### HINTS AND TIPS
>
> #### CARBOHYDRATE NOMENCLATURE
>
> Six-carbon carbohydrates are also known as 'hexose' sugars. 'Pentose' sugars are five-carbon carbohydrates. 'Triose' sugars are three-carbon carbohydrates.

CARBOHYDRATE DIGESTION

Carbohydrates are degraded by two groups of enzymes: amylases and disaccharidases. Amylases hydrolytically degrade polysaccharides into disaccharides, whereas disaccharidases break down disaccharide molecules into their component monosaccharides. Monosaccharides are absorbable, whereas the larger polymers are not, hence the need for enzymatic digestion. Glucose and galactose are absorbed across the brush border of the small intestine by glucose–sodium cotransport, whereas fructose is absorbed by facilitated diffusion.

Mouth

Salivary amylase is mixed with food by chewing. This commences carbohydrate digestion in the buccal cavity. Polysaccharides (e.g. starch) are hydrolytically degraded to oligosaccharides and disaccharides (e.g. sucrose, lactose, maltose).

Stomach

The low pH of the gastric lumen then arrests amylase activity, effectively pausing carbohydrate digestion until food material enters the small intestine.

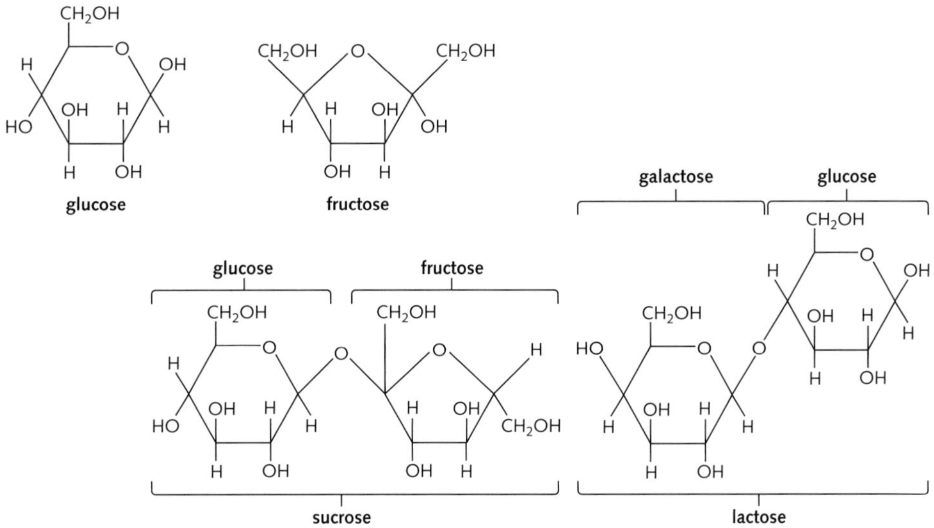

Fig. 5.1 Monosaccharides. These all share the formula $C_x(H_2O)_y$. Glucose and fructose monosaccharides are shown. The disaccharides lactose and sucrose are also illustrated.

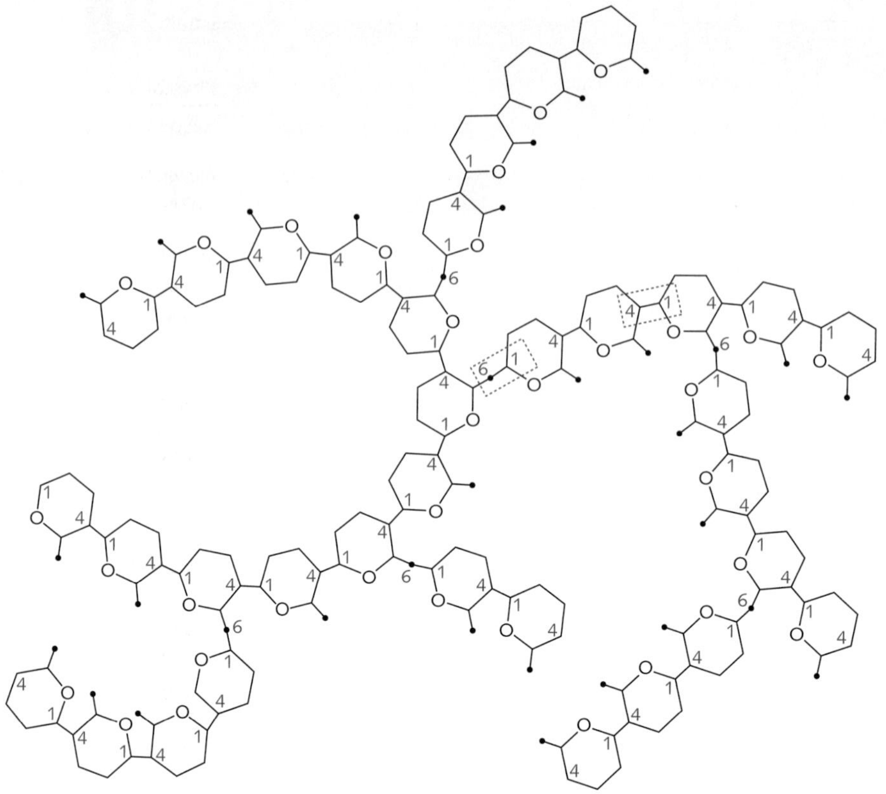

Fig. 5.2 Macroscopic structure of glycogen. Each hexagon represents a glucose monomer. Note that both (1–4) and (1–6) carbon-to-carbon bonds are present (examples shown within the *dotted boxes*). These bonds are shown in more detail in Fig. 5.11.

Duodenum

Pancreatic amylase resumes hydrolysis of any polysaccharides not already degraded by salivary amylase, generating further oligosaccharides and disaccharides.

Small intestine

Disaccharidases (such as sucrase, lactase and maltase) split their specific substrate disaccharides into their monosaccharide components.

GLUCOSE ENTRY INTO CELLS

Glucose (or its derivatives, such as glucose-6-phosphate (Glc-6-P)) participates in all the carbohydrate pathways of metabolism. As phospholipid bilayers are impermeable to polar molecules, glucose cannot directly diffuse across plasma cell membranes. To allow glucose to move into and out of cells, specialized transporter structures span the membranes. Regulating transporter function therefore allows regulation of glucose traffic across the cell membrane.

Facilitated diffusion

In certain environments, extracellular glucose exceeds intracellular glucose. The concentration gradient is thus favourable for glucose to passively enter the cell. However, a route across the phospholipid bilayer is necessary. This is provided by the GLUT transporters, which enable facilitated diffusion. The different characteristics of the most important GLUT transporters are shown in Table 5.1.

Secondary active transport

When the extracellular glucose is lower than the intracellular glucose, glucose entry is coupled to sodium transport, via the sodium–glucose cotransporter (also called 'symport', known as the SGLT-1 transporter; see Chapter 1). This allows the transmembrane Na^+ gradient to 'power' intracellular import of glucose *against* the prevailing concentration gradient. This mechanism predominates at the brush border epithelial cells lining the gastrointestinal tract.

Table 5.1 Glucose transporters. High-affinity transporters permit more rapid glucose traffic across membranes

Subtype	Transported sugar(s)	Tissue sites	Affinity	Insulin sensitivity	Physiological role
GLUT-1	Glucose only	Blood–brain barrier endothelia, erythrocytes and astrocytes (adults) Widespread (fetus)	High	No	Responsible for basal glucose intracellular import in the fetus. Allows bloodstream glucose to access the central nervous system tissue across the blood–brain barrier.
GLUT-2	Glucose, fructose or galactose	Luminal face of gut enterocytes	Low	No	Allows digested carbohydrate (monomeric hexose sugars) absorption into enterocytes.
		Pancreatic beta cells			Low-affinity, high-capacity characteristics permit the intracellular glucose of beta cells to closely mirror plasma glucose, permitting appropriate regulation of insulin secretion.
		Hepatocytes			Main access route for bloodstream glucose entry into hepatocytes.
GLUT-3	Glucose only	Neurons Placenta	High	No	Permits continual glucose access into neurons and placental (and thus the fetus) independent of insulin.
GLUT-4	Glucose only	Cardiac myocytes, skeletal myocytes, adipocytes	High	Yes GLUT-4 expression proportional to blood insulin	This transporter accounts for the sensitivity of glucose uptake to insulin levels.
GLUT-5	Fructose only	Basolateral face of gut enterocytes	High	No	

GLYCOLYSIS

Overview

Glycolysis is catabolism of glucose and the equation is as follows ($CH_3COCOOH$ is the formula of pyruvate):

$$C_6H_{12}O_6 + 2NAD^+ + 2ADP + 2HPO_4^{2-}$$
$$\rightarrow CH_3COCOOH + 2NADH + H^+ + 2ATP$$

Glycolysis occurs in the cytoplasm of all cells. It occurs in both aerobic and anaerobic environments. A glucose molecule is sequentially oxidized via 10 specific reactions, ultimately forming two molecules of pyruvate (Table 5.2).

During glycolysis, two adenosine triphosphate (ATP) molecules are generated via substrate-level phosphorylation (in fact, four are generated, but two are consumed by the pathway). Two NADH+H$^+$ are also generated, each representing approximately 2.5 ATP in energy equivalents. The net ATP yield of glycolysis is therefore 7 ATP per oxidized molecule of glucose:

$$2\,ATP + 2(\sim 2.5\,ATP) = 7\,ATP$$

Much of the pyruvate generated in glycolysis is subsequently decarboxylated, forming acetyl-coenzyme A (CoA). Recall that acetyl-CoA may enter the tricarboxylic acid (TCA) cycle and undergo further oxidation (see Chapter 3), generating further ATP and NADH+H$^+$, or participate in other synthetic pathways.

Glycolysis: the reaction pathway

Each reaction is detailed in Table 5.1 and the pathway is divided into two phases as follows.

'Energy investment' phase

The energy investment phase is so-called because during this first segment of the glycolysis pathway ATP is consumed (rather than generated):

- Reaction 1: Glucose is phosphorylated, forming Glc-6-P. ATP donates the phosphoryl group.
- Reaction 2: Glc-6-P isomerizes to form fructose-6-phosphate (Fru-6-P).
- Reaction 3: Fru-6-P is phosphorylated, generating fructose-1,6-bisphosphate (Fru-1,6-BP). Again, ATP is the phosphoryl donor.

Table 5.2 Reactions of glycolysis. Enzymes shown in bold represent key regulation points of the pathway

Reaction	Enzyme	Type of reaction	Reaction equation
1	**Hexokinase** (HK)[a]	Phosphorylation	Glucose + ATP → Glucose-6-phosphate + ADP + H^+
2	**Phosphoglucoisomerase**	Isomerization	Glucose-6-phosphate ↔ Fructose-6-phosphate
3	**Phosphofructokinase**	Phosphorylation	Fructose-6-phosphate + ATP → Fructose-1,6-bisphosphate + ADP + H^+
4	**Aldolase**	Cleavage	Fructose-1,6-bisphosphate ↔ dihydroxyacetone phosphate + glyceraldehyde-3-phosphate
5	**Triose phosphate isomerase**	Isomerization (ketose → aldose)	Dihydroxyacetone phosphate ↔ glyceraldehyde-3-phosphate
6	**Glyceraldehyde-3-phosphate dehydrogenase**	Oxidation, phosphorylation	Glyceraldehyde-3-phosphate + NAD^+ + HPO_4^{2-} ↔ 1,3-bisphosphoglycerate + NADH+H^+
7	**Phosphoglycerate kinase**	Substrate-level phosphorylation	1,3-Bisphosphoglycerate + ADP ↔ ATP + 3-phosphoglycerate
8	**Phosphoglycerate mutase**	Isomerization	3-Phosphoglycerate ↔ 2-phosphoglycerate
9	**Enolase**	Dehydration	2-Phosphoglycerate ↔ phosphoenolpyruvate + H_2O
10	**Pyruvate kinase**	Substrate-level phosphorylation	Phosphoenolpyruvate + ADP → pyruvate + ATP

[a] Hexokinase is substituted for by glucokinase in hepatocytes and pancreatic islet cells.
Enzymes in bold represent the targets of pathway regulation.
ATP, Adenosine triphosphate; ADP, adenosine diphosphate; NAD, nicotinamide adenine dinucleotide.

- Reaction 4: Fru-1,6-BP is split into *two* three-carbon molecules, glyceraldehyde-3-phosphate (GAP) and dihydroxyacetone phosphate.
- Reaction 5: Dihydroxyacetone phosphate isomerizes, producing a second molecule of GAP.

'Energy generation' phase

It is important to understand that the following glycolysis reactions occur in duplicate, because the original six-carbon glucose molecule is split into two three-carbon molecules, each of which progresses through reactions 6–10:

- Reaction 6: The three-carbon GAP undergoes dehydrogenation and phosphorylation to form 1,3-bisphosphoglycerate (1,3-BPG), with nicotinamide adenine dinucleotide (NAD^+) reduced to NADH+H^+ as the redox partner.
- Reaction 7: 1,3-BPG donates a phosphate group to adenosine diphosphate (ADP), forming a molecule of 3-phosphoglycerate (3-PG) and a molecule of ATP. This is a substrate-level phosphorylation.
- Reaction 8: 3-PG is isomerized; the phosphate group is transferred from the third to the second carbon atom, forming 2-phosphoglycerate (2-PG).
- Reaction 9: 2-PG is dehydrated, forming phosphoenolpyruvate (PEP).
- Reaction 10: The final step of glycolysis is the transfer of the phosphoryl group from PEP to ADP. This generates pyruvate and ATP and represents the

second substrate-level phosphorylation of glycolysis (Fig. 5.3).

Glycolytic intermediates as biosynthetic precursors

The glycolysis pathway also acts as an essential source of intermediates for other pathways, which rely on glycolytic intermediates for substrate provision (Fig. 5.4). These include:

- The TCA cycle (see Chapter 3)
- The PPP (see 'The pentose phosphate pathway' section)
- Gluconeogenesis (i.e. synthesis of glucose from noncarbohydrate precursors; see the 'Gluconeogenesis' section)
- Lipid synthesis (see Chapter 7)
- Synthesis of several nonaromatic amino acids (see Chapter 9)
- Synthesis of aromatic amino acids (see Chapter 9)

Regulation of glycolysis

The enzymes catalysing reactions 1, 3 and 10 of the pathway function as glycolysis regulation points, because these reactions are all highly exergonic (i.e. are essentially irreversible).

Reaction 1: glucose phosphorylation

Reaction 1 of glycolysis is catalysed by hexokinase (HK). This enzyme is allosterically inhibited by the reaction product Glc-6-P. Insulin upregulates HK transcription, whereas

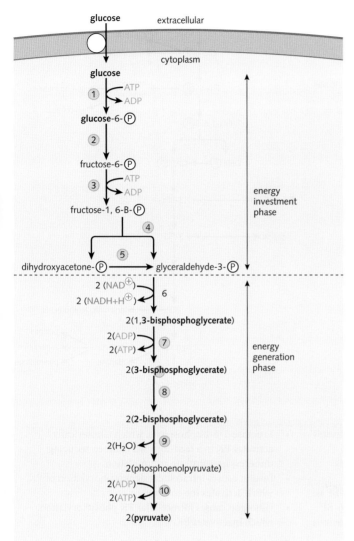

Fig. 5.3 The glycolysis pathway. Circled numbers represent enzymes given in Table 5.2. This example is shown with a facilitated diffusion transport mechanism. Note the conceptual division into the energy investment and energy generation phases shown by the *dotted line*. *ADP,* Adenosine diphosphate; *ATP,* adenosine triphosphate; *NAD,* nicotinamide adenine dinucleotide.

glucagon downregulates HK transcription. Insulin and glucagon thus comprise the main hormonal regulation of this reaction.

Note that glucokinase (the isoform of HK present in liver, pancreatic beta cells and hypothalamic cells) is insensitive to product inhibition by Glc-6-P. Glucose phosphorylation will persist in these locations even when the remainder of the pathway is less active, resulting in Glc-6-P accumulation. Isoform affinity also differs; glucokinase will only catalyse glucose phosphorylation at very high intracellular glucose, whereas the more ubiquitous HK operates at any concentration, including much lower concentrations.

Reaction 3: fructose-6-phosphate phosphorylation

Phosphofructokinase (PFK), the enzyme catalysing this reaction is an important site of glycolysis regulation, because reaction 3 is the principal rate-limiting step of the pathway.

Accelerating this reaction therefore accelerates the overall rate of glycolysis. Various factors influence PFK-1 activity, including:

- ATP: ATP allosterically inhibits PFK-1. When ATP is abundant, reflecting high cellular energy status, PFK-1 operates at a lower rate.
- Citrate: This is not a direct product of reaction 3, but the final pathway product, pyruvate, is decarboxylated to acetyl-CoA, which then combines with oxaloacetate to form citrate. Citrate allosterically inhibits PFK-1. When glycolysis is highly active, citrate is abundant and has an inhibitory effect on the pathway.
- Adenosine monophosphate (AMP) and ADP: These allosterically activate PFK-1. They are abundant in cells where the energy status is low, reflecting a requirement for more ATP to be generated.

Fig. 5.4 Participation of the glycolytic intermediates in other anabolic pathways. *1,3-BPG,* 1,3-Bisphosphoglycerate; *2,3-BPG,* 2,3-bisphosphoglycerate; *2-PG,* 2-phosphoglycerate; *3-PG,* 3-phosphoglycerate; *CoA,* coenzyme A; *DHA,* dihydroxyacetone phosphate; *Fru-1,6-BP,* fructose-1,6-bisphosphate; *Fru-6-P,* fructose-6-phosphate; *Glc-1-P,* Glucose-1-phosphate; *GAD,* Glyceraldehyde phosphate; *Glc-6-P,* glucose-6-phosphate; *PEP,* phosphoenolpyruvate.

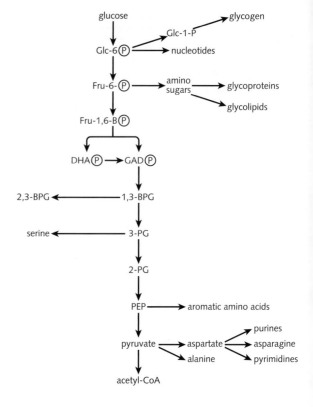

- Fru-6-P (a reaction 3 substrate) allosterically activates PFK-1; accumulation of substrate feed-forward positively on PFK-1 activity, increasing glycolysis.
- Fructose-2,6-bisphosphate (Fru-2,6-BP): This allosterically activates PFK-1. Note that Fru-2,6-BP is synthesized by PFK-2, not PFK-1. When Fru-2,6-BP is high, glycolysis predominates over gluconeogenesis (see the 'Gluconeogenesis' section).
- Insulin: Insulin regulates glycolysis by increasing synthesis of PFK-1. More enzyme means that glycolysis activity runs at a greater rate in high insulin physiological settings.
- Glucagon: Glucagon regulates glycolysis, by decreasing synthesis of PFK-1. This means that glycolysis operates at a lower rate where glucagon is predominant.

Reaction 10: Phosphoenolpyruvate → pyruvate

Pyruvate kinase (PK) catalyses reaction 10 of glycolysis. It is influenced by:

- ATP, which allosterically inhibits PK by decreasing the affinity of the enzyme for its substrate PEP. When cellular energy status is high and ATP is abundant, PK is less active.
- Acetyl-CoA, which allosterically inhibits PK. Acetyl-CoA reflects high cellular energy status; in this context PK is less active.

- Fructose-1-6-bisphosphate, which allosterically activates PK in a feed-forward manner, reducing unnecessary substrate accumulation.
- Insulin causes intracellular dephosphorylation of PK, which activates the enzyme.
- Glucagon causes intracellular PK phosphorylation, which inactivates PK.

The role of fructose-2,6-bisphosphate

PFK-1 is an enzyme of the glycolysis pathway. By contrast, PFK-2 does not participate directly in glycolysis but produces Fru-2,6-BP, which powerfully influences glycolysis via its effect on PFK-1. Importantly, however, Fru-2,6-BP also inhibits one of the enzymes of the gluconeogenesis pathway. This ensures that glucose is not degraded and synthesized simultaneously. Fig. 5.5 elaborates this concept.

THE INSULIN:GLUCAGON RATIO INFLUENCE ON GLYCOLYSIS

Insulin is secreted when blood glucose is high (i.e. in the 'fed' state). When glucose is abundant, the oxidation of glucose generating ATP (via glycolysis) is advantageous. Insulin promotes glycolysis by various effects on key regulatory enzymes. Glucagon, by contrast, is released into the bloodstream when blood glucose is low (i.e. in the 'fasting'

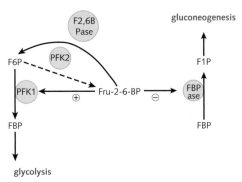

Fig. 5.5 Dual role of fructose-2,6-bisphosphate (Fru-2,6-BP) as a regulator of glycolysis and gluconeogenesis. *F6P,* fructose-6-phosphate; *FBP,* fructose bisphosphate; *FBPase,* fructose bisphosphatase; *PFK,* phosphofructokinase.

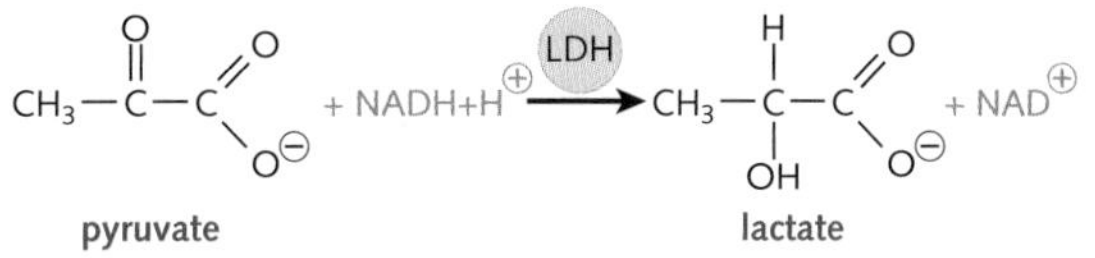

Fig. 5.6 Lactate production. *LDH,* Lactate dehydrogenase; *NAD⁺,* nicotinamide adenine dinucleotide.

state). It has the converse effect on the regulatory enzymes of glycolysis; it suppresses (rather than promotes) glycolytic pathway activity.

Physiologically, insulin and glucagon are usually released by the pancreas reciprocally. This means that the release of one is usually combined with suppression of the other. The relationship between the two is reflected in the insulin:glucagon ratio. If insulin is high and glucagon low, this ratio is high, and likewise vice versa. In health, the response of the pancreas to changes in blood glucose is swift. Thus the insulin:glucagon ratio both reflects the nutritional state of the organism in terms of carbohydrate intake and determines the metabolic fate of glucose.

Regarding glycolysis, when the insulin:glucagon ratio is high ('fed' state), pathway activity is also high. When the ratio is low ('fasting' state), glycolysis activity is low (see Chapter 6).

AEROBIC GLYCOLYSIS VERSUS ANAEROBIC GLYCOLYSIS

Glycolysis occurs regardless of whether oxygen is present or absent. It is the only pathway capable of producing ATP in the absence of oxygen, and therefore is of paramount importance in cells lacking mitochondria, such as erythrocytes, and in hypoxic (low-oxygen) environments such as in ischaemic tissue or rapidly contracting skeletal muscle (see Chapter 6).

The key difference between aerobic and anaerobic glycolysis is that in the presence of oxygen (aerobic environment) the NADH+H⁺ generated during glycolysis transfers electrons to the mitochondrial electron transport chain, where the oxidative phosphorylation takes place (see Chapter 4), producing approximately 2.5 ATP

per NADH+H⁺. However, when oxygen is not present to act as a terminal electron acceptor, oxidative phosphorylation cannot occur. In anaerobic conditions, NADH+H⁺ is reoxidized to NAD⁺ as a redox partner for the reaction converting pyruvate to lactate (Fig. 5.6). This reaction is catalysed by lactate dehydrogenase and yields no ATP. This lowers the ATP yield of glycolysis in anaerobic conditions to 2 ATP per glucose molecule, rather than the 7 ATP that would be generated in aerobic conditions. To compound the situation, because pyruvate is converted to lactate, pyruvate cannot enter the TCA cycle. In aerobic conditions this would yield a further 10 ATP per pyruvate molecule.

HYPERLACTATAEMIA

Cells cannot perform oxidative phosphorylation if they are not supplied with oxygen. Pathophysiologically, the state of insufficient oxygen supply is known as 'hypoxia', and is seen in many disease states, for example, ischaemia (impaired tissue perfusion local to the supply territory of a compromised blood vessel) and shock (global failure of tissue perfusion which may arise due to many disease scenarios). In such anaerobic environments, intracellular pyruvate is converted to lactate, which enters the bloodstream. An elevated plasma lactate (hyperlactataemia) is a useful indicator of widespread tissue hypoxia and is pathological (unless appearing transiently during intense exercise).

Elevated lactate levels combined with an increase in H⁺ generation during hypoxia lead to the formation of lactic acid accompanied by a blood pH < 7.35 ([H⁺]> 44 nmol/L) (acidaemia) and are particularly worrisome. This condition is known as 'lactic acidosis'. All the following scenarios will cause hyperlactaemia and acidosis:

- Hypovolaemic shock resulting from haemorrhage, dehydration or distributive shock
- Cardiogenic shock
- Hypoxaemic tissue hypoxia

HEREDITARY RED CELL ENZYMOPATHIES

Mutations in the gene coding for one of the glycolysis enzymes are known as 'inherited red cell enzymopathies'.

These conditions are extremely rare; however, among these glycolytic enzyme deficiencies, PK deficiency is the most common. Inheritance is autosomal recessive for all but enolase (autosomal dominant) and phosphoglycerate kinase (X-linked recessive) deficiencies.

Deficiencies in glycolytic enzymes damage red blood cells, which, lacking mitochondria, rely solely on glycolysis for ATP generation. Unable to produce sufficient ATP to maintain necessary intracellular processes, in particular membrane integrity, their lifespan is dramatically shortened. This manifests clinically with symptoms of anaemia due to chronic haemolysis.

THE PYRUVATE → ACETYL-CoA REACTION

Acetyl-CoA is formed from pyruvate (Fig. 5.7). This is an irreversible oxidative decarboxylation, catalysed by pyruvate dehydrogenase (PDH). This reaction is important, because it allows the final common product of carbohydrate catabolism (pyruvate) to access to the TCA cycle. Note that this reaction also reduces NAD^+ to $NADH+H^+$, which can generate further ATP via oxidative phosphorylation in the presence of oxygen (see Chapter 4).

PYRUVATE DEHYDROGENASE

PDH is in fact a trio of enzymes (E1, E2 and E3) that are all spatially associated. It is located in the mitochondrial matrix. There are five steps in the pyruvate → acetyl-CoA reaction, which are not essential to learn for medicine (however, it does explain why so many coenzymes are necessary!). These coenzymes are:

- Thiamine pyrophosphate (TPP)
- Lipoic acid
- CoA
- Flavin adenine dinucleotide (FAD)
- NAD^+

TPP is deficient in thiamine-deficient states, resulting in failure of the pyruvate → acetyl-CoA reaction and thus accumulation of pyruvate. Because excess pyruvate is

converted to lactate, hyperlactataemia may be associated with thiamine deficiency (see Table 12.2).

Regulation of PDH

PDH mediates the reaction pyruvate → acetyl-CoA, also generating $NADH+H^+$. Both these reaction products allosterically inhibit the PDH complex via negative feedback. PDH activity is also regulated by phosphorylation: phosphorylation *inactivates* PDH, whereas dephosphorylation *activates* the enzyme. PDH phosphorylation (inactivation) is mediated by a physically associated kinase enzyme, itself allosterically activated by acetyl-CoA and $NADH+H^+$, whereas PDH dephosphorylation (activation) is mediated by a physically associated phosphatase enzyme (Fig. 5.8), which is itself activated by insulin.

GLUCONEOGENESIS

Gluconeogenesis is the production of glucose from noncarbohydrate sources. It mainly takes place in hepatocytes, but also occurs in renal cortical cells. Most gluconeogenesis reactions occur in the cytoplasm, but two of the reactions occur within mitochondria. The substrate molecules for the gluconeogenesis pathway are derived from breakdown of either lipids, carbohydrates or protein.

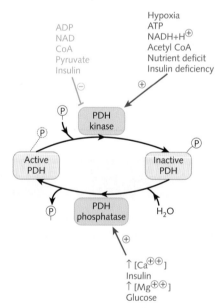

Fig. 5.8 Regulation of pyruvate dehydrogenase (PDH) activity. This occurs primarily by phosphorylation/ dephosphorylation, mediated by PDH kinase and PDH phosphatase. Factors influencing these enzymes are illustrated. *ADP,* Adenosine diphosphate; *ATP,* adenosine triphosphate; *CoA,* coenzyme A; *NAD,* nicotinamide adenine dinucleotide.

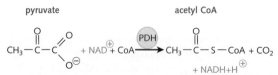

Fig. 5.7 Formation of acetyl-coenzyme A (acetyl-CoA) from pyruvate. *NAD+,* Nicotinamide adenine dinucleotide; *PDH,* pyruvate dehydrogenase.

Recall that glycolysis includes several reactions that are essentially irreversible. In gluconeogenesis, reactions mediated by different enzymes bypass these steps; therefore gluconeogenesis is not a simple molecular backtracking of the glycolysis pathway. Gluconeogenesis is overall an energy-consuming pathway: 6 ATPs are consumed per molecule of glucose produced. This energetic 'expense' is justified by the physiological importance of glucose.

PLASMA GLUCOSE CONCENTRATION MUST BE MAINTAINED ABOVE CRITICAL LEVEL

Even when fasting, blood glucose must not fall below 3 mmol to avoid serious, particularly neurological, complications of hypoglycaemia (see Chapter 6). Blood glucose is maintained over 3 mmol in healthy individuals by a combination of three main ways:

- Intake of exogenous glucose (eating)
- Endogenous release of stored glucose (glycogenolysis)
- Endogenous synthesis of glucose (gluconeogenesis)

TIMESCALE OF GLYCOGENOLYSIS VERSUS GLUCONEOGENESIS

Glycogen breakdown (glycogenolysis) is the 'first-line' mechanism exploited physiologically to prevent blood glucose falling below the normal range. However, glycogen reserves in the liver, kidney and skeletal muscle are quickly exhausted by exercise or fasting for a short time. The body metabolism must therefore be able to compensate (when immediate eating is not a viable option) by converting other metabolic substrates into glucose (i.e. gluconeogenesis).

GLUCONEOGENIC SUBSTRATES

Various types of macronutrient molecules may be degraded to provide substrates for gluconeogenesis. These include:

- Carbohydrates: Glycolysis under anaerobic conditions ultimately generates lactate, which can be reconverted back to pyruvate by lactate dehydrogenase. Pyruvate is also a gluconeogenic substrate.
- Proteins: Catabolism of proteins forms amino acids, some of which (the 'glucogenic' amino acids) can participate in gluconeogenesis. The most important gluconeogenic precursor is alanine.

- Lipids: Mobilized fat stores (lipolysis) or ingested fats (triacylglycerols) are hydrolysed to release glycerol and fatty acids (see Chapter 7). Glycerol and propionyl-CoA (a product of the β-oxidation of odd-numbered fatty acids; see Chapter 7) can enter the gluconeogenesis pathway and be converted into glucose. Note that fatty acids cannot be converted into glucose, although ketones *derived* from fatty acids (see Chapter 7) may be oxidized in the mitochondria and thus are an alternative acetyl-CoA precursor in starvation.

SEQUENCE OF GLUCONEOGENESIS

This is best illustrated as a diagram (Fig. 5.9).

KEY DIFFERENCES BETWEEN GLUCONEOGENESIS AND GLYCOLYSIS

- The conversion of pyruvate to PEP in gluconeogenesis is a two-step reaction, rather than the single PEP → pyruvate reaction seen in glycolysis (reaction 10, see Fig. 5.3 and Table 5.2). Furthermore, this conversion requires both ATP and guanosine triphosphate. The responsible enzymes are mitochondrial pyruvate carboxylase and cytoplasmic PEP carboxykinase.
- Between these first two reactions, oxaloacetate 'leaves' the mitochondria and 'enters' the cytoplasm via the malate–aspartate shuttle (see Chapter 4).
- Fru-1,6-BP is converted to Fru-6-P via a hydrolytic reaction catalysed by fructose-1,6-bisphosphatase, with no involvement of ADP or ATP in contrast to reaction 3 of glycolysis (see Fig. 5.3).
- The final reaction of gluconeogenesis is the dephosphorylation of Glc-6-P, catalysed by glucose-6-phosphatase in a hydrolytic reaction. There is no involvement of ADP or ATP in contrast to reaction 1 of glycolysis.
- Gluconeogenesis occurs only in cells possessing the appropriate enzymes (i.e. in hepatocytes and renal cortical cells).
- Some reactions of gluconeogenesis occur in the cytoplasm and others in the mitochondria, as opposed to the purely cytoplasmic glycolysis pathway.
- As one might expect, the activity of gluconeogenesis tends to be reciprocal to glycolysis (i.e. high glycolytic activity is associated with low gluconeogenetic activity).

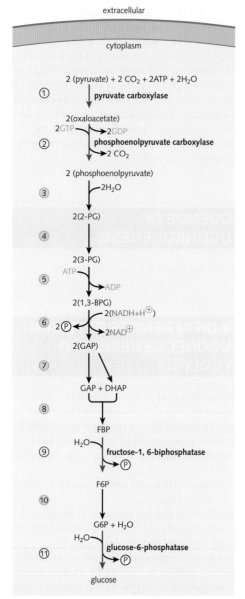

Fig. 5.9 The gluconeogenesis pathway. The reactions differing from glycolysis (reactions 1, 2, 9 and 11) are catalysed by enzymes shown in *red circles*. Please note that *two* three-carbon pyruvate molecules enter the pathway. *1,* Pyruvate carboxylase; *2,* phosphoenolpyruvate carboxylase; *3,* enolase; *4,* phosphoglycerate mutase; *5,* phosphoglycerate kinase; *6,* glyceraldehyde-3-phosphate dehydrogenase; *7,* triose phosphate isomerase; *8,* aldolase A; *9,* fructose-1,6-bisphosphatase; *10,* phosphoglucoisomerase; *11,* glucose-6-phosphatase. *1,3-BPG,* 1,3-bisphosphoglycerate; *2-PG,* 2-phosphoglycerate; *3-PG,* 3-phosphoglycerate; *ADP,* adenosine diphosphate; *ATP,* adenosine triphosphate; *DHAP,* dihydroxyacetone phosphate; *FBP,* Fructose bisphosphate *F6P,* fructose-6-phosphate; *G6P,* glucose-6-phosphate; *GAP,* glyceraldehyde-3-phosphate; *GDP,* guanosine diphosphate; *GTP,* guanosine triphosphate; *NAD,* nicotinamide adenine dinucleotide.

REGULATION OF GLUCONEOGENESIS

In physiological contexts that necessitate endogenous glucose production (e.g. fasting, starvation, prolonged exercise and low-carbohydrate diets), gluconeogenesis appropriately increases. Gluconeogenesis is *inappropriately* activated in the setting of pathological insulin deficiency, that is, type 1 diabetes (see Chapter 6).

Bearing in mind the reciprocity between glycolysis and gluconeogenesis, it follows that the conditions that inhibit one pathway would promote the other.

The reactions of gluconeogenesis (reactions 1, 2, 9 and 11) that differ from glycolysis are highly exergonic and thus essentially irreversible. The enzymes catalysing these reactions therefore function as points of regulation for gluconeogenesis.

Reaction 1: pyruvate → oxaloacetate (carboxylation)

Pyruvate carboxylase is allosterically activated by acetyl-CoA. Remember that acetyl-CoA *inhibits* PK (glycolysis reaction 10). A high acetyl-CoA therefore promotes gluconeogenesis but inhibits glycolysis. Acetyl-CoA is generated by β-oxidation of fatty acids (see Chapter 7), is maximal during fasting, and therefore is an appropriate activator of gluconeogenesis.

Reaction 2: oxaloacetate → phosphoenolpyruvate (decarboxylation)

PEP carboxykinase expression is enhanced by glucagon and inhibited by insulin. A low insulin:glucagon ratio therefore inhibits glycolysis, but promotes gluconeogenesis.

Reaction 9: fructose-1,6-bisphosphate → fructose-6-phosphate (hydrolysis)

AMP and Fru-2,6-BP both promote glycolysis (by activating PFK) but inhibit gluconeogenesis (by allosteric inhibition of fructose-1,6-bisphosphatase).

Reaction 11: Glc-6-P → glucose (hydrolysis)

Glucose-6-phosphatase is allosterically activated in a feed-forward fashion by the reaction substrate Glc-6-P. Remember that Glc-6-P also inhibits HK. A high Glc-6-P thus promotes gluconeogenesis but inhibits glycolysis (Fig. 5.10).

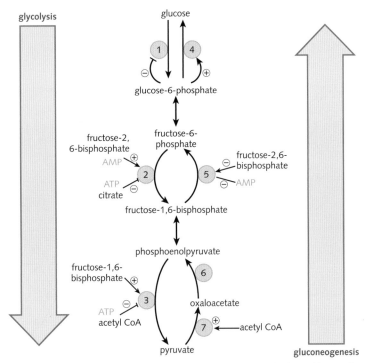

Fig. 5.10 Regulation of gluconeogenesis and glycolysis. *1*, Hexokinase; *2*, phosphofructokinase; *3*, pyruvate kinase; *4*, glucose-6-phosphatase; *5*, fructose-1,6-bisphosphatase; *6*, phosphoenolpyruvate carboxykinase; *7*, pyruvate carboxylase; *ADP*, adenosine diphosphate; *ATP*, adenosine triphosphate; CoA, coenzyme A.

GLYCOGEN METABOLISM

Glycogen is a polysaccharide: a polymer consisting of glucose monomers. It is stored in intracellular granules in the liver and muscle cell cytoplasm. Glycogen is synthesized from excess dietary glucose.

Glycogen breakdown (glycogenolysis) allows rapid mobilization of glucose. Glycogenolysis can therefore function to delay hypoglycaemia until gluconeogenesis increases to an appropriate level or until the next meal takes place (see Chapter 6). It also provides an intracellular depot of glucose for muscle contraction. Adrenaline and glucagon stimulate glycogenolysis, whereas insulin stimulates glycogen synthesis (glycogenesis).

GLYCOGEN STORES

Liver glycogen accounts for 10% of the liver's total mass. Liver glycogen functions as a systemic reserve allowing maintenance of blood glucose levels during fasting. Once released into the blood, the glucose liberated from hepatic glycogen can be taken up and oxidized by any tissue of the body.

Muscle, however, lacks the necessary enzyme (glucose-6-phosphatase) to convert Glc-6-P (generated by glycogenolysis) to free glucose. Because Glc-6-P cannot cross cell membranes, it remains intracellular and is then available exclusively to the cell containing the glycogen it originated from. The role of muscle glycogen is to provide glucose for oxidation in glycolysis when glucose demand exceeds its supply from the circulation, for example, during rapid muscle contraction.

GLYCOGEN STRUCTURE

Glycogen consists of chains of glucose molecules, linked by glycosidic bonds between the C1 of one glucose and the C4 of the next. The polymer is branched; a branch point occurs every 8–12 glucose units (residues). Branch bonds are between the C6 of a main strand residue and C1 of the terminal glucose of the branch (Fig. 5.11).

Such branched structure presents a large number of 'ends' (termini). Enzymes that degrade glycogen can only operate on these termini; thus the more available termini there are, the more rapidly the glycogen molecule can be degraded. The structure thus permits rapid mobilization of glucose in acute situations requiring glucose supply, for example, the adrenaline-fuelled 'fight-or-flight' response.

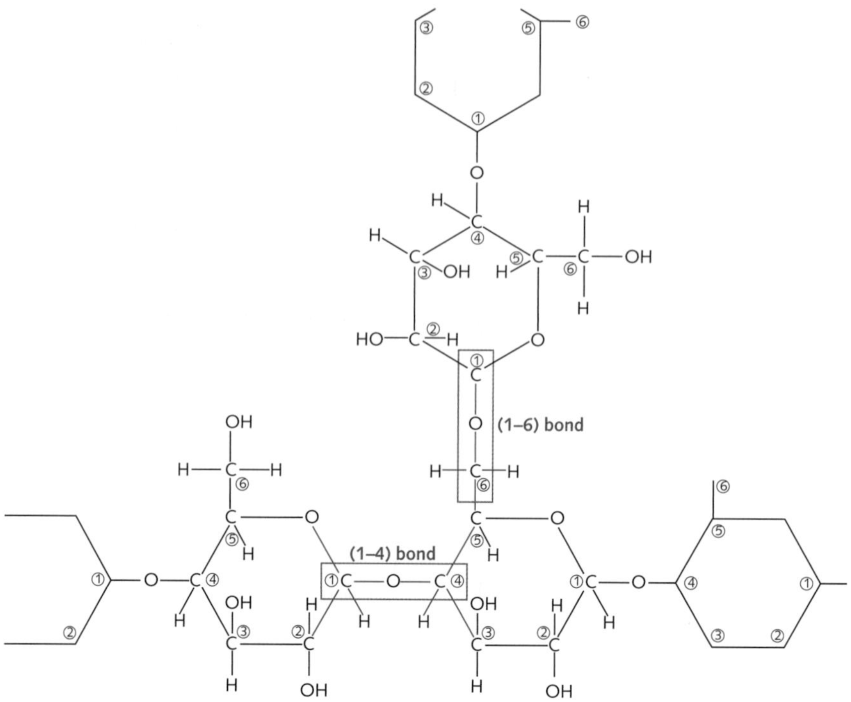

Fig. 5.11 Glycogen structure. The (1–4) and (1–6) linkages are *highlighted*. *Ringed numbers* illustrate the numbering of the carbon atoms within each glucose monomer.

GLYCOGEN SYNTHESIS (GLYCOGENESIS)

This occurs in the cytoplasm. The process requires:

- UDP–glucose, which acts as the glucose donor. UDP is uridine diphosphate (a nucleotide). It is required to 'activate' glucose molecules so they are recognizable to the glycogenetic enzymes.
- Four enzymes: phosphoglucomutase, glycogen synthase, branching enzyme)amylo (1,4→1,6) transglycosylase) and uridyl transferase.
- ATP.
- A preexisting glycogen chain to link additional glucose molecules to; in its absence, glycogenin (a molecular 'primer') must be present instead for the additional glucose molecules to link with.

Stage 1: formation of glucose-1-phosphate

Glc-6-P is converted to glucose-1-phosphate (Glc-1-P) by phosphoglucomutase.

Stage 2: formation of 'activated' glucose (UDP–glucose)

UDP–glucose is synthesized from Glc-1-P and uridine triphosphate (UTP) by uridyl transferase (also called 'UDP–glucose pyrophosphorylase'). Glucose in this form is now 'eligible' to join the growing glycogen chain.

Stage 3: Elongation

Glycogen synthase now transfers the glucose from UDP–glucose to the C4 of the terminal glucose in an existing glycogen strand (Fig. 5.12). It is linked via a (1–4) glycosidic bond. Elongation requires presence of a strand of four or more glucose residues before elongation can occur; else the protein glycogenin (primers) must be present for additional glucose to be incorporated.

Stage 4: Branch formation

Glycogen synthase can only lengthen strands; it cannot create branches. For this, branching enzyme is required. This enzyme cleaves off a length from a growing glycogen strand (typically approximately 7 residues in length) and transfers this to another strand (Fig. 5.13). This generates a branch point. A (1–6) bond is formed (between the C1 of the incoming fragment and the C6 of the 'branch' residue on the main strand).

GLYCOGEN BREAKDOWN (GLYCOGENOLYSIS)

This also occurs in the cytoplasm. It is stimulated by glucagon (in liver) and adrenaline (in liver and muscle). There

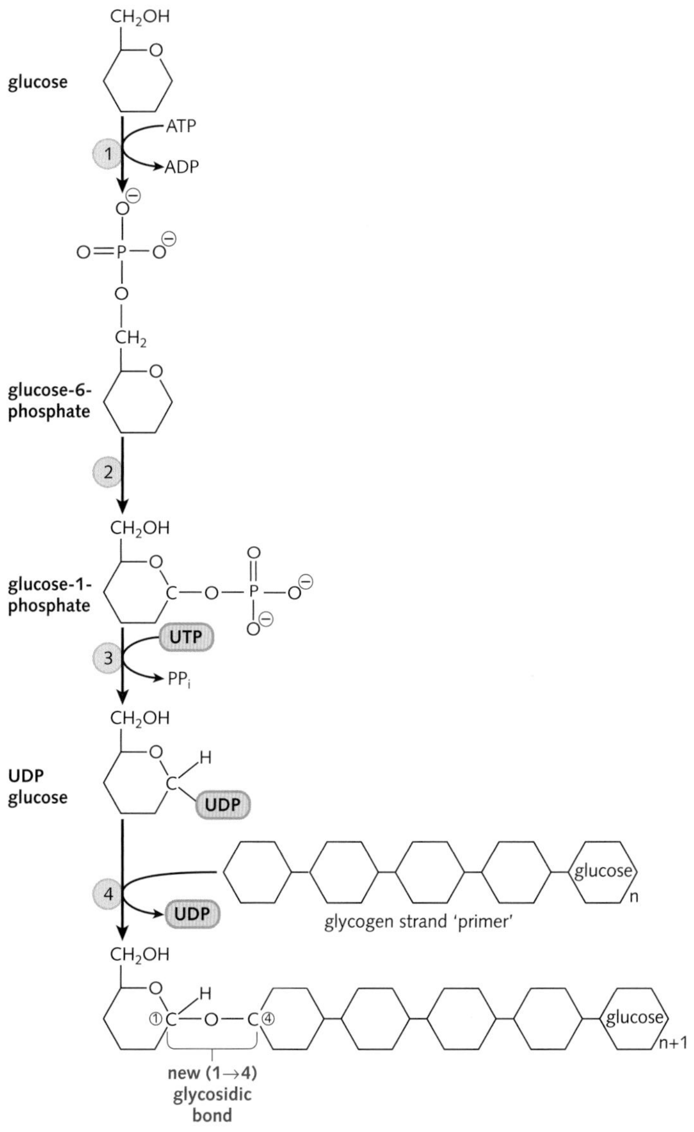

Fig. 5.12 Synthesis of the glycogen polymer: chain elongation. Each *hexagon* represents a glucose residue; for clarity, only the main carbon skeleton structure is shown in this illustration. Please refer to Fig. 5.1 for the precise structure. ADP, adenosine diphosphate; ATP, adenosine triphosphate; *PP$_i$*, pyrophosphate; *UDP*, uridine diphosphate; *UTP*, uridine triphosphate; *1*, hexokinase; *2*, phosphoglucomutase; *3*, UDP glycogen pyrophosphorylase; *4*, glycogen synthase. Note that glycogenin can replace the existing strand of residues as the 'primer' where an existing strand is not available.

are two elements to glycogenolysis; strand shortening and branch removal. The enzymes involved are glycogen phosphorylase (which requires pyridoxal phosphate as a cofactor), debranching enzyme (also called (1,4)→(1,4) glucan transferase) and amylo-α-1,6-glucosidase.

Strand shortening

Glucose units are cleaved off strand termini, one by one. The cleavage of the (1→4) glycosidic bond linking terminal and penultimate units is performed by glycogen phosphorylase (phosphorolysis), and within lysosomes by lysosomal α-1,4-glucosidase. Glc-1-P is released.

Unhelpfully, glycogen phosphorylase will only remove units if the chain is four residues or more in length. It also cannot process branch-point residues. Thus this enzyme

stops short when the strand/branch diminishes to four residues in length (not including the 'branch' unit). This leaves a number of remnant 'stubs' (Fig. 5.14).

Glc-1-P released by glycogenolysis may be converted by phosphoglucomutase to Glc-6-P, which can enter glycolysis. In hepatocytes, Glc-6-P may be converted to glucose by hepatocyte glucose-6-phosphatase.

Branch removal

Once a branch has been shortened to the final four units of a branch (stemming from a 'branch' unit), the distal three units of this branch are trimmed off by the debranching enzyme, which hydrolyses the (1→4) glycosidic bond. These three units are then attached to another strand elsewhere in the polymer. This leaves the 'branch' unit of the main

47

Fig. 5.13 Synthesis of the glycogen polymer: branch formation. Each hexagon represents a glucose residue. *Stage 1*, Excision of terminal six residues of an existing strand via hydrolysis of a (1→4) bond; *stage 2*, transfer to a proximal residue and formation of a (1→6) glycosidic bond. Residues of the transferred segment are *shaded*.

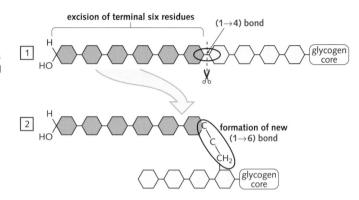

excision of terminal six residues

(1→4) bond

glycogen core

formation of new (1→6) bond

glycogen core

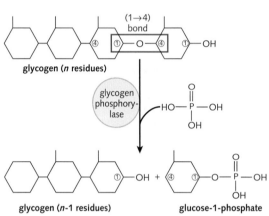

(1→4) bond

glycogen (*n* residues)

glycogen phosphory-lase

glycogen (*n-1* residues) glucose-1-phosphate

Fig. 5.14 Glycogenolysis. The strand/branch is shortened via sequential phosphorolysis. The *ringed numbers* indicate carbon numbers within each individual glucose residue.

strand with just one remaining unit (step 1, Fig. 5.15). This protruding unit requires amylo-α-1,6-glucosidase to hydrolyse the (1→6) glycosidic bond, releasing free glucose (step 2, Fig. 5.15).

REGULATION OF GLYCOGEN METABOLISM

The activity of the key synthesis and degradation enzymes (glycogen synthase and glycogen phosphorylase, respectively) is controlled via hormonal and allosteric mechanisms.

Hormonal control

Hormones regulate these enzymes via phosphorylation. Glycogen phosphorylase is activated by phosphorylation, whereas glycogen synthase is deactivated by phosphorylation. Refer to Fig. 5.10.

- The same kinase enzyme (protein kinase A; PKA) phosphorylates both enzymes.
- PKA itself is activated by cyclic AMP (cAMP).

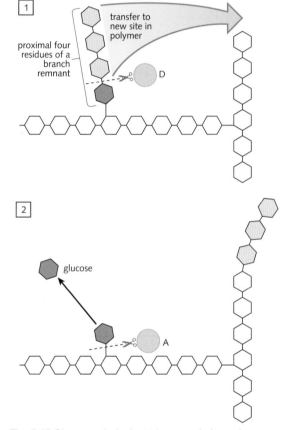

transfer to new site in polymer

proximal four residues of a branch remnant

D

glucose

A

Fig. 5.15 Glycogenolysis: branch removal. *A*, amylo-α-(1→6)-glucosidase; *D*, debranching enzyme; *stage 1*, excision of three of the proximal four residues of a branch remnant; *stage 2*, release of the remaining branch residue. Note that H_2O is required for this reaction, but is omitted from the diagram for simplicity. For clarity, the unit that initially bears the branch is *shaded heavily*, whereas the three transferred residues are *shaded lightly*.

- Intracellular cAMP is elevated after adrenaline or glucagon bind to their respective membrane adenylate cyclase-associated receptors. Adenylate cyclase synthesizes cAMP from ATP.

- Glucagon and adrenaline therefore elevate intracellular cAMP, activating PKA, which phosphorylates (deactivates) glycogen synthase and (activates) glycogen phosphorylase.
- This activates glycogenolysis and inhibits glycogen synthesis.
- Insulin has the opposite effect, because insulin binding to its membrane receptors generates a signal leading to upregulation of intracellular protein phosphatase-1 (PP-1). This dephosphorylates the two enzymes, with the opposing outcome: glycogen synthesis is activated and glycogenolysis is inhibited.

ALLOSTERIC REGULATION

The scenario differs according to the location of glycogen: hepatocytes or muscle cells.

Hepatic glycogen

Glucose allosterically inhibits glycogen phosphorylase, inhibiting glycogenolysis. Glucose binds to glycogen phosphorylase, causing a conformational change that exposes its phosphate group. This phosphate group is the target for hydrolytic cleavage by PP-1. Thus glucose binding increases the probability of dephosphorylation (i.e. deactivation) of glycogen phosphorylase, and inhibition of glycogenolysis. Conversely, glucose allosterically activates glycogen synthase, promoting glycogen synthesis. Glc-6-P too allosterically inactivates phosphorylase and activates synthase.

Muscle glycogen

Ca^{2+} ions, intracellularly elevated during skeletal muscle contraction, allosterically activate glycogen phosphorylase. Thus glycogenolysis is promoted in a context where glucose mobilization is desirable. Similarly, AMP, plentiful in active cells undergoing high levels of ATP hydrolysis, allosterically activates glycogen phosphorylase.

GLYCOGEN STORAGE DISEASES

This term describes genetic diseases arising from deficiencies of one of the enzymes of either glycogen synthesis or degradation. They result in clinical manifestations reflecting the resulting abnormalities of glycogen synthesis or degradation (Table 5.3).

Table 5.3 Glycogen storage diseases

Type	Name	Defective enzyme	Pathology	Clinical features
I	von Gierke disease	Glucose-6-phosphatase (G-6-P) *or* debranching enzyme	G-6-P derived from hepatic gluconeogenesis/glycogenolysis cannot be converted to free glucose, and thus remains trapped within the liver and renal cortical cells where it accumulates.	Hepatomegaly and enlarged kidneys. Fasting hypoglycaemia due to inability to release glucose generated by gluconeogenesis (G-6-P deficiency) or glycogenolysis (debranching enzyme deficiency).
II	Pompe disease	Lysosomal α-(1-4)-glucosidase (also called 'maltase')	Glycogen strands cannot be shortened intralysosomally, thus accumulation of glycogen occurs, particularly within the heart, skeletal muscle and the central nervous system.	Hepatomegaly, cardiomegaly, neuromuscular symptoms. Inheritance follows an autosomal recessive pattern.
III	Cori disease	Debranching enzyme	The final four residues of shortened branches cannot be removed from main strands. These 'branchlets' persist.	Hepatomegaly, fasting hypoglycaemia, late-onset muscle weakness and cardiomyopathy. Inheritance follows an autosomal recessive pattern.
IV	Andersen disease	Branching enzyme	Glycogen synthesis is abnormal, with accumulation of long unbranched strands. These structures are less soluble than normal glycogen.	Accumulation of relatively insoluble abnormal glycogen, most pronounced in cardiac muscle and the liver. Heterogeneous genetic abnormalities can lead to defective branching enzyme; inheritance varies according to the particular abnormal gene.

(Continued)

Table 5.3 Glycogen storage diseases—cont'd

Type	Name	Defective enzyme	Pathology	Clinical features
V	McArdle disease	Glycogen phosphorylase (muscle isoform)	Muscle cells are unable to perform glycogenolysis, thus are reliant on glucose absorbed from the bloodstream.	Decreased exercise tolerance, hallmarked by muscle fatigue and cramping. Hypoglycaemia is absent, because the liver isoform of glycogen phosphorylase is functional.
VI	Hers disease	Glycogen phosphorylase	Impaired glycogenolysis results in accumulation of glycogen in liver and muscle.	Hepatomegaly, fasting hypoglycaemia; 75% of cases are X-linked recessive, 25% are autosomal recessive.
VII	Tarui disease	Phosphofructokinase (muscle isoform)	Abnormally active glycogen synthase results in accumulation of glycogen within muscles.	Haemolytic anaemia, myoglobinuria, poor exercise tolerance and muscle cramps.

THE PENTOSE PHOSPHATE PATHWAY

The PPP, also called the 'hexose monophosphate shunt', is a primarily anabolic pathway that utilizes Glc-6-P as its initial substrate. The PPP generates $NADPH+H^+$, pentose sugars and other intermediates. $NADPH+H^+$ is vital for fatty acid and cholesterol synthesis (see Chapter 7: Cholesterol metabolism) and also for glutathione regeneration. Pentose sugars are required for synthesis of nucleotides and nucleic acids. The PPP also allows conversion of dietary pentose sugars into hexose and triose intermediates, which can then enter glycolysis for oxidation.

REACTIONS OF THE PPP

The pathway (Fig. 5.16) has two stages:

- An initial oxidative phase: Three exergonic reactions ultimately generate ribulose-5-phosphate, CO_2 and two molecules of $NADPH+H^+$ for every molecule of Glc-6-P oxidized.
- A reversible nonoxidative phase, consisting of a series of reactions converting ribulose-5-phosphate into intermediates with varying carbon numbers.

REGULATION OF THE PPP

The main regulatory influence is exerted at the Glc-6-P → 6-phosphogluconolactone reaction. The substrate:product ratio drives the reaction forward; the higher the $NADP^+$ (substrate) relative to the $NADPH+H^+$ (product), the greater the pathway activity. Higher activity results in more Glc-6-P entering the PPP (and therefore less Glc-6-P participation in glycolysis).

Demand for intermediates (generated during the second, nonoxidative phase) determines which products are predominantly generated. For example, if ribose-5-phosphate is withdrawn from the PPP to enter nucleic acid synthesis, it will not be able to combine with xylulose-5-phosphate and progress along the PPP to produce downstream intermediates (Fig. 5.16).

GLUCOSE-6-PHOSPHATE DEHYDROGENASE DEFICIENCY; THE FAILURE OF THE PPP

Glucose-6-phosphate dehydrogenase (G6PD) deficiency is an X-linked recessive condition, affecting over 400 million persons worldwide, making it the most common enzymopathy. Because inheritance is X linked and recessive, females are rarely severely affected, as they still have one normal copy of the G6PD gene.

The absence of functional G6PD results in failure of the PPP. The mitochondrial citrate shuttle (see Chapter 7) is the only other mechanism that generates $NADPH+H^+$. Erythrocytes, however, lack mitochondria, and so cannot compensate for the abnormal $NADPH+H^+$ deficit. This leads to failure of glutathione regeneration (see following section) and leaves erythrocytes unable to survive oxidative assaults, dramatically shortening their lifespan. This manifests clinically as haemolysis in situations of oxidative stress.

Precipitating factors

There are a number of factors that are known to enhance cellular oxidative stress and precipitate haemolysis in G6PD-deficient patients. These include:

- Ingestion of broad beans (fava beans), which contain high levels of vicine compounds (powerful intracellular oxidants)

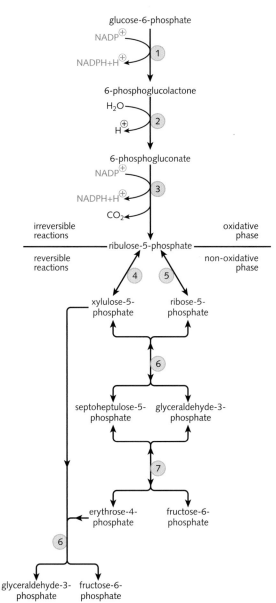

Fig. 5.16 The pentose phosphate pathway. *1*, glucose-6-phosphate dehydrogenase; *2*, gluconolactonase; *3*, 6-phosphogluconate dehydrogenase; *4*, ribulose-5-phosphate-3-epimerase; *5*, ribulose-5-phosphate isomerase; *6*, transketolase; *7*, transaldolase; *NADP⁺*, nicotinamide adenine dinucleotide phosphate.

GLUTATHIONE

Glutathione is a tripeptide, a trio of amino acids (glutamate, cysteine and glycine). It is the primary intracellular antioxidant, neutralizing harmful intracellular reactive oxygen species (ROS; see Chapter 2) and limiting oxidative damage. This function is particularly important in immune cells. Glutathione also plays fundamental roles in many vital metabolic processes, including enzyme activation, protein synthesis, DNA synthesis and DNA repair.

Mechanism of antioxidant action of glutathione

Glutathione neutralizes ROS by donating H^+ from the thiol group of the cysteine residue to the unstable ROS. In donating reducing equivalents, glutathione is itself oxidized, and becomes unstable. It then rapidly reacts with another (unoxidized) glutathione molecule, forming glutathione disulphide, which is inactive in terms of its antioxidant role. To regenerate glutathione to its active, unoxidized form, $NADPH+H^+$ is required (Fig. 5.17).

Role of glutathione in drug metabolism

Glutathione is of key importance in the hepatocytes. They require a constant supply of active (unoxidized) glutathione for participation in the conjugation (excretion) of numerous foreign compounds – including drugs and toxins. If active glutathione is unavailable, these substances accumulate to toxic levels. Because a constant supply of $NADPH+H^+$ is required to regenerate glutathione, the intact PPP is largely responsible for the liver's function in drug metabolism.

Glutathione in erythrocytes

When high levels of ROS are present in a context of cellular oxidative stress, the cytochrome b_5 reductase system (which normally maintains haemoglobin in the reduced state (Fe^{2+})) becomes overwhelmed. Glutathione protects against oxidation of haemoglobin to a nonfunctional methaemoglobin (Fe^{3+}), and allows erythrocytes to continue performing

- Acute infection, particularly pneumonia
- Numerous drugs, for example, sulphonamide derivatives, nitrofurantoin (for a list of unsafe drugs in this condition, and also for a list of drugs *safe* to use in these patients, please see www.g6pd.org)

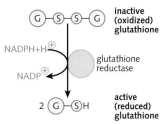

Fig. 5.17 Glutathione regeneration. *NADP⁺*, nicotinamide adenine dinucleotide phosphate.

their oxygen-carrying role. In this way, the PPP is also very important in the context of oxidative stress in erythrocytes, because NADPH+H$^+$ generated in PPP production ensures that sufficient glutathione is available to maintain normal haemoglobin activity (i.e. oxygen carriage).

Glutathione: the γ-glutamyl cycle

The γ-glutamyl cycle is a mechanism for importing various amino acids into cells (see Chapter 9). Glutathione is needed for this process to operate.

FRUCTOSE METABOLISM

Fructose is a hexose ($C_6H_{12}O_6$). This formula is the same as glucose; however, fructose differs in structure. Its main dietary source is the disaccharide sucrose. Gut sucrase hydrolyses sucrose to glucose and fructose. Absorption of fructose into gut enterocytes is via the GLUT-5 transporter. Fructose then leaves the enterocytes into the portal vein blood (this time via GLUT-2; Fig. 5.18).

Fructose is phosphorylated by hepatocyte fructokinase, forming fructose-1-phosphate. This is further metabolized to GAP by aldolase B, which enters glycolysis or gluconeogenesis according to cellular energy status (Fig. 5.10). In muscle, fructose is phosphorylated to Fru-6-P by HK (like glucose) and enters glycolysis.

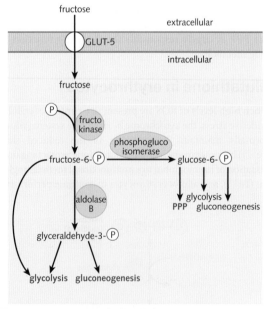

Fig. 5.18 Fructose metabolism in hepatocytes. In myocytes (muscle cells), hexokinase would perform the first phosphorylation instead of fructokinase. *PPP,* Pentose phosphate pathway.

Role of fructose-6-phosphate

Recall that Fru-6-P participates in glycolysis; PFK-1 adds a second phosphate, generating Fru-1,6-BP. In the liver, Fru-6-P can also participate in gluconeogenesis or the PPP, after conversion to Glc-6-P by phosphoglucoisomerase.

In erythrocytes, fructose-derived Glc-6-P enters the PPP or glycolysis (gluconeogenesis does not occur in erythrocytes), allowing NADPH+H$^+$ production.

GENETIC DEFICIENCIES OF FRUCTOSE METABOLISM

The two main enzymopathies of fructose metabolism are fructokinase deficiency and fructose-1-phosphate aldolase deficiency. Both are autosomal recessive conditions.

Fructokinase deficiency

Deficiency of fructokinase results in failure of hepatic fructose catabolism. Fructose therefore can only be degraded by muscle HK. This leads to increased plasma fructose, and elevated urinary fructose. This is clinically asymptomatic.

Fructose-1-phosphate aldolase deficiency (aldolase B deficiency)

Also called 'hereditary fructose intolerance', this results from aldolase B deficiency and leads to accumulation of fructose-1-phosphate and failure of dietary fructose to be diverted to glycolysis or gluconeogenesis. Fructose-1-phosphate elevation is toxic, because high intracellular concentration sequesters intracellular phosphate. Enzymes reliant on phosphorylation for their activation thus fail. For instance, glycogen phosphorylase (required for glycogen mobilization) is inhibited. Gluconeogenesis is also inhibited. Therefore the two mechanisms for maintaining plasma glucose concentration during fasting fail and fasting hypoglycaemia occurs following fructose exposure in deficient individuals. Treatment is by complete dietary exclusion of anything containing fructose, including sucrose.

GALACTOSE METABOLISM

Galactose is also a hexose and shares the $C_6H_{12}O_6$ formula with fructose and glucose. The main dietary source is the disaccharide lactose, found in milk products. Gut lactase hydrolyses lactose to its components glucose and galactose. Absorption into enterocytes is via the sodium–glucose symport. Like glucose, entry into the bloodstream from the enterocytes is via the GLUT-2 transporter. Galactose is converted into Glc-6-P, which can enter gluconeogenesis (in the liver), glycolysis or the PPP (Fig. 5.19).

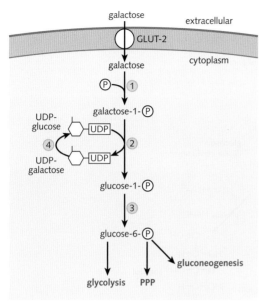

Fig. 5.19 Galactose metabolism. *1*, Galactokinase; *2*, galactose-1-phosphate uridyltransferase; *3*, phosphoglucomutase; *4*, galactose-6-phosphate epimerase; *PPP*, Pentose phosphate pathway; *UDP*, uridine diphosphate.

Galactose → Glucose-6-phosphate

This occurs in several stages:

- Galactose is converted to galactose-1-phosphate by galactokinase
- Galactose-1-phosphate then reacts with UDP–glucose, forming Glc-1-P and UDP–galactose. This is catalysed by galactose-1-phosphate uridyl transferase
- Glc-1-P is then converted to Glc-6-P by phosphoglucomutase
- The UDP–galactose is reconverted to UDP–glucose by galactose-6-phosphate epimerase

GALACTOSAEMIA

This is a rare, autosomal recessive condition, arising from deficiency of either galactose-1-phosphate uridyl transferase, galactokinase or galactose-6-phosphate epimerase. Failure of galactose catabolism results in toxic accumulation of galactose or galactose-1-phosphate in various tissues, particularly the liver, kidney, lens and central nervous system (CNS). These serious and irreversible events occur soon after feeding commences postpartum; even breast-feeding galactosaemic infants exposes them to galactose. Treatment is complete exclusion of all galactose-containing foods from the diet. Incidence is approximately 1 in 36,000 births in Europe; however, in the Irish Traveller community its incidence is approximately 1 in 450 births.

SORBITOL METABOLISM

Sorbitol (also called 'glucitol') is a sugar alcohol, produced endogenously from excess glucose via the polyol pathway. It can also be obtained from the diet. Tissues containing sorbitol dehydrogenase (such as the liver or sperm cells) oxidize sorbitol to fructose. This reaction uses NAD^+ as a redox partner, thus generating $NADH+H^+$, which can then participate in oxidative phosphorylation. The fructose may ultimately feed into glycolysis or the PPP (or gluconeogenesis in the liver; Fig. 5.20).

At high plasma glucose, such as is seen in poorly controlled diabetes for example, aldose reductase upregulates. As this enzyme is part of the sorbitol synthesis (polyol) pathway, this results in enhanced sorbitol production. This is significant for two reasons:

- The polyol pathway utilizes $NADPH+H^+$ as a redox partner in the glucose → sorbitol reduction, resulting in lesser availability of $NADPH+H^+$ for regeneration of glutathione. This renders cells less able to survive oxidative assaults.
- Certain tissues lack sorbitol dehydrogenase and cannot divert sorbitol into glycolysis via fructose. Sorbitol accumulates and exerts a pathological osmotic effect, leading to structural damage and impaired function. This is seen particularly in Schwann cells and retinal cells.

ETHANOL METABOLISM

Ethanol (C_2H_5OH) is a component of alcoholic beverages. It binds to numerous CNS receptors, including acetylcholine, serotonin, γ-aminobutyric acid and glutamate receptors, with an overall depressant effect on neuronal activity. Clinically, CNS depression associated with significant acute ethanol intake can lead to loss of airway reflexes, aspiration of stomach contents and death.

Ethanol catabolism

Ethanol detoxification occurs primarily in liver cells. Two sequential oxidations culminate in the less toxic ethanoic acid (also called 'acetic acid').

Ethanol → Ethanal conversion

There are two main mechanisms underpinning this oxidation reaction:

- Cytoplasmic oxidation by alcohol dehydrogenase (main mechanism)
- Microsomal ethanol oxidizing system: CYP2E1 of the P450 enzyme

This first ethanol oxidation reaction produces the even more toxic aldehyde ethanal (also called 'acetaldehyde').

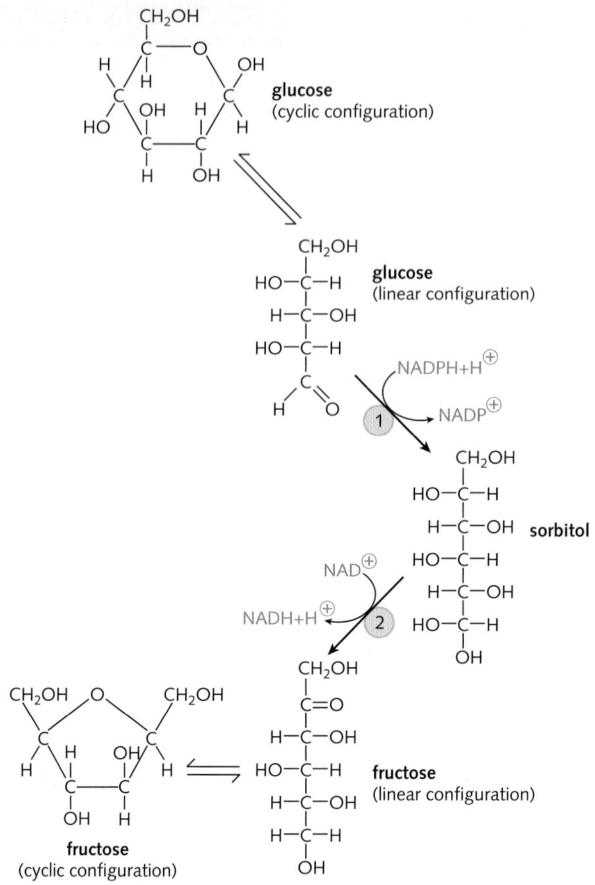

CH₂OH

glucose
(cyclic configuration)

$$CH_2OH$$
$$HO-C-H$$
$$H-C-OH$$
$$HO-C-H$$
$$C=O$$
$$H$$

glucose
(linear configuration)

NADPH+H⊕

1

NADP⊕

$$CH_2OH$$
$$HO-C-H$$
$$H-C-OH$$
$$HO-C-H$$
$$H-C-OH$$
$$HO-C-H$$
$$OH$$

sorbitol

NAD⊕

NADH+H⊕

2

$$CH_2OH$$
$$C=O$$
$$H-C-OH$$
$$HO-C-H$$
$$H-C-OH$$
$$H-C-H$$
$$OH$$

fructose
(linear configuration)

CH₂OH   CH₂OH

fructose
(cyclic configuration)

Fig. 5.20 The polyol pathway. *1,* Aldose reductase; *2,* sorbitol dehydrogenase; *NAD⁺*, nicotinamide adenine dinucleotide; *NADP⁺*, nicotinamide adenine dinucleotide phosphate.

Ethanal → Ethanoate conversion

Ethanal (produced by one of the aforementioned mechanisms) then enters the mitochondria, where it is further oxidized to ethanoate (acetate) by mitochondrial aldehyde dehydrogenase. A cytoplasmic isoform of this enzyme also exists. The generated acetate may then react with CoA in a reaction catalysed by acetyl-CoA synthetase, forming acetyl CoA.

Ethanal toxicity

Aldehydes are highly reactive, and react promiscuously with numerous biological molecules. The aldehyde ethanal arising from ethanol catabolism is responsible for many of the unpleasant effects of ethanol consumption. Interestingly, approximately 50% of Oriental people lack the mitochondrial isoform of aldehyde dehydrogenase. With only the cytoplasmic isoform available to deal with an ethanal load following ethanol consumption, degradation is retarded, leading to accumulation of ethanal. After a relatively small ethanol consumption, such individuals experience symptoms and signs of ethanal toxicity such as flushing, nausea and vomiting.

CLINICAL NOTES

DISULFIRAM

The unpleasantness of ethanol accumulation symptoms is exploited by disulfiram (Antabuse), a drug used to deter recovering alcoholics from consuming alcohol. Disulfiram inhibits aldehyde dehydrogenase (mitochondrial and cytoplasmic), resulting in rapid ethanal accumulation following ethanol consumption. The unpleasant symptoms of ethanal toxicity act as a deterrent against repeated consumption.

CLINICAL NOTES

ETHANOL TOXICITY

Signs of ethanol toxicity are seen following excessive ethanol consumption. These are usually seen when individuals consume excessively and exceed their own personal capacity for maintaining ethanal below the symptomatic oncentration. Nausea, vomiting, flushing, dizziness, elevated heart rate, headache and shortness of breath are seen.

IMPACT OF ETHANOL CATABOLISM

Both reactions of ethanol catabolism consume NAD^+ (Fig. 5.21). This depletes the NAD^+ available to act as a redox partner in numerous metabolic pathway reactions with widespread detrimental consequences. Pathways/reactions affected in particular include:

- Glycolysis: Reduced NAD^+ availability impairs pathway progression. Less glucose oxidation therefore occurs, with the consequence of less ATP production.
- Pyruvate → acetyl-CoA reaction: Recall that NAD^+ is a cofactor for the PDH enzyme complex. When scarce, pyruvate is instead converted to lactate, causing hyperlactataemia, and reducing availability of the entry substrate (acetyl-CoA) for the TCA cycle.
- The TCA cycle: As well as reduced acetyl-CoA availability, reduced NAD^+ availability leads to less generation of $NADH+H^+$, ultimately resulting in less ATP generation.

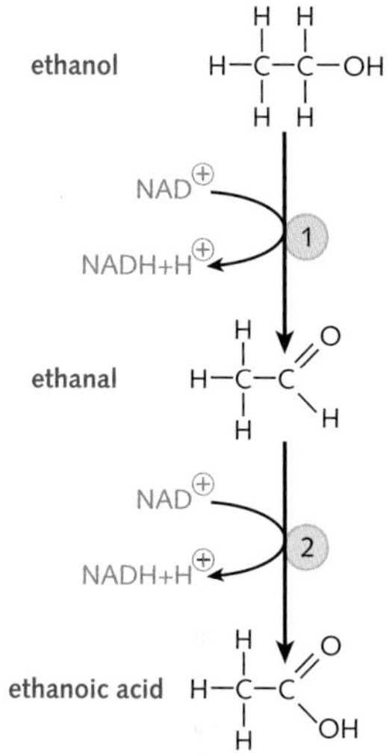

Fig. 5.21 Ethanol catabolism. *1,* Alcohol dehydrogenase; *2,* aldehyde dehydrogenase; *NAD^+*, Nicotinamide adenine dinucleotide.

- Gluconeogenesis: Because of reduced NAD^+ availability, impaired gluconeogenesis results in fasting hypoglycaemia (once glycogen reserves are exhausted).
- Fatty acid oxidation: This is depressed (like the TCA cycle, glycolysis and gluconeogenesis).

CLINICAL NOTES

GOUT

Lactate and urate compete for the same cellular excretion apparatus in the renal tubules. Thus excess lactate is associated with a proportionate retention of urate. The urate may be deposited as crystals in connective tissue, leading to a local inflammatory reaction (gout), which is associated with excessive ethanol intake. For further details, please see Chapter 10.

Overabundant acetyl-CoA is diverted towards lipogenesis

Acetyl-CoA (which would otherwise be consumed by the TCA cycle) is diverted into de novo fatty acid synthesis (see Chapter 7). This results in increased hepatic triglyceride synthesis and very-low-density lipoprotein assembly, which contributes to the pathogenesis of alcoholic hepatic steatosis. The overabundance of acetyl-CoA in this context is further compounded by acetyl-CoA generated directly from the ethanoate (acetate) formed by the oxidation of ethanal.

Ethanol impact on drug metabolism

Regular or high ethanol consumption causes an upregulation in synthesis of alcohol-detoxifying enzymes. This includes CYP2E1. However, this enzyme is also responsible for the metabolism of many individual therapeutic drugs. An alcohol-induced increase in CYP2E1 leads to excessive metabolism of its normal substrate drugs, which can result in subtherapeutic drug concentrations and clinical inefficacy. This can occur with any drugs predominantly metabolized by CYP2E1, but warfarin is an often-used example.

Warfarin is metabolized via CYP2E1. An increase in usual alcohol intake leads to an alcohol-induced upregulation of CYP2E1 expression. The usual warfarin dose will now be more rapidly degraded by the increased CYP2E1. The blood warfarin may therefore fail to reach the desired therapeutic level. If the patient relies on warfarin-mediated anticoagulation to prevent thrombotic events, this can be catastrophic.

Chapter Summary

- Carbohydrates are essential macronutrients, defined by a ratio of their constituent atoms: C:H:O = 1:2:1.
- Digestion of dietary carbohydrates is performed by different enzymes present at specific points in the gastrointestinal tract (the mouth, stomach and small intestine).
- Absorbed glucose entry into cells from the bloodstream may be by facilitated or secondary active transport.
- Glycolysis is a catabolic pathway occurring in all cells, because it takes place in the cytoplasm and therefore is not restricted to mitochondria-containing cells.
- Glycolysis utilizes glucose as a substrate, ultimately generating pyruvate, which can then progress towards the tricarboxylic acid cycles via acetyl-coenzyme A (acetyl-CoA). Regulation occurs at reactions 1, 3 and 10 of the pathway.
- Conversion of pyruvate to acetyl-CoA or lactate depends on whether intracellular conditions are aerobic (acetyl-CoA) or anaerobic (lactate).
- Gluconeogenesis is an endergonic, anabolic pathway responsible for the synthesis of glucose from noncarbohydrate substrates. This pathway becomes prominent during prolonged fasting. Gluconeogenesis pathway regulation occurs at reactions 1, 2, 9 and 11.
- Glycogen is a multibranched polymer of glucose monomers, and as such functions as a glucose storage molecule. It is present in intracellular granules, primarily within the liver and muscle.
- Glycogen is degraded to maintain blood glucose during the initial stages of fasting. Disorders of glycogen synthesis or catabolism result in the glycogen storage disorders.
- The pentose phosphate pathway is the main source of $NADPH+H^+$, which is a vital substrate required for normal fatty acid and cholesterol metabolism and arguably most importantly, glutathione regeneration.
- Fructose, galactose and sorbitol are other examples of carbohydrates of significance, each with specific metabolic pathways.
- Ethanol catabolism relies on intact alcohol and aldehyde dehydrogenation enzymes. Sustained intake impacts a whole host of metabolic pathways, with a variety of damaging consequences, particularly nicotinamide adenine dinucleotide depletion.

Glucose homeostasis and diabetes mellitus

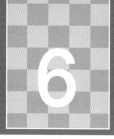

6

HORMONAL ASPECTS OF GLUCOSE REGULATION

Normal metabolic function is dependent on the tight control of blood glucose, known as 'glucose homeostasis'. Homeostasis is primarily accomplished by the balance between the actions of two pancreatic hormones: glucagon and insulin. The main changes elicited by glucagon and insulin are summarized in Table 6.1.

Insulin

Insulin release

Insulin is a peptide hormone secreted from pancreatic β cells in response to a rise in blood glucose. Postprandially (i.e. the 'fed' state), β cells respond to elevations in blood glucose when glucose enters these cells (via GLUT-2; see Table 5.1). Glucose is metabolized, generating adenosine triphosphate (ATP) and increasing the intracellular ATP.

Table 6.1 A summary of the contrasting effects of insulin and glucagon on macromolecule metabolism

Pathway	Insulin	Glucagon
Carbohydrate metabolism		
Glycogen synthesis	↑ (muscle and liver)	↓
Glycogenolysis	↓	↑
Glycolysis	↑	↓
Gluconeogenesis	↓	↑
Peripheral cellular glucose uptake	↑	↔
Pentose phosphate pathway	↑	↔
Lipid metabolism		
Lipolysis	↓	↑
β-Oxidation	↓	↑
Ketogenesis	↓	↑
Lipogenesis	↑	↓
Protein metabolism		
Amino acid uptake	↑ (peripheral tissues)	↑ (liver only)
Protein synthesis	↑	↓
Proteolysis	↓	↑

ATP-sensitive K^+ channels open, depolarizing the β cell. Depolarization activates voltage-gated calcium channels, allowing influx of extracellular Ca^{++}. Intracellular Ca^{++} elevation leads to exocytosis of stored insulin and an accompanying peptide (C-peptide) – a remnant of the insulin precursor, proinsulin.

Cellular effects of insulin

Insulin released into the bloodstream binds to cell surface insulin receptors. These receptors are members of the superfamily of tyrosine kinase receptors. Insulin binding activates an array of intracellular pathways, including in particular synthesis of storage macromolecules such as glycogen and triglycerides.

Overall metabolic response to insulin

Insulin-induced changes are all physiologically and energetically advantageous in the context of the glucose-abundant fed state. Energy-consuming pathways such as gluconeogenesis and catabolic pathways such as glycogenolysis and lipolysis (which are necessary during the fasting state to maintain circulating glucose and fatty acid levels) are suppressed by insulin. Blood glucose falls primarily due to an ATP-dependent insertion of GLUT-4 receptors at peripheral cell membranes, which increases cellular glucose uptake.

Glucagon

Glucagon is a peptide hormone secreted by pancreatic α cells. Glucagon is released into the bloodstream in response to the fall in blood glucose that occurs in the fasting state. Glucagon release is also stimulated by exercise and dietary protein consumption.

Glucagon binds to specific G-protein-coupled receptors on the hepatocyte cell surface. Activated G proteins then stimulate adenylate cyclase, a membrane-bound enzyme that catalyses the conversion of ATP to cyclic adenosine monophosphate (cAMP). cAMP in turn activates protein kinase A, which (by phosphorylation) activates a number of enzymes including glycogen phosphorylase.

Glucagon upregulates gluconeogenesis, and also promotes the catabolism of storage macromolecules, including:

- Liver, muscle and renal glycogen
- Adipocyte lipolysis

The overall effect of this is that in the absence of abundant blood glucose tissues are provided with substrates for cellular catabolism and ATP generation. These substrates are derived from endogenous stores (e.g. fatty acids from lipids and triglycerides glucose from glycogen). These changes are needed during fasting, because these molecules are no longer being assimilated from ingested food and yet blood glucose must be maintained. Cellular responses similar to glucagon are elicited by adrenaline, noradrenaline and cortisol.

Gluconeogenesis in the context of glucose homeostasis

Details of the gluconeogenesis pathway are outlined in Chapter 5. Gluconeogenesis represents a source of glucose for maintenance of blood glucose once glycogen reserves are exhausted (e.g. following fasting or intense/prolonged exercise). The main gluconeogenic substrates include glycerol (see Chapter 7), the 'glucogenic' amino acids (see Chapter 9) particularly alanine, lactate and certain tricarboxylic acid (TCA) cycle intermediates (see Chapter 5).

Gluconeogenesis also indirectly stimulates ketogenesis via oxaloacetate depletion. This causes an accumulation of acetyl CoA (see Chapter 3). The accumulated acetyl CoA is diverted towards ketone synthesis.

Ketogenesis in the context of glucose homeostasis

Ketogenesis is a metabolic pathway that generates ketones. It is described in detail in Chapter 7. Ketones are an important energy source for certain tissue types, particularly the brain, during fasting and starvation.

Ketogenesis is upregulated by various factors:

- Hypoglycaemia, that is, low blood glucose
- Glycogen depletion
- Glucagon
- Insulin deficiency (as seen in type 1 diabetes)

INTEGRATED GLUCOSE HOMEOSTASIS

The overall messages of the following sections are summarized in Table 6.2. The stages following a meal are subdivided by the length of time elapsed postprandially (i.e. 'after eating', or following a meal).

The 'fed' (absorptive) state

Immediately during and after a meal, ingested carbohydrates are digested in the gastrointestinal tract. The absorbable products of digestion (e.g. glucose) begin to be absorbed. This process tails off and stops after about 4 hours following the meal. This period is referred to as the 'fed' or 'absorptive' state.

Absorbed glucose travels first to the liver, via the portal vein. Absorbed glucose in excess of the liver's demands ultimately enters the systemic circulation, that is, the blood glucose begins to rise. This elevation in blood glucose triggers increased insulin secretion from pancreatic β cells. Insulin promotes liver glycogen synthesis, using absorbed glucose as a substrate. Glucose usually enters the glycolysis pathway and any additional glucose over and above the demand of these pathways is converted to fatty acids, incorporated into triacylglycerols and dispatched via very-low-density lipoprotein (VLDL) particles to adipocytes for storage.

The increased insulin levels and decreased glucagon levels define the 'fed' state as an overall anabolic state.

Under the influence of insulin, all tissues increase their uptake of glucose via insulin-dependent GLUT-4 upregulation. Insulin increases lipoprotein lipase (see Chapter 7) activity and triglyceride uptake from VLDL in the bloodstream. Muscle and liver cells also increase their glucose uptake and direct glucose towards glycogenesis for replenishment of stores. Note that glucose uptake in the liver is insulin independent.

Table 6.2 A summary of glucose homeostasis during the various physiological states following a meal

State	Period following eating[a]	Predominant macromolecule catabolized[b]	Hormonal profile
Fed/Absorptive	0–4 h	Glucose (absorbed)	High insulin:glucagon ratio
Fasting/Postabsorptive	4–12 h	Glucose (glycogenolysis → gluconeogenesis)	Lower insulin:glucagon ratio
Early starvation	12 h to 16 days	Glucose (gluconeogenesis) = Fatty acids Ketones (lipid catabolism)	Very low insulin:glucagon ratio
Late starvation	≥16 days	Ketones (proteolysis) >> Glucose (Gluconeogenesis; proteolysis)	Extremely low insulin:glucagon ratio

[a] Please note that the periods are approximate and will vary between individuals.
[b] Brackets indicate the main mechanism from which the macromolecule is derived.

The 'fasting' (postabsorptive) state

Once the input of absorbed glucose from the gut begins to slow and stops, the body enters the 'fasting' state. This occurs during the period approximately 4–12 hours following eating.

Glucagon release by pancreatic α cells begins to increase, and insulin secretion from β cells begins to decline. These changes are enhanced in proportion to the length of time elapsed from the last meal. Onset of these changes marks the physiological shift from the absorptive to the postabsorptive state. The decreased insulin:glucagon ratio causes several important changes, which overall result in store depletion rather than replenishment.

Glycogenolysis activity begins to outweigh glycogen synthesis, until there is net consumption of glycogen stores. This maintains the blood glucose despite no further glucose entering the circulation from gut absorption.

Following progressive depletion of glycogen reserves, the blood glucose beings to fall, which further increases glucagon release and decreases insulin release from the pancreas. This situation promotes an increase in liver gluconeogenesis, which increases until the blood glucose levels are being maintained by gluconeogenesis rather than by glycogenolysis. Gluconeogenic substrates are released peripherally as catabolism progressively begins to outweigh the synthesis of glycogen, triacylglycerols and protein.

The progressive switch from glycogenolysis to gluconeogenesis as a means of maintaining blood glucose defines the postabsorptive state. At this point, the brain is still completely reliant on glucose as its primary energy substrate.

Starvation

Prolonged fasting (early starvation)

Once over 12 hours has passed from the last meal, the body enters an early starvation state. The basal metabolic rate (see Chapter 8) falls in response to prolonged fasting, reducing total energy expenditure and the tissue demands on blood glucose.

Catabolism of lipid stores, primarily from adipocytes, begins to increase. Lipolysis of triacylglycerols liberates fatty acids and glycerol (see Chapter 7). Fatty acids undergo β-oxidation (see Chapter 7) and become the main energy substrate (as described in Chapters 3–5). Excess acetyl CoA (generated by β-oxidation begins to be diverted towards ketone synthesis (see Chapter 7) rather than the TCA cycle.

Ketones are vital because, unlike fatty acids, they can cross the blood–brain barrier and access the central nervous system (CNS). Normally exclusive CNS reliance on glucose as a metabolic fuel begins to change as the CNS starts to increase its ability to catabolize ketones (see Chapter 7) instead.

During early starvation, protein catabolism also slowly increases, releasing amino acids which may enter gluconeogenesis.

Fat metabolism increases progressively until the fat reserves are completely exhausted. In a person of normal body composition and weight, this usually takes approximately 16 days. The body then shifts from an 'early starvation' setting to a 'late starvation' setting.

Late starvation

Proteins now represent the predominant source of metabolic energy. However, there are no specific 'stores' of proteins as such. Instead proteins that play functional or structural roles are now catabolized, releasing amino acids into the circulation. These are diverted towards ketogenesis and gluconeogenesis, allowing continuing brain survival. However, protein loss has serious consequences for organ function and the person as a whole (see Chapter 9). Ketogenesis allows some sparing of protein catabolism, as it provided a substitute energy substrate (instead of glucose) for muscle and brain ATP generation.

GLUCOSE HOMEOSTASIS DURING EXERCISE

During exercise, the ongoing energy demands of the contracting tissue require not only a sustained delivery of oxygen, but also a continued supply of ATP to fuel ATP-dependent muscle contraction.

Initially, phosphocreatine functions as a phosphate donor to adenosine diphosphate (see Chapter 4). This enables immediate ATP generation via substrate-level phosphorylation. Soon after, glycogenolysis supplies glucose, which enables glycolysis to generate some ATP directly. The quantity of ATP generated from glucose depends on whether sufficient oxygen is present (see later discussion). Note that initially glycogen 'fuels' exercise. The respiratory quotient is typically ~1.0 during carbohydrate catabolism.

HINTS AND TIPS

THE RESPIRATORY QUOTIENT

This parameter describes the ratio between O_2 utilized and CO_2 generated. It is of clinical relevance as a component of cardiopulmonary exercise testing, as well as an important metabolic parameter coarsely indicative of the basal metabolic rate (see Chapter 8 for definition and discussion).

Once glycogen reserves are exhausted, increases in glucagon, noradrenaline and adrenaline promote lipolysis, liberating fatty acids and glycerol into the bloodstream.

The fatty acids are taken up by muscle cells, where they undergo β-oxidation, generating ATP. The same hormones also promote gluconeogenesis which (as discussed earlier) utilizes glycerol as a substrate, releasing glucose into the bloodstream. In contrast to the fasting and starvation states, during exercise, ketogenesis is not prominent. Once the principal ATP generation mechanism has shifted away from carbohydrate catabolism and towards fat metabolism, the respiratory quotient shifts towards a value of ~0.7.

Aerobic exercise

In the presence of sufficient oxygen ('aerobic' exercise), significantly more ATP generation can occur when pyruvate (generated by glycolysis) is oxidized further via the TCA cycle and oxidative phosphorylation. Recall that oxidative phosphorylation requires an adequate supply of oxygen, which is the terminal electron acceptor (see Chapter 4). However, efficient glycolysis/TCA/oxidative phosphorylation depends on sufficient oxygen delivery. Long distance running is a good example of aerobic metabolism.

Anaerobic exercise

Sufficient oxygen delivery relies on cardiac output, systemic vascular resistance, blood oxygen carrying capacity and several other factors. However, these variables are all finite. Once muscle contraction occurs at an intensity or frequency at which the oxygen *demand* of the tissues outstrips oxygen *supply*, the scenario is termed 'anaerobic' exercise. Sprinting or weightlifting are examples of anaerobic exercise.

The relative tissue hypoxia means that glycolysis is the only viable ATP generation mechanism during anaerobic exercise. Glycolysis is significantly less efficient in anaerobic conditions because of the inability to exploit downstream ATP generation pathways (see Chapter 5). Pyruvate generated by glycolysis is converted to lactate (see Chapter 5) rather than to acetyl CoA (see Chapter 5). This lactate dehydrogenase-mediated reaction also permits regeneration of nicotinamide adenine dinucleotide (NAD^+) from $NADH + H^+$, which enables glycolysis activity to continue (see Fig. 5.6).

The Cori cycle allows blood lactate (released during anaerobic exercise) to be converted to pyruvate by the liver. Pyruvate then enters gluconeogenesis.

METABOLIC SYNDROME

Metabolic syndrome refers to a cluster of abdominal obesity, hypertension, hypercholesterolaemia and impaired glucose tolerance or frank diabetes.

DIABETES MELLITUS

Diabetes is a chronic multisystem endocrine disorder resulting from absolute (type 1 diabetes mellitus (T1DM)) or a relative (type 2 diabetes mellitus (T2DM)) lack of pancreatic insulin secretion.

Lack of insulin impairs cellular import of glucose from the bloodstream and causes disturbances in normal macronutrient metabolism. There is hyperglycaemia. The hyperglycaemia causes progressive damage to cells, organs and vasculature, which leads to health complications that are ultimately disabling and life-threatening. Around 418 million adults are living with diabetes worldwide.

Metabolic features of diabetes

The cardinal metabolic features of diabetes (both T1DM and T2DM) are fasting hyperglycaemia and failure of the normal insulin-induced suppression of catabolic pathways. The outcome of this latter feature is an inappropriate breakdown of carbohydrate, protein and lipid stores despite dietary intake of glucose.

CLINICAL NOTES

WORLD HEALTH ORGANIZATION DEFINITION OF DIABETES

A fasting blood >7.0 mmol *or* a blood glucose >11.1 mmol 2 hours post an oral glucose tolerance test (OGTT). An OGTT consists of an oral administration of 75-g glucose in a fasted patient, with a blood glucose measurement taken at a preset times following the load (usually 1 hour and 2 hours postingestion). HbA1c equal to or above 6.5% (48 mmol/mol) is also diagnostic for diabetes.

Classification of type 1 or type 2 diabetes mellitus

Diabetes is clinically classified by whether there is a *failure* of insulin secretion by pancreatic β cells (T1DM) or *insufficient secretion* of insulin to maintain normal metabolism in a context of peripheral insulin resistance (T2DM). Both T1DM and T2DM are managed differently, and it is important to be clear about their differences.

Glycated haemoglobin

'Glycated haemoglobin', also known as 'haemoglobulin A1c (HbA1c)' is now used for both diagnosing and biochemical monitoring of diabetes. Glucose binds to the haemoglobin within red blood cells. Red blood cells therefore become glycosylated in proportion to the blood glucose. The amount of glycated haemoglobin present is therefore directly related to the average blood glucose during the red cell's lifespan of approximately 120 days, that is, the 3 months prior to the measurement. For this reason, the HbA1c is in fact superior to measuring blood glucose for the monitoring of diabetes, because it is not subjective to the acute rises and falls of blood glucose, which can confound the relevance of an individual measurement.

This parameter is recommended by the World Health Organization to use in diagnosis of diabetes:

HbA1c equal to or above 6.5% (48 mmol/mol) is also diagnostic for diabetes.

However, note that HbA1c less than 6.5% (48 mmol/mol) cannot *exclude* diabetes.

Overview of T1DM

T1DM is the result of loss of functional pancreatic β cells, rendering the patient incapable of producing insulin. The mechanism of β-cell destruction is usually autoimmune. This may be precipitated by many events (e.g. viral illness) and may be more likely in certain genetically predisposed individuals.

Various diseases can also cause pancreatic damage including β-cell islet destruction – this is known as secondary diabetes. This is clinically indistinguishable from T1DM and is managed identically. Type 1 diabetics require lifelong subcutaneous insulin replacement. It is required for survival.

Metabolic picture of T1DM

The primary metabolic consequence of insulin hyposecretion is a failure of intracellular import of glucose from the bloodstream. In T1DM insulin secretion is absent, therefore the metabolic consequences are highly pronounced. Blood glucose is abnormally high (hyperglycaemia).

The altered hormonal balance in each case (between insulin and the blood glucose-elevating hormones) leads to increased catabolism of storage macromolecules (i.e. carbohydrates, proteins and lipids), with the following outcomes:

- Glycogen reserves are catabolized, releasing glucose into the bloodstream and exacerbating hyperglycaemia.
- Adipocyte triacylglycerol hydrolysis (lipolysis) releases fatty acid and glycerol into the circulation.
- Activation of gluconeogenesis, the endogenous glucose generation pathway (see Chapter 5). This exacerbates the hyperglycaemia by releasing glucose into the bloodstream.
- Upregulation of ketogenesis (see Chapter 7) generating ketones.

This additional glucose release and synthesis would be appropriate in the normal insulin-deficient context of starvation. In the fed state, however, it is unnecessary, pathological and energetically costly.

Significant hyperglycaemia exceeds renal glucose re-absorption thresholds, leading to glycosuria. This causes osmotic diuresis, resulting in polyuria and thirst and dehydration. A metabolic acidosis may develop due to accumulation of the ketone bodies, the end products of ketogenesis.

Clinical presentation of T1DM

T1DM may present acutely with diabetic ketoacidosis (DKA) or with a short history of sudden unintentional weight loss, fatigue, polyuria and polydipsia.

Clinical management of T1DM

Subcutaneous insulin replacement is the key intervention in T1DM. Various insulin preparations are available, with different durations of action. An integrated multidisciplinary approach with regular communication between disciplines is important to address the multiple aspects of managing the patient's lifelong condition. This will typically include diabetologist/endocrinologist, the patient's general practitioner, diabetic nurse specialists and dieticians.

TYPE 2 DIABETES MELLITUS

T2DM is far more common than T1DM. It represents an enormous public health burden and its incidence and prevalence are increasing dramatically. It is usually adult onset, although worrying is that its incidence is now rising in children. It may be treated initially with diet and lifestyle modification, and if this approach is unsuccessful, oral medications and ultimately insulin are required.

Overview of T2DM

The exact cause of T2DM is not yet established. Multiple risk factors predisposing to T2DM have been clearly identified. These include:

- Obesity
- Insufficient exercise
- Older age
- Poor nutrition
- Certain genetic features
- Genetic background/family history of diabetes
- Personal history of gestational diabetes

In T2DM, symptom onset is insidious, in contrast to T1DM, as symptoms reflect a progressive failure of sufficient insulin effect than a relatively abrupt absolute deficit of insulin as in T1DM. T2DM may go undiagnosed for years.

Metabolic picture of T2DM

T2DM is hallmarked by progressive development of insulin resistance. 'Insulin resistance' is the term used to describe a blunting of normal cellular response to a given insulin dose. Insulin resistance provokes the pancreas to secrete higher than usual amounts of insulin to maintain normal glucose homeostasis. Initially, increased insulin secretion compensates for insulin resistance. This stage is known as 'impaired glucose tolerance' and is of variable duration. It is asymptomatic and frequently undetected.

CLINICAL NOTES

IMPAIRED GLUCOSE TOLERANCE (IGT)

The World Health Organization criteria diagnoses IGT when 2 hours post an oral glucose tolerance test, the blood glucose is in the range 7.8–11.1 mmol. Fasting blood glucose should not exceed 7.0 mmol. If blood glucose exceeds these ranges/values, diabetes should be considered rather than IGT.

Insulin resistance is progressive, so as it worsens, ever-increasing amounts of insulin must be released to maintain glucose homeostasis. Ultimately, the pancreas is unable to secrete enough insulin to compensate for the insulin resistance, and glucose homeostasis becomes disrupted. This is termed 'relative insulin hyposecretion'. The features of diabetes then begin to manifest. At this point, the patient will meet the diagnostic criteria for diabetes.

Their metabolic landscape resembles that of T1DM: impaired cellular glucose uptake causes hyperglycaemia, and glycosuria with thirst and polyuria and possible dehydration via the same mechanisms as described earlier. However, the key difference is that insulin-induced suppression of lipid catabolism and ketogenesis is far more pronounced in T2DM than T1DM, so the chronic hyperglycaemia is the more prominent metabolic derangement in T2DM, rather than the ketoacidosis and lipid catabolism as in T1DM.

Clinical presentation of T2DM

Fatigue, polyuria and polydipsia usually develop insidiously in contrast to the sudden onset seen in T1DM. The patient may even be asymptomatic. In these patients, if the glycosuria and hyperglycaemia are not detected incidentally or through screening, the diagnosis may be made too late to prevent development of chronic complications of diabetes.

Clinical management of T2DM

Initially, lifestyle modification, including weight loss, a healthy diet and regular exercise, is trialled. If hyperglycaemia persists despite these measures, first oral medications (oral hypoglycaemics; Table 6.3) are commenced, with recourse to parenteral hypoglycaemics Table 6.4 and ultimately subcutaneous insulin if insufficient glycaemic control is achieved.

Table 6.3 Oral hypoglycaemic drugs used in type 2 diabetes mellitus[a]

Drug class	Example	Mechanism of action	Advantages	Disadvantages
Biguanides 'insulin sensitizers'	Metformin	Increase insulin-induced peripheral glucose uptake, decrease gluconeogenesis	Unlikely to cause weight gain Low risk for hypoglycaemia Insulin sparing when used in combination therapy Highly efficacious Low cost	Gastrointestinal disturbance Rarely, B12 malabsorption → deficiency Rarely, biguanides may cause lactic acidosis. The risk is greater in patients with heart, lung, liver and kidney disease and therefore biguanides are contraindicated in this patient population.
Thiazolidinediones (glitazones): 'insulin sensitizers'	Pioglitazone	Activate nuclear receptor PPAR-γ influencing gene expression. Ultimately promote adipogenesis and fatty acid uptake in peripheral adipocytes, forcing other cells to retain normal reliance on carbohydrate (rather than lipid) metabolism.	Low risk for hypoglycaemia Safe in renal impairment Highly efficacious Well tolerated (minimal side effects)	Water retention Weight gain Allergic reactions Macular oedema Exacerbation of impaired cardiac function, liver failure Sustained efficacy Multiple contraindications Maximal effect takes several months to achieve
Sulphonylureas 'insulin secretagogues'	Gliclazide	Activate the ATP-sensitive K^+ channels in β cells, promoting endogenous insulin release	Once-daily dosing possible Highly efficacious Safest in renal impairment Low cost	Relatively high risk for hypoglycaemia Weight gain Efficacy may decline with use
Meglitinides 'insulin secretagogues'	Nateglinide, repaglinide	Promote insulin release by activating ATP-sensitive K^+ channels (as for sulphonylureas) but in addition open Ca^{++} channels, further promoting β-cell release of insulin.	Well tolerated (minimal side effects) High efficacy	Moderate risk of hypoglycaemia GI intolerance Skin reactions Liver problems
Gliptins 'incretin mimetics'	Sitagliptin, vildagliptin, sitagliptin, saxagliptin	DPP-IV inhibition (↑ endogenous GLP-1 release) ↑ Insulin secretion ↓ Glucagon secretion	Hypoglycaemia is uncommon	Skin reactions GI intolerance Skin reactions Pancreatitis
Sodium-glucose cotransporter 2 (SGLT2) inhibitors	Dapagliflozin, canagliflozin	Inhibition of renal sodium-coupled glucose reuptake, that is, impairing glucose reabsorption and increasing glucose loss in urine	Weight loss Beneficial effect on fat mass redistribution May attenuate hypertension	Increased frequency of urinary tract and genital fungal infection Dehydration and hypovolaemic hypotension Hyperkalaemia Hypoglycaemia when used in combination with insulin or sulfonylurea
Glucosidase inhibitors	Acarbose	Retards GI starch hydrolysis thus reducing GI glucose absorption	Hypoglycaemia is uncommon	Significant GI intolerance

[a] For full details of side effects and contraindications, please refer to https://www.diabetes.co.uk/diabetes-medication/
ATP, Adenosine triphosphate; GI, gastrointestinal; PPAR-γ, peroxisome proliferator-activated receptor-γ.

Table 6.4 Parenteral hypoglycaemic treatment

Drug	Examples	Mechanism of action	Advantages	Disadvantages
Insulin[a]	Rapid (ultrashort) acting: NovoRapid, Humalog Apidra Humulin S Short acting: Humulin-R Intermediate acting: Humulin-N, Hypurin isophane Long acting: Lantus, Levemir	As for endogenous insulin: ↑ cellular glucose uptake, ↓ gluconeogenesis, ketogenesis, lipolysis and glycogenolysis	Highly effective	Accurate dosing relative to carbohydrate intake/exercise level challenging: overdosing → hypoglycaemia, underdosing risks DKA Regular self-monitoring of BM necessary Self-injection necessary. Large dose-related weight gain
Incretin mimetics	Exenatide, Liraglutide	GLP-1 Glucagon-like peptide-1 (GLP-1) agonist ↑ Insulin secretion ↓ Glucagon secretion	Moderate dose-related weight loss Low risk of hypoglycaemia	Dose-related GI intolerance Pancreatitis Self-injection necessary

[a] Note that insulin is used as the mainstay of treatment in type 1 diabetes mellitus.
BM, Body mass; DKA, diabetic ketoacidosis; GI, gastrointestinal.

GESTATIONAL DIABETES MELLITUS

During normal pregnancy, there is a physiological increase in insulin resistance, which ensures normoglycaemia is maintained despite the additional demand of fetal glucose consumption. However, when insulin resistance increases excessively leading to persistent hyperglycaemia, gestational diabetes mellitus (GDM) is diagnosed. Approximately one in seven births worldwide is affected by GDM. The metabolic derangements resemble T2DM rather than T1DM. As with T2DM, GDM can be treated initially with diet and lifestyle modification. If this approach is unsuccessful, oral medications and ultimately insulin are introduced.

If symptoms develop, and the hyperglycaemia is more marked, diabetes mellitus (DM) is diagnosed (Table 6.5). In these circumstances, the diagnosis is 'diabetes mellitus in pregnancy', although this effectively represents pre-pregnancy diabetes that is first identified in pregnancy.

GDM is most commonly diagnosed after the 24th week of pregnancy. Both these clinical entities, in addition to pre-existing diabetes in women who become pregnant, convey the following increased risks:

- These women are at greater risk for preeclampsia.
- Their babies are at risk for adverse outcomes.
- These women are at greater risk for developing T2DM in later life.

Effective control of hyperglycaemia can attenuate these risks significantly.

Table 6.5 Investigation results discriminating gestational diabetes mellitus from diabetes mellitus in pregnancy (as per World Health Organization criteria)

Test	Diabetes mellitus in pregnancy	Gestational diabetes mellitus
Fasting blood glucose	≥7 mmol/L	5.1–6.9 mmol/L
Blood glucose 2 h postglucose load during OGTT[a]	≥11.1 mmol/L	8.5–11.1 mmol/L
Random blood glucose	≥11.1 mmol/L AND symptoms consistent with diabetes	

[a] OGTT, Oral glucose tolerance test. This consists of an oral administration of 75-g glucose and monitoring of blood glucose after a standardized interval.

CLINICAL NOTES

COMPLICATION OF GESTATIONAL DIABETES AND DIABETES MELLITUS IN PREGNANCY

The risk for preeclampsia (hypertension, proteinuria and placental compromise), obstructed labour, shoulder dystocia and birth trauma is all greater in gestational diabetes mellitus and diabetes mellitus in pregnancy. Furthermore, there are often complications for the baby, including intrauterine growth retardation, postdelivery hypoglycaemia, macrosomia, polyhydramnios, shoulder dystocia and even perinatal death.

ACUTE COMPLICATIONS OF DIABETES

Hypoglycaemia

Hypoglycaemia is a common problem that can occur in both T1DM and T2DM. It often develops secondary to the *treatments* used to lower blood glucose (insulin in T1DM and hypoglycaemic drugs with or without insulin in T2DM).

In diabetics reliant on subcutaneous insulin injections (all T1DM and some T2DM patients) hypoglycaemia develops due to a mismatch between insulin requirement and the patient's carbohydrate intake. This scenario can develop where carbohydrate intake is insufficient or excessive insulin is self-administered.

Hypoglycaemia can also occur following exercise, if the individual has not increased their carbohydrate intake adequately prior to activity. However, overall, exercise is known to reduce the insulin resistance that characterizes T2DM, and is therefore an important component of self-management of the condition.

Hypoglycaemic symptoms manifest at different blood glucose levels in different individuals. This minimum threshold can be quite variable. Hypoglycaemic symptoms include:

- Autonomic symptoms: sweating, tremor, nausea, hunger, tachycardia, postural hypotension
- Neuroglycopenic symptoms: anxiety or irritability, poor concentration, headache and reduced/loss of consciousness

Diabetes UK recommends that a blood glucose <4 mmol *in a* diabetic is treated urgently (Make four the floor). In a conscious and compliant patient, oral glucose tablets or a sugary drink or sweet biscuit will correct the symptoms. In a vomiting or unconscious or noncompliant patient, intravenous dextrose (e.g. 250 mL of 10% dextrose providing 25 g of glucose) should be used instead.

Some patients are 'silent hypoglycaemics' (i.e. they do not experience the warning symptoms and cannot administer/be administered glucose in a timely manner). They may fall into hypoglycaemic coma with little or no warning. This is often a consequence of advanced autonomic neuropathy as a complication of the diabetes.

Acute complications specific to T1DM: diabetic ketoacidosis (DKA)

DKA consists of the triad of hyperglycaemia, ketosis and metabolic acidosis. DKA is almost always a feature of uncontrolled T1DM, but very rarely can occur in T2DM in certain circumstances. It is life-threatening and must be promptly treated. Treatment must include insulin replacement, intravenous rehydration, avoidance of hypokalaemia during treatment and treatment of any acute illness(es) that may have precipitated the episode.

> ### RED FLAG
> Acute management of diabetic ketoacidosis: The priorities are resuscitation, rehydration, and insulin replacement. An insulin infusion must be commenced immediately. The dose/infusion rate is weight-determined initially. Aggressive intravenous rehydration is given according to national guidelines and includes up to 1.5 L over the first hour. The patient should also be catheterized to accurately assess fluid balance and will need hourly finger pricks for blood ketones and glucose. Serial venous blood gases are useful for monitoring metabolic acidosis and guiding electrolyte replacement. Intravenous potassium replacement is usually necessary, and phosphate and rarely bicarbonate may also be necessary. Resolution is indicated by normalization of blood pH and blood ketones.

Once the patient has recovered from the acute episode, they will need in-patient review by the hospital multidisciplinary diabetes team.

Causes

DKA is often the first presentation of new T1DM, but is also frequently seen as a complication of acute illness in a type 1 diabetic. Acute infection, myocardial infarction and ischaemic stroke are possible precipitating causes. DKA may also occur due to noncompliance with regular insulin injections.

Clinical features

Symptoms, signs and investigation findings consistent with DKA are presented in Table 6.6.

Mechanism

The effects of the extreme insulin deficit in DKA are wide ranging, affecting numerous metabolic pathways. The metabolic landscape is essentially that of untreated T1DM. The main features and their clinical markers are illustrated in Fig. 6.1.

Acute complications specific to T2DM: hyperosmolar, hyperglycaemic, nonketotic syndrome (HHNS)

HHNS is a complication specific to T2DM. HHNS typically occurs in elderly patients with multiple comorbidities. Incidence is rare, less than 1% of T2DM patients; however; the mortality is between 10% and 20%.

Table 6.6 Symptoms, signs and investigation findings in DKA

Symptoms	Thirst, polyuria, nausea, vomiting, confusion, abdominal pain
Signs	Unwell Severe dehydration (see Table 14.2) 'Pear-drops' breath odour (due to acetone) ↑ RR and depth of breathing ("Kussmaul respiration") Signs of organ hypoperfusion (shock): • ↑ HR, ↑ CRT, ↓ BP • Mental status change, coma • Acute renal impairment
Investigation findings	Urinary glucose and ketones +++ Blood glucose >11 mmol ↑ Blood ketones Metabolic acidosis: pH < 7.3, (H⁺ > 50 nmol/L) HCO₃⁻ ≤ 15 mmol, pCO₂ < 4 kPa ↑ Anion gap ↑ Urea, ↑ creatinine in proportion to prerenal impairment K⁺ likely to fall during treatment ↓ PO₄²⁻ (hypophosphataemia)

BP, Blood pressure; CRT, C-reactive protein; DKA, diabetic ketoacidosis; HCO3–, bicarbonate; HR, heart rate; pCO2, partial pressure of carbon dioxide; RR, respiratory rate.

As with DKA, patients are very unwell at presentation, and HHNS represents a medical emergency. It shares the following features with DKA:

• Hyperglycaemia (typically more pronounced than DKA)
• Severe dehydration
• Serum hyperosmolality (typically more pronounced than DKA)
• Presentation with confusion or coma (more likely than DKA) due to neuroglycopenia

However, metabolic acidosis and elevated blood ketones are *not* a feature of hyperosmolar, hyperglycaemic, nonketotic coma. The reason for this is that the suppression of lipid catabolism requires much less (about 1/10) insulin than the levels needed to maintain glucose. In T2DM, whilst the secreted insulin is insufficient to maintain normal glucose, it *is* able to supress lipid catabolism. For this reason, because suppression of lipid catabolism is intact, fatty acid diversion to ketogenesis is not prominent, therefore ↑ blood ketones and acidosis are not features of HHNS.

Treatment hinges on:

• Intravenous rehydration (to limit the severe dehydration that often characterizes HHNS) with careful normalization of serum osmolality

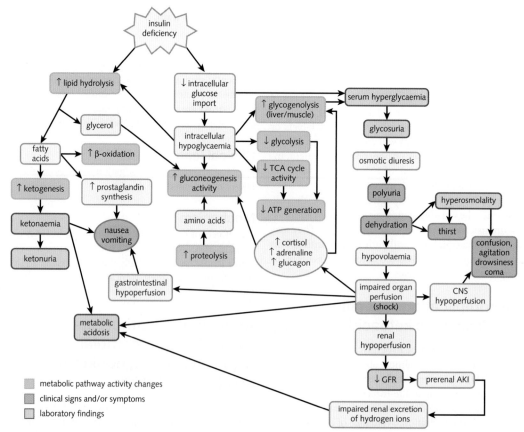

Fig. 6.1 Metabolic disturbances seen in diabetic ketoacidosis (DKA). *AKI*, Acute kidney injury; *ATP*, adenosine triphosphate; *CNS*, central nervous system; *GFR*, glomerular filtration rate; *TCA*, tricarboxylic acid.

- Insulin replacement to restore a degree of glucose homeostasis

As with DKA, in HHNS it is extremely important to avoid disturbance of serum potassium, because restoration of insulin powerfully stimulates intracellular movement of K^+ ions. This leads to hypokalaemia and all the consequent complications (see Chapter 13). Once the acute episode is resolved, the HHNS patient will need review by the hospital multidisciplinary diabetes team.

CHRONIC COMPLICATIONS OF DIABETES

Whilst the acute complications of diabetes are life-threatening, it is the long-term complications that represent the bulk of the disease burden. These are briefly summarized by system in the following sections. Chronic hyperglycaemia is the underlying mechanism causing most of the pathological manifestations. Excellent blood glucose control is the most effective method of reducing the onset and intensity of complications, but to some degree many are ultimately inevitable.

Cardiovascular complications

Diabetics experience an increased incidence of atherosclerosis relative to nondiabetics. This translates to higher incidence of ischaemic heart disease, peripheral vascular disease and cerebrovascular disease, which together account for approximately 65% of diabetic mortality.

CLINICAL NOTES

PERIPHERAL VASCULAR DISEASE

This leads to limb ischaemia (in combination with the predilection to ulcer formation), delayed wound healing and increased susceptibility to infection, creating the perfect storm in terms of distal tissue damage and destruction. Peripheral vascular disease in diabetics represents the leading cause of nontraumatic lower limb amputations.

Endothelia lining large (macrovascular) and small (microvascular) blood vessels are rendered dysfunctional by chronic hyperglycaemia leading to macrovascular and microvascular changes, respectively. Multiple factors associated with absolute or relative insulin deficiency exacerbate diabetic endothelial dysfunction, with the final outcome of increased occurrence of atherosclerosis and accelerated progression of established plaques. Hypertension prevalence is also significantly elevated in diabetes and further increases cardiovascular risk.

Renal complications

Diabetic microvascular disease leads to glomerular failure. This is known as diabetic nephropathy. Diabetes nephropathy is one of the most common causes of renal disease and represents the leading cause of new end-stage renal failure in the UK. Renal impairment exacerbates hypertension, which is far more common in diabetics. Caution must be exerted when prescribing potentially nephrotoxic drugs in diabetics, because their resilience of their kidneys is greatly reduced.

Peripheral neuropathy

Neuropathy in diabetes is multifactorial. Microangiopathy leads to cumulative ischaemic nerve damage. Persistently raised blood glucose is also directly neurotoxic. As with the other complications, the likelihood of occurrence and severity of diabetic neuropathy are inversely related to therapeutic efficacy in terms of normalizing hyperglycaemia. The 'glove and stocking' distribution of sensory neuropathy is classical, but mononeuritis multiplex, painful sensory neuropathy and autonomic neuropathy can occur. Peripheral neuropathy often leads to the patient failing to recognize minor foot trauma, which increases the chance of ulcer formation, which may also be unrecognized until advanced.

Autonomic neuropathy

The presence of autonomic neuropathy is indicative of advanced diabetes. Autonomic neuropathy is thought to be responsible for the phenomenon of painless (silent) myocardial infarction which may be seen in diabetic patients. Other pathological complications are highly likely to be well established if autonomic neuropathy is present.

Any or all functions of the autonomic nervous system may be impaired, including normal bowel motility, bladder emptying, temperature regulation, sweating, erectile function, salivation, visual accommodation and appropriate variation of cardiac output in response to changes in metabolic demand. The latter is suggested by resting tachycardia, fixed heart rate and postural hypotension.

General anaesthesia is particularly hazardous for patients with autonomic neuropathy due to gastroparesis, intraoperative hypothermia, excessive lability of blood pressure and an impaired ability to maintain sufficient blood pressure in the context of volatile maintenance agents-induced vasodilation.

Immune impairment

Diabetic patients are more susceptible to infections. This applies to both trivial infections (e.g. thrush) and more severe systemic infections. *Candida albicans* (the fungus responsible for thrush) thrives particularly in diabetics, which is thought to be attributable to increased glucose in vaginal secretions.

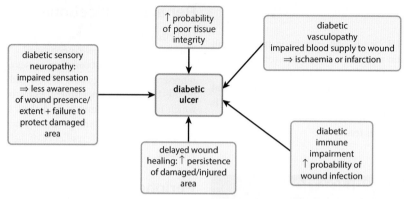

Fig. 6.2 Mechanisms underlying persistent and complicated ulcer formation in diabetics.

Once infected, infections are more challenging to treat effectively. Importantly, acute severe infection also places diabetic patients at risk for metabolic decompensation and may provoke DKA (mainly in T1DM, but rarely in T2DM) or HHNS in T2DM.

Delayed wound healing

Vascular disease of large and small vessels exacerbates wound ischaemia, impairing nutrient and oxygen delivery to damaged tissues when their demand is greatest. Coexisting immune dysfunction further impairs wound recovery by increasing the risk for infection and colonization.

Diabetic eye disease

Diabetic retinopathy leading to vision impairment including blindness is an important cause of disability in the diabetic population. Proliferative neovascularization on a background of diabetic retinopathy further complicates vision impairment. Diabetic patients must attend regular screening optometry examinations and retinal photography, with timely referral to diabetic eye clinics.

Ulcers

Approximately 15% of diabetic patients experience foot ulcers, which are a common primary cause of lower limb amputations that represent significant morbidity. Foot ulcers are the leading cause of hospital admissions in diabetics. Increased incidence, persistence and complication rate are multifactorial (summarized in Fig. 6.2).

Meticulous foot care is extremely important in diabetics, and all diabetic in-patients should have dependent and pressure areas carefully examined throughout admissions as they may not feel pain usually associated with such features themselves due to sensory neuropathy.

This also may delay recognition and appropriate treatment.

● Chapter Summary

- Glucose and insulin are the key regulatory hormones regulating the relevant pathways underpinning normal glucose homeostasis (ketogenesis and gluconeogenesis).
- Different metabolic pathways sustain glucose homeostasis in the fed, fasting and starvation contexts.
- Type 1 and type 2 diabetes mellitus both represent disorders of glucose homeostasis, but their underlying pathophysiology differs as do their clinical features and most acute complications.
- The chronic sequelae of diabetes are legion and include cardiovascular, renal, neuropathic, immune, eye disease and ulcers.
- Disruption of glucose homeostasis specific to pregnancy, that is, gestational diabetes mellitus (GDM), has specific diagnostic criteria. Diagnosis is important as many secondary fetomaternal complications can arise as a result of GDM.

LIPIDS: AN INTRODUCTION

Definition

Lipids are a large group of diverse molecules ranging from waxes to sterols. In this chapter the term 'lipids' is used synonymously with 'fats', that is, referring to fatty acids (FAs) and their derivatives. Lipid molecules all have the same general structure, shown in Fig. 7.1.

Lipid roles

Lipids have varied physiological roles – both structural and metabolic. In anabolism, triacylglycerol (TAG, also known as 'triglyceride') molecules are the major form of energy storage. TAGs consist of three FAs linked to a glycerol backbone by ester bonds. Fig. 7.2 shows an example. During catabolism, lipid stores are mobilized, releasing FAs and glycerol, which enter the bloodstream and act as substrates for oxidation by distant tissues, generating energy.

Fatty acids: archetype lipids

FAs are excellent examples for illustrating lipid structure: a carboxylate head linked to a long unbranched hydrocarbon tail (Fig. 7.3).

Fatty acids in metabolism

FAs are required as substrates for lipogenesis, that is, synthesis of TAGs, energy-dense storage molecules. FA are synthesized from acetyl-coenzyme A (acetyl-CoA). When acetyl-CoA is abundant (i.e. the fed state), the chemical energy intrinsic to acetyl-CoA can be 'stored' as TAGs.

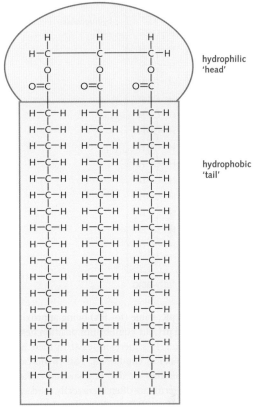

Fig. 7.2 Tristearin: a triacylglycerol (triglyceride).

Conversely, FA can be released into the bloodstream from TAGs (stored in adipose tissue) by lipolysis; once released they can be catabolized to release energy. The long hydrocarbon tails of FA molecules are incredibly efficient in terms of energy storage, because they contain fully reduced carbon and release plenty of energy on oxidation (catabolism). FA catabolism is via β-oxidation, which both generates $FADH_2$ (reduced flavin adenine dinucleotide) and $NADH + H^+$ (reduced nicotinamide adenine dinucleotide) and releases acetyl-CoA. Acetyl-CoA can enter the tricarboxylic acid (TCA) cycle for oxidation, and reducing equivalents can undergo oxidative phosphorylation, releasing energy.

Fatty acids: the suffixes '-ic acid' and '-ate'

Note that FAs all have molecular formula 'R–COOH', that is, 'something' carrying a carboxylic acid group (the 'something' in this case is a hydrocarbon chain). Chemically, FAs are weak acids:

$$R - COOH \leftrightarrow R - COO^- + H^+$$

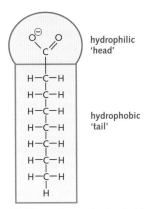

Fig. 7.1 General lipid structure: a hydrophobic 'tail' composed of a hydrocarbon chain (C and H) and a hydrophilic 'head' consisting of C, H and O.

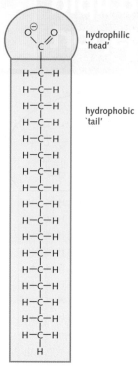

Fig. 7.3 Stearate: a fatty acid.

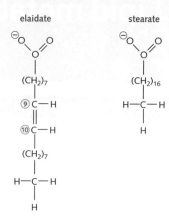

Fig. 7.4 Saturated and unsaturated fatty acids: stearate versus elaidate. The *ringed numbers* illustrate the carbon number. Appreciate that stearate is the same molecule as in Fig. 7.3; however, for brevity not every single carbon and bond have been drawn.

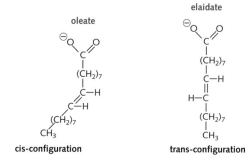

Fig. 7.5 Stereoisomerism: cis (oleate) and trans (elaidate) configuration of $CH_3(CH_2)_7CH = CH(CH_2)_7COO^-$.

Due to the average pK_a value (for FA) being approximately 4.5, at physiological pH, the equilibrium position lies to the right of the equation. FAs therefore exist in their anionic form under physiological conditions. This is indicated by the suffix '-ate' rather than '-ic acid' (e.g. stear*ate* rather than stear*ic acid*). These terms are often incorrectly used synonymously. In this text, the suffix '-ate' is used, as this represents the physiological charged status of these molecules.

Saturated versus unsaturated

FAs are described as 'saturated' or 'unsaturated'. *Un*saturated FAs contain a double bond at some location within the hydrocarbon tail, whereas saturated FAs contain no double bonds. In saturated FAs, there are no double bonds within the hydrocarbon chain, and so no opportunity for any new bonds to be formed; the molecule is 'saturated' with hydrogen atoms. 'Polyunsaturated' FAs have more than one double bond, whereas 'monounsaturated' FAs have only a single double bond (Fig. 7.4).

Stereoisomerism: cis and trans configurations of the C=C double bond

Double bonds within an unsaturated FAs may adopt one of two stereoisomeric configurations: *cis* or *trans*. The nature of a C=C double bond can have significant consequences for molecular properties, for example structure and chemical characteristics. The *cis* configurations impose a sharp bend in the hydrocarbon chain, whereas the *trans* configurations

do not. Most naturally occurring unsaturated FAs possess C=C bonds in the *cis* configuration (Fig. 7.5).

Naming organic molecules

Carbon counting in organic chemistry

Carbon counting in chemistry begins from the carbon attached to the main functional group of the molecule (in FAs this is the carboxyl group). The carbon bearing this functional group is designated carbon-1 (C1). C1 is also sometimes called the 'alpha' carbon, and C2 the 'beta' carbon. This explains why Greek letters are part of the names of biochemical molecules; for example, α-ketoglutarate (this tells us that the keto (C=O) functional group originates from the alpha carbon of glutarate).

With unsaturated FAs, the number of carbons as well as the number, position and nature of the double bonds must be communicated by the notation.

This is illustrated using the example of palmitoleate (16:1cΔ9) and arachidonate (20:4cΔ5,8,11,14) in Fig. 7.6.

- The number before the colon describes the total number of carbons in the molecule (16).

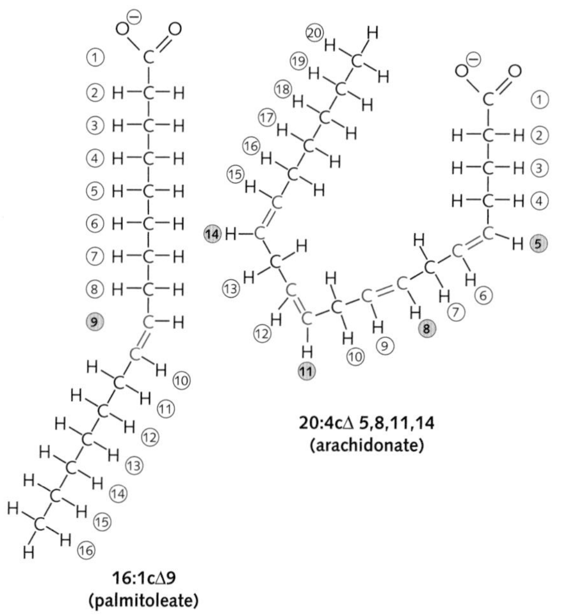

Fig. 7.6 Fatty acid nomenclature: palmitoleate (16:1c∆9) and arachidonate (20:4c∆5,8,11,14). *Ringed numbers* indicate the carbon numbering.

- The number directly after the colon describes the number of double bonds – in this case (1).
- The 'c' indicates that the configuration of that double bond is cis (as opposed to trans).
- The '∆' symbol is followed by a number representing the carbon atom at which the double bond starts.

Omega-3 fatty acids

Omega-3 FAs are a family of FA molecules with a common structural feature: a double bond between the third and fourth carbon counted from the end of the hydrocarbon tail. The final carbon in the hydrocarbon tail is the 'omega' carbon, irrespective of whether it is C5 or C25. This final carbon is at the opposite end of the molecule to the carboxyl group. Whilst confusing that this naming system counts from the other end to the functional group, it is used because the proximity of the first unsaturation (C=C double bond) to the terminal (omega) carbon has more influence on molecular properties of the FA than its proximity to the carboxylate group at the other end of the molecule.

FATTY ACID BIOSYNTHESIS

Introduction

Although FAs are accessible from dietary fats (from hydrolysis of ingested TAGs), the bulk of human energy intake occurs in the form of carbohydrates. Carbohydrate storage (as glycogen) is limited; thus a process for conversion of carbohydrate to fat is required. This process is FA synthesis; acetyl-CoA derived from pyruvate (a glycolysis product) is incorporated into new FA molecules. These may then be esterified, forming TAGs for storage in adipose tissue.

Location of FA synthesis

FA synthesis occurs in cytoplasm. It occurs mainly in specialized fat cells (adipocytes), but also in the liver, kidney and of course the lactating mammary glands. It requires various substrates but the most important ones to remember are acetyl-CoA and $NADPH + H^+$.

Overview of fatty acid synthesis

FA synthesis consists of a number of stages:

1. Transport of acetyl-CoA to the cytoplasm (where the synthetic enzymes are located)
2. Activation; synthesis of malonyl-CoA and binding to FA synthase homodimers
3. A sequence of condensation, reduction, dehydration and a second reduction
4. Addition of a 2-carbon unit (derived from another C3 malonyl-CoA molecule)
5. Repeat of stages 3 and 4

The number of 'repeats' determines the length of the hydrocarbon chain. In the example of palmitate (16:0), after the initial process (stages 1 through 4), this would repeat a further six times. Note that this process generates a saturated FA, with no double bonds (hence the '0' in 16:0). Synthesis of unsaturated FAs requires a saturated FA to first be synthesized and then enzymatically modified.

Details of fatty acid synthesis

Transport of acetyl-CoA from mitochondria to cytoplasm

This is via a mechanism known as the 'citrate shuttle', also known as the 'pyruvate–malate' cycle (Fig. 7.7).

- Acetyl-CoA condenses with oxaloacetate (in the mitochondrial matrix) forming citrate, catalysed by citrate synthase.
- Citrate is then exported from matrix → cytoplasm in exchange for malate.
- Here the citrate reacts with adenosine triphosphate (ATP) and CoA to form oxaloacetate and acetyl-CoA. This is catalysed by citrate lyase. The acetyl-CoA is now located in the cytoplasm and able to participate in FA synthesis.
- The oxaloacetate is reduced to malate by malate dehydrogenase, using $NADH + H^+$ as a redox partner.
- Malate is decarboxylated to pyruvate by malic enzyme, using nicotinamide adenine dinucleotide phosphate ($NADP^+$) as a redox partner. This generates $NADPH + H^+$, which can then participate in FA

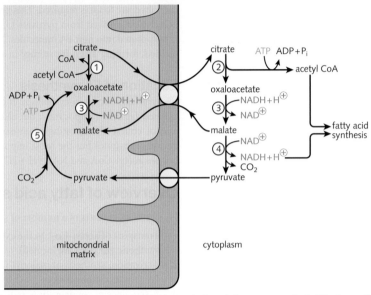

Fig. 7.7 The citrate shuttle mechanism for mitochondrial import of acetyl-coenzyme A. *1*, Citrate synthase; *2*, citrate lyase; *3*, malate dehydrogenase; *4*, malic enzyme; *5*, pyruvate carboxylase. *ADP*, adenosine diphosphate; *ATP*, adenosine triphosphate; *CoA*, coenzyme A; *NAD+*, nicotinamide adenine dinucleotide; *P_i*, inorganic phosphate.

synthesis, or return to the mitochondrial matrix in exchange for citrate.

- Pyruvate then reenters the mitochondria, where it may either be used to regenerate oxaloacetate or acetyl-CoA, completing the circuit. Fig. 7.7 illustrates the entire process.

Conversion of acetyl-CoA to malonyl-CoA

This is the irreversible rate-limiting step of FA synthesis. Carboxylation of acetyl-CoA is mediated by acetyl-CoA carboxylase (requiring biotin as a cofactor). The reaction is shown in Fig. 7.8.

Getting it together: assembly of malonyl and acetyl groups on acyl carrier protein

Acyl carrier protein (ACP) is a component of FA synthase. ACP accepts acyl groups, such as the acetyl and malonyl groups of acetyl-CoA and malonyl-CoA, thus anchoring them to the enzyme in preparation for FA synthesis. The CoA components are released and the acyl components bind to the terminal sulphur atom of the

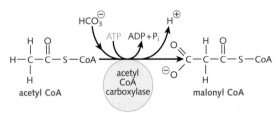

Fig. 7.8 Conversion of acetyl-CoA to malonyl-CoA. *ADP*, Adenosine diphosphate; *ATP*, adenosine triphosphate; *CoA*, coenzyme A; *P_i*, inorganic phosphate.

phosphopantetheine moiety (Fig. 7.9). This reaction is mediated by acetyl transacylase and malonyl transacylase. Note that two ACPs are present; this is because FA synthase exists as a homodimer.

Fatty acid synthase

This enzyme is a homodimer, consisting of two copies (a 'dimer') of identical (homo) enzymatic units. The units themselves are also composed of a number of subunits, each fulfilling various enzymatic roles in the reactions of FA synthesis.

Condensation

The ACP-anchored acetyl group is cleaved off and transferred to the protruding end of the malonyl group (bound to the other ACP molecule). This transfer displaces the carboxyl group, liberating CO_2. This condensation reaction is catalysed by β-ketoacyl-ACP synthase and results in a saturated four-carbon chain, still attached to the ACP. This forms the basic skeleton of an FA.

Reduction, dehydration, reduction…

The nascent FA has a C=O double bond at the C3 position, which is now removed. Two new bonds are created for C3: one with –H and one with –OH. $NADPH + H^+$ is oxidized as the redox partner. This reduction reaction is mediated by β-ketoacyl-ACP reductase.

A double bond is then introduced between C2 and C3. This releases H_2O (dehydration) and is catalysed by 3-hydroxyacyl-ACP dehydratase.

Finally, this double bond is removed by saturation of C2 and C3 with H atoms. This second reduction reaction is mediated by enoyl-ACP reductase, and the redox partner again

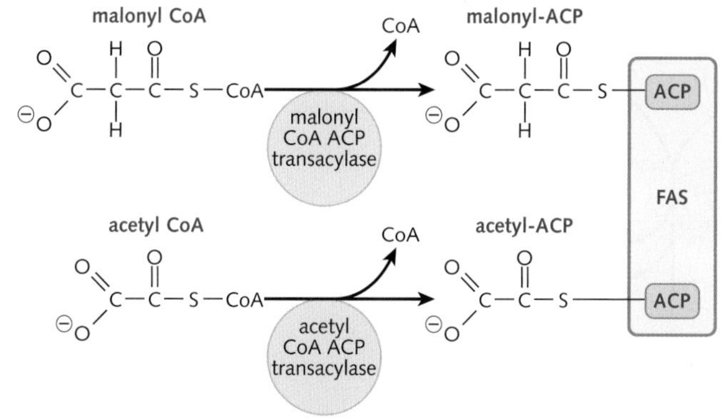

Fig. 7.9 Synthesis of acetyl-ACP and malonyl-ACP. *ACP,* Acyl carrier protein; *CoA,* coenzyme A; *FAS,* fatty acid synthase.

is NADPH+H$^+$. This has generated a four-carbon acyl group, which remains attached to its ACP anchor (Fig. 7.10).

'Site switch' of the growing chain
β-Ketoacyl-ACP synthase now transfers the four-carbon acyl chain from ACP onto the sulphur atom on one of its own cysteine residues. This leaves the ACP free to receive further incoming malonyl-CoA (Fig. 7.10).

Addition of further malonyl-CoA
Further malonyl-CoA (produced by conversion of acetyl-CoA) arrives, sheds its CoA and binds to the available ACP in a condensation reaction, forming malonyl-ACP (Fig. 7.9). Malonyl-ACP is now ready to receive the growing acyl chain, which is currently attached to a Cys residue within β-ketoacyl-ACP synthase.

Transfer of the lengthened acyl chain onto malonyl-ACP
The enzyme β-ketoacyl-ACP synthase catalyses the transfer (condensation) of the nascent acyl chain from itself onto the malonyl-ACP. This marks the start of a new cycle of FA synthesis (Fig. 7.10).

Elongation to palmitate
At this point, the developing FA undergoes six further cycles of condensation/reduction/dehydration/reduction/site switch/transfer (seven times in total). This produces an acyl chain, 16 carbon atoms in length. A thioesterase then cleaves off the acyl chain from where it is bound to the ACP, releasing a 16-carbon saturated FA (palmitate; Fig. 7.11). This may later then be further elongated (via a different mechanism) or undergo further reactions to introduce double bonds, generating an unsaturated FA (Fig. 7.12).

Elongation of fatty acids beyond 16 carbons
FA synthase can only manufacture FAs up to 16 carbons in length. Additional enzymes are required to lengthen 16-carbon FA. These are located within the *mitochondria* and the *endoplasmic reticulum*. The process is complex and

is not addressed in this text; however, it is important to be aware that further elongation occurs in the endoplasmic reticulum and in mitochondria.

Desaturation of fatty acids
Introduction of a double bond (to a saturated fatty acyl-CoA) occurs in the smooth endoplasmic reticulum and requires oxygen and NADH+H$^+$. A monounsaturated equivalent fatty acyl-CoA is generated, along with nicotinamide adenine dinucleotide (NAD$^+$) and two H$_2$O molecules (Fig. 7.12). Three enzymes are required:

- NADH-cytochrome b$_5$ reductase
- Cytochrome b$_5$
- Fatty acyl-CoA desaturase

Essential fatty acids
In mammals, double bonds can only be introduced at positions Δ4, Δ5, Δ6 and Δ9 due to enzyme availability; there are four subtypes of desaturases, each responsible for introduction of a double bond at these positions. However, FA with double bonds at the ω-6 and ω-3 positions are also physiologically required (e.g. for eicosanoid synthesis (including prostaglandins)). As these cannot be synthesized, they must be obtained in the diet and are therefore termed 'essential FAs'. Linoleate (18:2cΔ9,12 – double bond at the ω-6 carbon) and α-linolenate (18:3cΔ9,12,15 – double bonds at ω-6 and ω-3) are the two essential unsaturated FAs that cannot be endogenously synthesized in humans. Some plants possess desaturases capable of introducing the double bond at the ω-6 and ω-3 locations, hence the presence of ω-6 and ω-3 oils in plant seed oil.

Regulation of fatty acid synthesis
Substrate availability: malonyl-CoA
Malonyl-CoA availability is directly related to acetyl-CoA availability. Acetyl-CoA is abundant following carbohydrate intake (high glycolysis activity → high pyruvate → high acetyl-CoA). Initially, elevated acetyl-CoA drives the

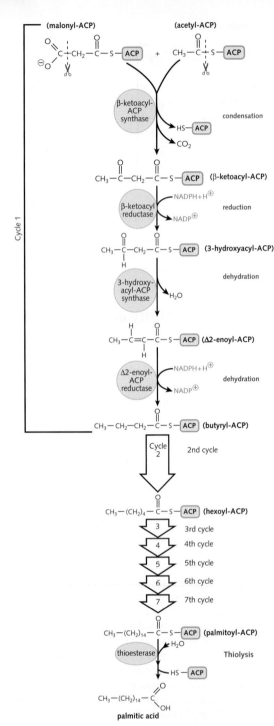

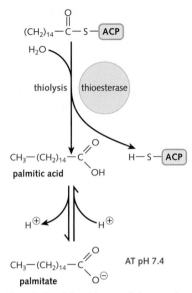

Fig. 7.11 Hydrolysis of the thioester linkage: release of palmitic acid and conversion to palmitate under physiological conditions. *ACP,* Acyl carrier protein.

Fig. 7.12 Conversion of saturated fatty acids to unsaturated forms (desaturation). This example illustrates introduction of a cis double bond at the C9 position. *1,* NADH-cytochrome b_5 reductase; *2,* cytochrome b_5; *3,* fatty acyl-CoA desaturase. *Ringed numbers* indicate carbon numbering. *CoA,* Coenzyme A; *NADP+,* nicotinamide adenine dinucleotide phosphate.

Fig. 7.10 Fatty acid synthesis: the synthesis of palmitic acid. Malonyl-ACP and acetyl-ACP condense initially, followed by reduction, dehydration and another reduction. Note the role of NADPH + H+ as a hydrogen donor. This cycle then repeats; however, butyryl-ACP (rather than acetyl-ACP) then receives 'CH₂–C=O' units from malonyl-ACP. After seven cycles, thiolysis clips the developed palmitic acid of the ACP anchor, releasing palmitic acid. *ACP,* Acyl carrier protein; *NADP+,* nicotinamide adenine dinucleotide phosphate.

activity of the TCA cycle. Once TCA cycle products accumulate, they then inhibit cycle activity. At this point acetyl-CoA becomes available to participate in FA synthesis. Citrate (a TCA cycle intermediate; see Fig. 3.1) also allosterically activates the rate-limiting enzyme of FA synthesis – acetyl-CoA carboxylase.

Substrate availability: NADPH + H+

Recall that NADPH + H+ inhibits glucose-6-phosphate dehydrogenase, and in doing so slows flux through the pentose phosphate pathway (PPP; see Chapter 5). When FA synthesis occurs, NADPH + H+ is oxidized to NADP+, lifting the inhibition of glucose-6-phosphate dehydrogenase and increasing PPP activity. Thus FA synthesis activity promotes further NADPH + H+ synthesis. In addition, the citrate shuttle (which is highly active when acetyl-CoA is high) also generates more $NADPH + H^+$ when acetyl-CoA (and therefore malonyl-CoA) is abundant.

Substrate availability: hormonal regulation

Acetyl-CoA carboxylase is also subject to hormonal regulation. Insulin (a fed-state hormone) binding to its intracellular receptors activates a signalling cascade which includes activation of a phosphatase (which dephosphorylates acetyl-CoA carboxylase, activating it). Acetyl-CoA carboxylase is re-phosphorylated (inactivated) in cells exposed to glucagon or adrenaline (epinephrine; both fasting-state hormones). Acetyl-CoA carboxylase is of key regulatory importance because it mediates conversion of acetyl-CoA to malonyl-CoA, thereby controlling substrate provision for FA synthesis. FA synthesis is promoted by insulin but inhibited by glucagon. In addition, insulin promotes dephosphorylation (activation) of pyruvate dehydrogenase, which converts pyruvate to acetyl-CoA (Fig. 7.13) for incorporation into FAs.

Lipogenesis: triacylglycerol synthesis

TAG molecules, in medicine more commonly called 'triglycerides', consist of three FAs linked to glycerol by ester bonds. TAG synthesis allows FA storage in adipocytes (specialized fat storage cells). Synthesis from glycerol and FA (illustrated in Fig. 7.14) occurs in three stages:

1. Formation of glycerol-3-phosphate via one of two mechanisms. Either glycerol is phosphorylated at C3 by glycerol kinase using ATP as the phosphate donor, or the glycolytic intermediate dihydroxyacetone phosphate (DHAP; see Chapter 5) is reduced by glycerol-3-phosphate dehydrogenase.
2. FA activation. FA must react with CoA to undergo lipogenesis. Fatty acyl-CoA synthetase performs this reaction.
3. The three activated FAs are esterified to glycerol-3-phosphate in stages.

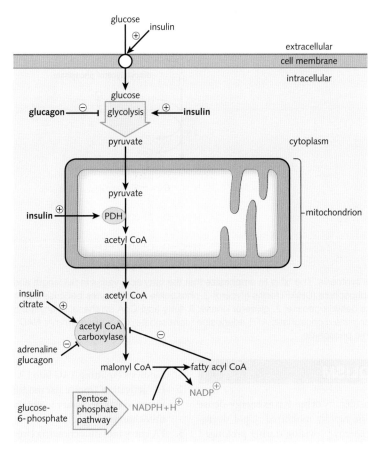

Fig. 7.13 Adipocyte: regulation of fatty acid synthesis. For simplicity, no shuttle mechanisms are shown, but recall that acetyl-CoA leaves the mitochondria via the citrate shuttle (Fig. 7.7). *CoA*, Coenzyme A; *NADP⁺*, nicotinamide adenine dinucleotide phosphate; *NADPH*, nicotinamide adenine dinucleotide phosphate (reduced form of NADP⁺); *PDH*, pyruvate dehydrogenase; *PPP*, pentose phosphate pathway.

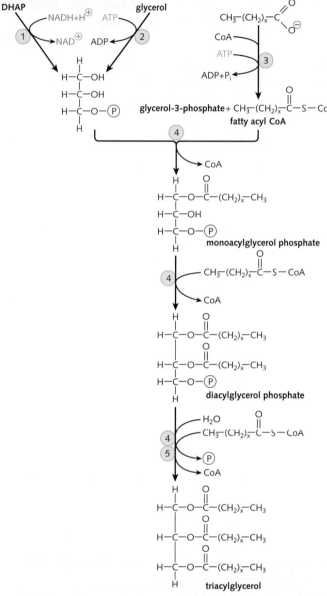

Fig. 7.14 Triacylglycerol synthesis. The 'x' is to emphasize that the fatty acid varies in tail length and saturation. Also note that dihydroxyacetone phosphate (DHAP) forms glycerol-3-phosphate in adipocytes because they lack glycerol kinase. *1*, Glycerol-3-phosphate dehydrogenase; *2*, glycerol kinase; *3*, fatty acyl-CoA synthase; *4*, acyltransferase; *5*, phosphatase; *ADP*, adenosine diphosphate; *ATP*, adenosine triphosphate; *CoA*, coenzyme A; *NAD+*, nicotinamide adenine dinucleotide; *Pi*, inorganic phosphate.

LIPID CATABOLISM

The major physiological identity of lipids is as energy-dense molecules, which can be rapidly mobilized. Lipid degradation releases FA for energy provision during prolonged exercise or when energy utilization exceeds dietary energy intake. Lipid breakdown includes the following stages:

1. Lipolysis (splitting TAG into FA and glycerol)
2. FA 'activation' (molecular modification of liberated FAs necessary to obtain access to the mitochondria)
3. FA entry into mitochondria (from the cytoplasm)
4. β-oxidation (oxidation, releasing energy)

Lipolysis

Lipolysis occurs in the cytoplasm, where TAGs are stored in droplets. A hormone-sensitive lipase (HSL) hydrolyses the ester bonds at C1 or C3, liberating one FA, leaving a diacyl glycerol, which comprises the glycerol backbone with two remaining FAs attached. Next, diacyl glycerol lipase removes a second FA, leaving monoacylglycerol. Monoacylglycerol lipase then cleaves off the remaining FA, freeing glycerol (Fig. 7.15).

Fate of liberated fatty acids

Newly freed FAs are released into the bloodstream, where they bind to albumin. They are taken up by muscle or liver cells and oxidized. They may also be taken up again by adipocytes and re-esterified to TAGs.

Fate of liberated glycerol

Intracellular glycerol is phosphorylated and oxidized to DHAP, which is then isomerized to glyceraldehyde-3-phosphate (see Chapter 5). This may then enter glycolysis. Alternatively, glycerol may be released into the bloodstream and enter hepatocytes, where it may participate in glycolysis or gluconeogenesis, depending on cellular energy status.

Fatty acid activation

Thiokinase converts FA to fatty acyl-CoA. This reaction requires ATP for generation of an adenylyl intermediate (Fig. 7.16). The second high-energy phosphoanhydride bond is also hydrolysed. Thus the equivalent of two ATP is consumed during FA activation. Now activated, fatty acyl-CoA is then ready to enter the mitochondrial matrix via the carnitine shuttle.

Accessing the mitochondrial matrix: the carnitine shuttle

Because of mitochondrial membrane impermeability to fatty acyl-CoA, a specialized mechanism exists to allow these molecules to access their site of catabolism (the matrix). This is the carnitine shuttle, which is best illustrated diagrammatically (Fig. 7.16).

β-Oxidation of fatty acids

This occurs in the mitochondrial matrix and is a four-stage process which repeats itself until the FA molecule is completely consumed.

(1) Oxidation by flavin adenine dinucleotide

The fatty acyl-CoA is oxidized by fatty acyl-CoA dehydrogenase. This enzyme exists in various isoforms, each specific for different length of FAs (long, medium and short).

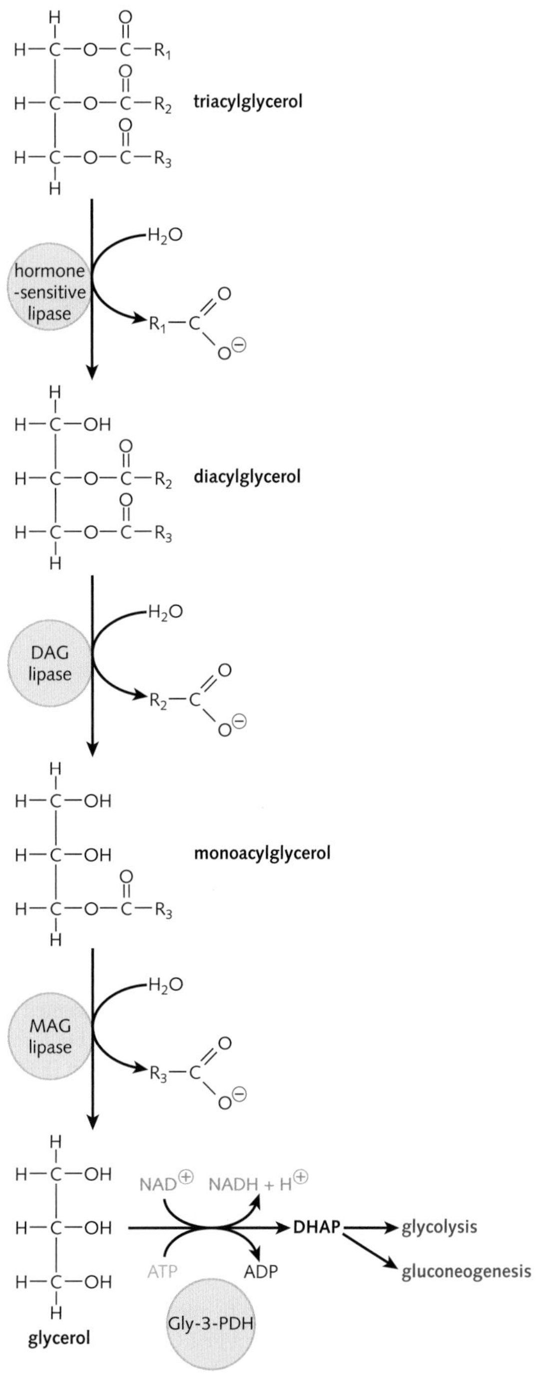

Fig. 7.15 Lipolysis of triacylglycerols. Please note that 'R' represents any acyl chain, for example $-(CH_2)x–CH_3$. *ADP,* Adenosine diphosphate; *ATP,* adenosine triphosphate; *DAG lipase,* diacylglycerol lipase; *DHAP,* dihydroxyacetone phosphate; *Gly-3-PDH,* glycerol-3-phosphate dehydrogenase; *MAG lipase,* monoacylglycerol lipase; *NAD+,* nicotinamide adenine dinucleotide.

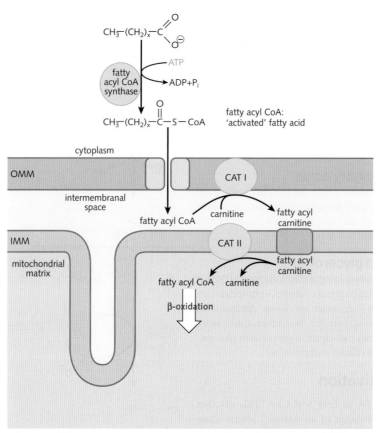

Fig. 7.16 Fatty acid activation and entry to the mitochondria: the carnitine shuttle. *ADP,* Adenosine diphosphate; *ATP,* adenosine triphosphate; *CAT,* carnitine acyltransferase (note the two isoforms: CAT I at the OMM and CAT II at the IMM); *CoA,* coenzyme A; *IMM,* inner mitochondrial membrane; *OMM,* outer mitochondrial membrane; *P$_i$,* inorganic phosphate.

Oxidation converts the single bond between C2 (the 'β' carbon) and C3 to a double bond. The H atoms are accepted by the redox partner flavin adenine dinucleotide (FAD), forming FADH$_2$. This enters the electron transport chain (ETC), generating approximately 1.5 ATP.

(2) Hydration

Enoyl-CoA hydratase introduces an O atom and two H atoms to the newly formed double bond between C2 and C3.

(3) Oxidation by NAD$^+$

β-Hydroxyacyl-CoA dehydrogenase mediates oxidation of the –OH group at C3, converting it to a C=O (ketone) group. This molecule is 3-ketoacyl-CoA. The two H atoms removed are transferred to NAD$^+$ (the redox partner) generating NADH+H$^+$. This enters ETC, generating approximately 2.5 ATP.

(4) Thiolysis: release of acetyl-CoA

Thiolase cleaves off the C1 and C2 from 3-ketoacyl-CoA, releasing acetyl-CoA. This shortens the fatty acyl chain by two carbons. Another CoA is required to 'cap' the newly shortened molecule. This molecule is a fatty acyl-CoA, but with two fewer carbons than the molecule in step 1.

Reiteration of 1→4

Steps 1 to 4 are repeated until the FA is almost completely degraded. The penultimate repeat leaves a four-carbon fatty acyl-CoA, which then undergoes steps 1→4 as before; however, this final 'round' of β-oxidation differs in that it produces two acetyl-CoA molecules rather than one. Note that this final step is only the case for FA with an *even* number of carbons (Fig. 7.17).

Odd-chain fatty acids

This final step differs for FAs with an odd number of carbons; the penultimate repeat leaves a five-carbon fatty acyl-CoA. This undergoes a final round of steps 1→4, but the final two products are one acetyl-CoA molecule and one three-carbon propionyl-CoA molecule (instead of two acetyl-CoA molecules; Fig. 7.18).

Propionyl-CoA

This molecule may be converted to succinyl-CoA in three steps. This requires 1 ATP and a bicarbonate ion (HCO$_3^-$). One of the requisite enzymes requires a vitamin B12-derived cofactor and another uses biotin as a cofactor.

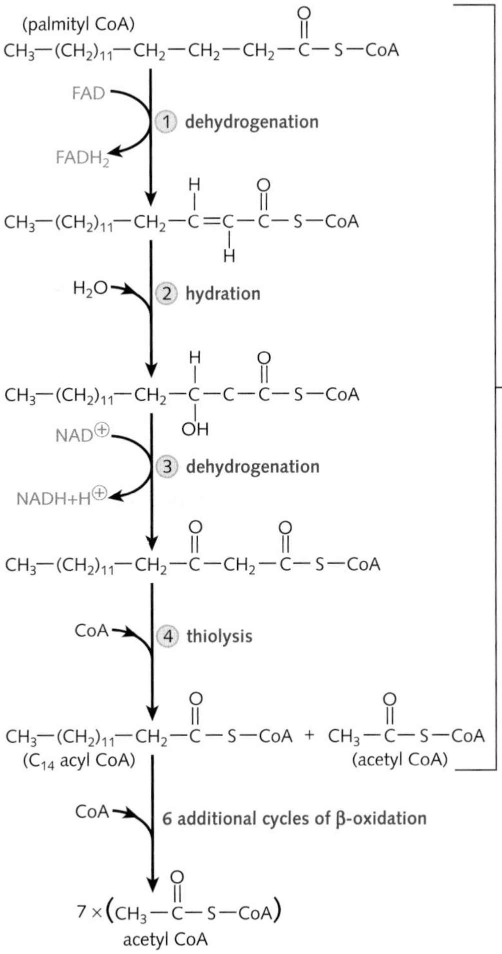

Fig. 7.17 β-Oxidation of fatty acids. Palmitate is used for illustration. *1,* fatty acyl-CoA dehydrogenase; *2,* enoyl-CoA hydratase; *3,* 3-hydroxyacyl-CoA dehydrogenase; *4,* thiolase; *CoA,* coenzyme A; *FAD,* flavin adenine dinucleotide; *NAD,* nicotinamide adenine dinucleotide.

Succinyl-CoA oxidation generates 1 NADH + H$^+$ (reduced nicotinamide adenine dinucleotide) and 1 FADH$_2$, reduced flavin adenine dinucleotide together yielding 4 ATP.

ATP yield from fatty acid oxidation

Every round of β-oxidation generates 1 FADH$_2$, 1 NADH + H$^+$ and 1 acetyl-CoA. Recall that full oxidation of one molecule of acetyl-CoA in the TCA cycle generates 10 ATP, and that FADH$_2$ and NADH + H$^+$ generate approximately 1.5 and 2.5 ATP per oxidized molecule, respectively. Therefore each round of β-oxidation yields 14 ATP.

Even-numbered fatty acids

To calculate the number of rounds of β-oxidation an even-numbered FA must undertake, divide the number of carbons by 2, and then subtract 1. In the example of the 16-carbon palmitate: (16 ÷ 2) – 1 = 7, so palmitate undergoes seven cycles of β-oxidation. Therefore 14 × 7 = 98 ATP molecules are produced from these seven rounds. However, remember that

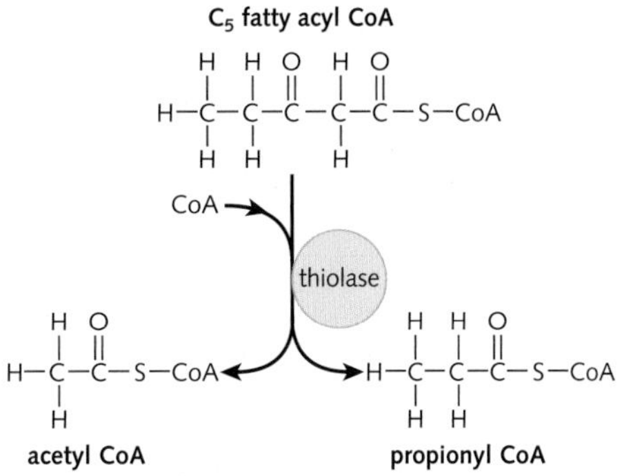

Fig. 7.18 Final round of β-oxidation of odd-numbered fatty acids. *CoA,* Coenzyme A.

the final round generates an extra acetyl-CoA, representing an additional 10 ATP; therefore 98 + 10 = 108 ATP molecules. In addition, remember that 2 ATP molecules are consumed during FA activation. Thus the net generation of ATP from the complete oxidation of palmitate is: 108 – 2 = 106 ATP.

Odd-numbered fatty acids

The final round of β-oxidation for an odd-numbered FA generates a propionyl-CoA rather than an acetyl-CoA. Propionyl-CoA is metabolized to succinyl-CoA, a TCA cycle intermediate (see Fig. 3.1). Entry to the TCA cycle and complete oxidation to oxaloacetate will yield one each of guanosine triphosphate (GTP), $FADH_2$ and $NADH + H^+$. This equates to 5 ATP; however, 1 ATP is consumed during conversion of propionyl-CoA to succinyl-CoA, so the energy yield represented by propionyl-CoA is in fact 4 ATP.

To calculate the number of rounds of β-oxidation an odd-numbered FA must undertake:

1. Subtract 1 from the number of carbons
2. Divide by 2
3. Then subtract 1

In the example of the 17-carbon margaric (heptadecanoic) acid: $17 - 1 = 16$. $(16 ÷ 2) - 1 = 7$, so margarate undergoes seven cycles of β-oxidation. Bearing this in mind, using margarate (C17) as an example, seven rounds of β-oxidation generate $14 × 7 = 98$ ATP. The final round generates propionyl-CoA, representing 4 ATP: thus $98 + 4 = 102$. Because activation consumes 2 ATP: $102 - 2 = 100$. Therefore total generation of ATP from complete oxidation of margarate is 100 ATP (Table 7.1).

Oxidation of unsaturated fatty acids

This process is slower than the oxidation of saturated FA, because the carnitine shuttle is retarded by the unsaturated

FA cargo. Catabolism is similar to that of saturated FA, however two extra enzymes are required:

- Enoyl-CoA isomerase converts the cis C=C bonds to the trans configuration, allowing the FA to be recognized by the enzymes of β-oxidation. Cis configurations are present in naturally occurring unsaturated FA, but the double bond introduced in β-oxidation is of the trans configuration.
- NADP-dependent 2,4-dienoyl reductase participates in metabolism of unsaturated FA with double bonds at both even- and odd-numbered carbon positions. For example, during the metabolism of the essential FA linoleate (18:2cΔ9,12; note the double bonds at 9 and 12), the intermediate 2,4-dienoyl-CoA is produced.

Peroxisomal β-oxidation

β-Oxidation occurs in peroxisomes as well as in mitochondria. Peroxisomes are intracellular membrane-bound structures. The relative contributions of mitochondrial and peroxisomal β-oxidation are unclear and appear to be influenced by numerous factors in health and disease. However, catabolism of all very-long-chain (24 or more carbons) FAs and branched chain FA occurs in mammalian peroxisomes. This is because these FAs are unable to use the carnitine shuttle and so cannot access the mitochondria. The actual process of β-oxidation is the same; however, be aware that:

- The enzymes differ; for example, a single peroxisomal enzyme performs hydration and oxidation.
- $FADH_2$ produced in the first oxidation cannot enter the ETC; $FADH_2$'s H^+ ions and electrons are instead transferred to molecular O_2, forming H_2O_2 and generating heat, rather than ATP.
- Acetyl-CoA produced by each round of β-oxidation must enter mitochondria to undergo oxidation in the TCA cycle.
- Once the fatty acyl-CoA is shortened to medium length (6–12 carbons), it is esterified to carnitine and then diffuses out from the peroxisome to the cytoplasm. It must enter the mitochondria (via the carnitine shuttle) for further β-oxidation.

Regulation of lipid breakdown

Control of lipid degradation operates at three levels. These are described in the following sections.

Regulation of lipolysis

Lipolysis controls oxidation of FAs by regulating FA availability. HSL is a major control point: remember, this enzyme catalyses the first step of TAG degradation, where the first FA is cleaved off the TAG. HSL is activated by phosphorylation, mediated by a cyclic adenosine monophosphate

Table 7.1 Comparison of adenosine triphosphate (ATP) yields

Six-carbon carbohydrate (glucose)	
	ATP yield
Glycolysis: 2 × ATP	$(2 × 1) = 2$
Glycolysis: 2 × $NADH+H^+$	$(2 × 2.5) = 5$
Glycolysis: 2 × pyruvate	$(2 × 2.5) = 5$
Glycolysis: 2 × acetyl-coenzyme A (acetyl-CoA)	$(2 × 10) = 20$
Total ATP	$2 + 5 + 5 + 20 = 32$ ATP
Six-carbon fatty acid (caproate)	
Cycles of β-oxidation:(6 / 2) – 1 = 2 cycles	
14 ATP per cycle	$(14 × 2) = 28$ ATP
Additional acetyl-CoA	10 ATP
ATP cost of fatty acid activation	−2 ATP
Total ATP	$28 + 10 - 2 = 36$ ATP

(cAMP)-dependent protein kinase. An increase in intracellular cAMP increases HSL phosphorylation. cAMP is synthesized from AMP by adenylate cyclase, which is activated by hormones adrenaline and glucagon. These hormones are released when mobilization of energy reserves is needed. Conversely, insulin lowers cAMP levels, by activating a cAMP-degrading phosphodiesterase. Insulin ultimately inhibits phosphorylation (activation) of HSL and is inhibitory to lipolysis (see Table 6.1).

Regulation of mitochondrial access

Oxidation of FAs is limited by the rate by which they can access their oxidation site, that is, the mitochondria, where β-oxidation of all short- and medium-chain FA occurs. Malonyl-CoA, which accumulates when FA synthesis is active, inhibits carnitine acyl transferase I and therefore FA import. This prevents simultaneous occurrence of synthesis and oxidation (a 'futile cycle').

Availability of NAD$^+$ and FAD

Both NAD$^+$ and FAD are required to function as redox partners in β-oxidation reactions. When these are scarce, due to cellular energy status being high (i.e. all the NAD$^+$ and FAD have been converted to NADH + H$^+$ and FADH$_2$), FA catabolism is inhibited due to lack of substrate availability. Conversely, when NAD$^+$ is plentiful, indicating low cellular energy status, FA catabolism is promoted.

Abnormalities of fatty acid metabolism

Deficiencies of the enzymes catalysing the first step of β-oxidation result in deficient FA oxidation. This imposes reliance upon catabolism of glucose and can cause life-threatening hypoglycaemia if exhaustion of both glycogen reserves and gluconeogenic substrates occurs. Individuals recovering from such metabolic crises can suffer permanent neurological impairment. Clinical severity varies depending on how severely β-oxidation is impaired. Severe phenotypes can cause sudden unexplained death in infants, leading to this being a valid clinical differential for sudden infant death syndrome (cot death).

Medium-chain acyl-CoA dehydrogenase deficiency

Medium-chain acyl-CoA dehydrogenase deficiency is the most common disorder of β-oxidation and (with an incidence of 1/4000–1/17,000) is one of the most common inborn errors of metabolism. Newborn screening (see Chapter 14) aims to identify individuals prior to clinical symptom development for appropriate management: avoidance of fasting and avoid metabolic decompensation when unwell by supplementation of simple carbohydrates.

CHOLESTEROL METABOLISM

Cholesterol is a 27-carbon molecule. It is an integral structural component of all cell membranes, conferring permeability and regulating fluidity, as well as being a precursor of a wide range of hormones and other signalling molecules. There is a continuous demand for this molecule, which is synthesized endogenously, but is also obtained in the diet from animal-derived fats.

Cholesterol is transported in the vascular system as a component of lipoprotein particles. Long-term excessively high serum cholesterol has potentially serious pathological consequences for cardiovascular health. Excessive consumption of high-cholesterol foods contributes to development of high cholesterol, but, interestingly, ingested saturated fats contribute more to blood cholesterol levels than actual cholesterol intake.

High-cholesterol foods

Full fat dairy products, animal fats, palm and coconut oil are all rich in saturated fat. They are therefore described as high-cholesterol foods, although the actual cholesterol level is variable.

Molecular features

Cholesterol is classed as a steroid because it contains a 17-carbon sterane core, a feature of all steroid molecules. Cholesterol contains 27 carbon atoms in total, all of which are derived from acetyl-CoA. It contains four fused ring structures, three cyclohexane and one cyclopentane (Fig. 7.19). Different steroids vary by virtue of different functional groups attached to these rings, and also via the oxidation state of the rings themselves.

Physiological roles of cholesterol

Cholesterol is a precursor of various important physiological molecules, including:

- Bile acids, which mediate fat solubilization in the gastrointestinal (GI) tract
- All steroid hormones (e.g. glucocorticoids, mineralocorticoids and sex hormones)
- Vitamin D (see Chapter 12)

Cholesterol synthesis

This occurs in the cytoplasm in most cells, mainly in the liver and intestine (Fig. 7.20). The process comprises three stages:

- Stage 1: formation of the basic isoprene unit
- Stage 2: progressive addition of isoprene units to form squalene
- Stage 3: conversion of squalene to lanosterol, and then lanosterol to cholesterol

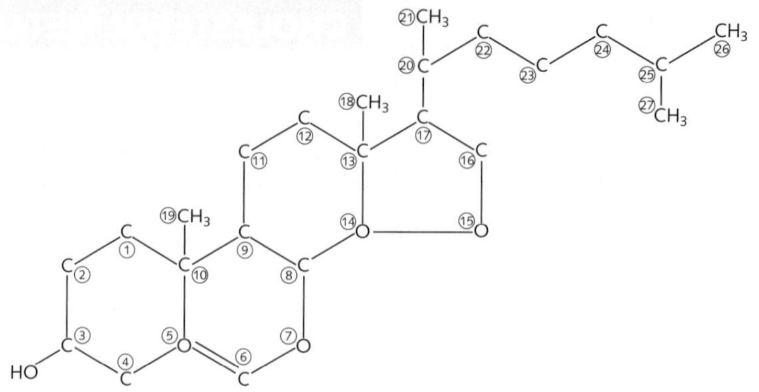

Fig. 7.19 Structure of cholesterol. Note that the hydrogen atoms are not detailed; appreciate that if a C atom is bonded to three other C atoms, one hydrogen atom fulfils the valence requirement. If bonded to two C atoms, two hydrogen atoms likewise fulfil the valence requirement, and so on.

Stage 1: formation of isopentyl pyrophosphate

The 3-hydroxy-3-methylglutaryl-CoA (HMG-CoA) is first synthesized. This involves:

- Condensation of a pair of acetyl-CoA molecules, generating the four-carbon acetoacetyl-CoA.
- HMG-CoA synthase catalyses incorporation of a third acetyl-CoA, generating HMG-CoA. This molecule is also an intermediate in ketogenesis, but the enzymes underpinning ketogenesis are mitochondrial, so cytoplasmic HMG-CoA cannot be diverted to ketogenesis.

HMG-CoA is then converted to isopentenyl pyrophosphate (IPP) in a two-step process:

- HMG-CoA is reduced to mevalonate by HMG-CoA reductase. $NADPH + H^+$ is the redox partner. This is the irreversible, rate-limiting step of cholesterol synthesis.
- Mevalonate is then phosphorylated and decarboxylated, forming IPP (the basic 5-carbon isoprene unit).

Stage 2: Progressive assimilation of isoprene units to form squalene

- IPP units are first isomerized to dimethylallyl pyrophosphate (DMAP).
- DMAP combines with another IPP, forming geranyl pyrophosphate (GPP), a 10-carbon molecule.
- GPP combines with another IPP unit, forming farnesyl pyrophosphate, a 15-carbon unit.
- Two FFPs now unite in a condensation reaction catalysed by squalene synthase. This generates squalene, a 30-carbon molecule. This reaction requires $NADPH + H^+$ as a redox partner.

Stage 3: Further conversions: squalene → cholesterol

- Squalene epoxidase recruits molecular oxygen and $NADPH + H^+$, oxidizing squalene to squalene epoxide.
- Lanosterol synthase converts squalene epoxide → lanosterol.
- Finally, lanosterol is converted to cholesterol. This conversion involves a complex series of reactions, many of which have yet to be characterized. In essence, three methyl (–CH$_3$) functional groups are removed, the double bond between C8 and C9 of lanosterol moves to between C5 and C6 (in cholesterol) and the double bond between C24 and C25 (of lanosterol) is opened (Fig. 7.20).

Regulation of cholesterol synthesis

Product-mediated inhibition

Cholesterol (the pathway product) allosterically inhibits the synthesis pathway's rate-limiting enzyme HMG-CoA reductase. Furthermore, HMG-CoA reductase synthesis is inversely proportional to intracellular cholesterol. Abundant intracellular cholesterol inhibits cholesterol synthesis by decreasing availability of the pathway's rate-limiting enzyme.

Hormonal regulation

The insulin:glucagon ratio also regulates cholesterol synthesis rate; the greater this ratio the greater pathway activity. To understand the mechanism, it is important to recognize that HMG-CoA reductase is activated by dephosphorylation and inactivated by phosphorylation. Insulin and glucagon influence phosphorylation in several ways. Insulin:

- Upregulates HMG-CoA reductase expression.
- Downregulates HMG-CoA reductase kinase.
- Upregulates phosphodiesterase, which lowers intracellular cAMP. This prevents cAMP-dependent

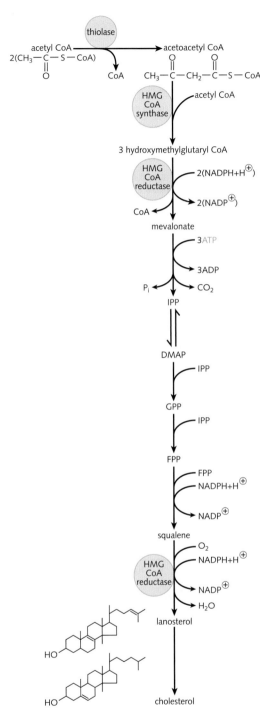

Fig. 7.20 Cholesterol synthesis. *ADP*, Adenosine diphosphate; *ATP*, adenosine triphosphate; *CoA*, coenzyme A; *DMAP*, dimethylallyl pyrophosphate; *FPP*, farnesyl pyrophosphate; *GPP*, geranyl pyrophosphate; *HMG-CoA*, 3-hydroxy-3-methylglutaryl-CoA; *IPP*, isopentyl pyrophosphate; *NADP+*, nicotinamide adenine dinucleotide phosphate; *NADPH*, nicotinamide adenine dinucleotide phosphate (reduced form of NADP +); *Pi*, inorganic phosphate.

protein kinase activation, which would phosphorylate (inactivate) HMG-CoA reductase, preventing it from promoting cholesterol synthesis.

Glucagon and adrenaline:

- Downregulate HMG-CoA reductase expression.
- Activate adenylate cyclase, increasing intracellular cAMP. This activates cAMP-dependent protein kinase, which then *in*activates HMG-CoA reductase.
- Endogenous cholesterol synthesis is thus reduced in situations where these hormones are elevated, such as fasting.

Statins

Statins are commonplace, important drugs. They reduce the risk for cardiovascular events such as myocardial infarction. Their mechanism of action is via inhibition of HMG-CoA reductase (the rate-limiting enzyme of cholesterol synthesis). This results in downregulated endogenous cholesterol synthesis, leading to reduced intracellular cholesterol. In response, cellular low-density lipoprotein (LDL)-receptor expression upregulates. This results in increased extraction of cholesterol from the bloodstream, lowering serum cholesterol. This in turn reduces the impact of raised cholesterol on atherogenesis (formation of atherosclerotic plaques) and thus cardiovascular health.

For statin treatment indication, please see below: Lipid lowering drugs, and Table 7.6.

LIPID TRANSPORT

Although lipids are technically amphipathic (both hydrophobic and hydrophilic), they are predominantly hydrophobic. This is because whilst the carboxyl group is hydrophilic, the hydrophobic tail represents the bulk of the molecule. The consequence of this is that lipids are insoluble in water. Therefore they require specialized transport vehicles to travel in the circulation, because blood is largely water, a polar solvent.

Lipoproteins

Lipid transport vehicles are known as 'lipoproteins'. A typical lipoprotein (Fig. 7.21) consists of:

- A hydrophilic surface shell, composed of a phospholipid monolayer (hydrophilic head groups orientated outwards).
- Cholesterol, present in both the surface shell (as free cholesterol) and the lipoprotein interior (as cholesterol esters).
- Apoproteins (Table 7.2): proteins that function as structural components, enzyme cofactors, and receptor binding sites for the lipoproteins.
- Hydrophobic interior, consisting of the lipid cargo. This includes TAG and esterified cholesterol.

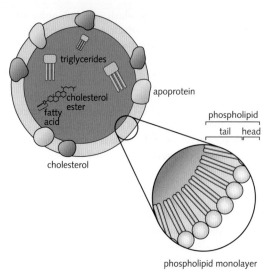

Fig. 7.21 Basic lipoprotein structure. Note phospholipid orientation; hydrophilic head groups orientated to the exterior of the structure and hydrophobic tail groups to the interior.

Table 7.2 Physiological roles of apoproteins

Apoprotein	Characteristics
A1	HDL shell protein Activates LCAT Interacts with ABCA1, receptor binding
AII	HDL shell protein, receptor binding
B48	CM structural component
B100	Major shell protein in VLDL, IDL, LDL particles. Binds to LDL receptors.
CI	CM apoprotein Activates LCAT and LPL
CII	Present in mature VLDL CM acquires CII from VLDL LPL cofactor
CIII	HDL particle apoprotein Inhibits LPL
D	HDL particle apoprotein Associated with LCAT
E	Features in mature VLDL, IDL, HDL and CM particles. LDL receptor binding

ABCA1, ATP-binding cassette transporter 1; CM, chylomicron; HDL, high-density lipoprotein; IDL, intermediate-density lipoprotein; LCAT, lecithin:cholesterol acetyltransferase; LDL, low-density lipoprotein; LPL, lipoprotein lipase; VLDL, very-low-density lipoprotein.

Lipoprotein classes

The different classes of lipoprotein are characterized by density, size, origin of lipid cargo, specific apoprotein array and their physiological role. The main properties are illustrated in Table 7.3.

Lipid processing

There are two main routes by which lipids are processed and access peripheral tissues, and these are differentiated by

the origin of the lipid; exogenous (from the diet) or endogenous (synthesized physiologically).

Lipid digestion

Hydrophobic lipids are poorly soluble in the aqueous environment of the GI lumen. The digestive enzymes that

Table 7.3 Lipoprotein particles

Lipoprotein	Density	Cargo origin	Apoproteins	Role
Chylomicrons	Lowest density	Dietary fatty acids, glycerol and fat-soluble vitamins	AI, AII, B48, CI CIII, ,E (mature chylomicrons additionally possess CII and E)	Transport of ingested absorbed dietary lipids from the GI tract to the liver and peripheral tissues
Very-low-density lipoproteins	Very low	Assembled in hepatocytes	B100, C1, CII, CIII, E	Transport cholesterol and lipids from the liver to the tissues
Intermediate-density lipoproteins	Intermediate (between VLDL and LDL) Also known as 'remnant particles'	VLDL particles	B100, C1, CII, CIII, E	IDLs evolve from VLDL as they progressively offload triglyceride cargo to the peripheral tissues
Low-density lipoproteins	Low	IDL particles	B100	LDLs evolve from IDL as they progressively offload triglyceride cargo to the peripheral tissues and liver
High-density lipoproteins	High	Assembled in Hepatocytes	AI, AII, C1, CII, CIII, D, E	Transport cholesterol and other lipids from tissues to the liver for biliary excretion

GI, gastrointestinal; IDL, intermediate-density lipoprotein; LDL, low-density lipoprotein; VLDL, very-low-density lipoprotein.

degrade lipid molecules are water soluble and thus can only operate at the surface of fat globules. Emulsification mediated by amphipathic bile salts reduces the volume of fat globules and increases their surface area:volume ratio. This optimizes the capacity of available water-soluble lipases to degrade lipids. The smaller, bile salt and phospholipid-coated globules are termed 'mixed micelles.' Micelles associate with the surfaces of enterocytes lining the GI lumen, where pancreatic lipase hydrolyses triglycerides, generating FAs and glycerol. These diffuse into enterocytes by simple diffusion.

EXOGENOUS LIPIDS

This describes the physiological digestion, absorption and transport of ingested lipids to tissue destination. Note that fat-soluble vitamins (see Chapter 12) are also absorbed via incorporation into chylomicrons (CMs).

1 Chylomicron formation

Lipases at the apical surface of enterocytes (in the GI tract) hydrolyse dietary TAG, generating free FAs and 2-monoacylglycerol. These are absorbed across the apical (luminal) surface of enterocytes. Once within the enterocyte cells, the products of lipid hydrolysis are assembled, along with apoprotein B48 and cholesterol (esterified and nonesterified), into CMs (Table 7.3). These are 'nascent' CMs at this stage.

2 Chylomicron circulation

CM particles are extruded from enterocytes into lacteals. Lacteals are blind-ending projections of the lymphatic system that protrude into intestinal villi. CM particles travel in the lymphatic system to the circulation via the thoracic duct. Once in the bloodstream, they acquire apoproteins CII and E from passing high-density lipoprotein (HDL) particles they encounter, and integrate them into the structure of their own surface shells. Following this acquisition, they are now termed 'mature' CMs.

3 Peripheral hydrolysis of chylomicron triacylglycerol cargo

Once CMs have acquired surface CII apoproteins, their role can now switch from transport mode to delivery mode. This is because the newly acquired surface CII apoproteins allow CM particles to react with the enzyme lipoprotein lipase (LPL), because CII functions as a cofactor for this enzyme. LPL is sited at the surface of endothelial cells throughout the entire vascular system. On contact with CM CII, LPL is activated and can perform its hydrolytic function on the

TAGs in the CM interior. These are hydrolysed to their FA and glycerol components.

The FA and glycerol then diffuse across the vascular lumenal surface into endothelial cells. From here they are able to access the body tissues, such as adipocytes, cardiac tissue or muscle cells. They may be reassembled into TAGs for storage or catabolized to produce energy.

4 Loss of CII apoproteins: remnant generation

Now that the TAG cargo has been delivered, the CM is greatly reduced in size. The CM now returns the 'borrowed' CII apoproteins to any passing HDL particles it encounters in the circulation. It does not, however, return the 'borrowed' E apoproteins. These smaller structures, with E but not CII apoproteins, are known as 'CM remnants'. Note that at no point have the CMs lost their B48 apoprotein; it has been present throughout and is retained in the remnants. When the remnants next traverse the hepatic circulation, they are endocytosed and degraded by hepatocytes (i.e. removed from the circulation; Fig. 7.21).

ENDOGENOUSLY SYNTHESIZED LIPIDS

This section describes the transport of TAGs synthesized in the liver to peripheral tissues (Fig. 7.22).

1 Very-low-density lipoprotein assembly

Very-low-density lipoproteins (VLDL) are assembled in hepatocytes from TAG, cholesterol and apoprotein B100. They are then released into the circulation. Like CM, VLDL particles 'steal' apoproteins CII and E from HDL particles they encounter in the bloodstream. Once these are acquired, VLDL are termed 'mature'; prior to acquisition of CII and E, they are termed 'nascent'. See stage 1 in Fig. 7.23.

2 LPL hydrolysis of VLDL cargo

Just as with CM, CII functions as a cofactor for endothelial LPL, allowing hydrolysis of VLDL TAG cargo and release of FA and glycerol. The only difference is that the TAG cargo of the VLDL is endogenously synthesized, rather than acquired from the diet (as in CM). See stage 2 in Fig. 7.23.

3 IDL and LDL formation

Progressive offloading of cargo leaves the VLDL reduced in size. Intermediate-density lipoproteins (IDL) now 'return'

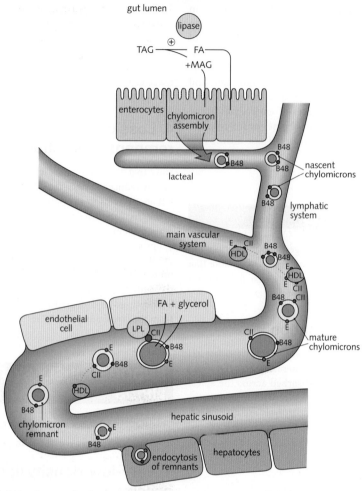

Fig. 7.22 Life cycle of chylomicrons: distribution of exogenous lipids. Endothelial lipoprotein lipase (LPL) hydrolyses CM TAG cargo to FA and glycerol, which enters the endothelial cells. *CM,* chylomicron; *FA,* fatty acid; *HDL,* high-density lipoprotein; *LPL,* lipoprotein lipase; *MAG,* monoacylglycerol; *TAG,* triacylglycerol.

CII (but not apoprotein E) to HDLs they encounter in the circulation, just like TAG-depleted CM. During this encounter, HDL also donate cholesterol esters (mediated by plasma cholesterol ester transfer protein), and in exchange receive phospholipids and TAG from the VLDL. The resulting lipoprotein is now known as VLDL 'remnants'.

Some remnants are endocytosed and dismantled by the liver, but those remaining in the circulation are further depleted of their TAG cargo, progressively reducing in size (and increasing in density). Further encounters with HDL particles result in further TAG depletion, further loss of CII and an increase in the cholesterol ester load. This results in remnants (IDL) progressively transforming into LDL. See stage 3 in Fig. 7.23.

HINTS AND TIPS

INTERMEDIATE-DENSITY LIPOPROTEIN

'Intermediate density' in this context refers to density intermediate between the 'very-low density' and 'low density', rather than intermediate between 'high density' and 'low density' They are also known as 'remnant particles'.

---

4 Cholesterol offloading at periphery

LDL apoprotein B100 binds to endothelial LDL receptors, mediating internalization of the entire particle (by endocytosis). Internalized LDL particles fuse with lysosomes and lysosomal enzymes dismantle the LDL, releasing cholesterol intracellularly. This may enter various synthetic pathways or may be esterified with FA to form cholesterol esters.

Note also that reduced intracellular cholesterol enhances transcription of the LDL receptor, increasing the amount of cholesterol the cell can assimilate via LDL capture. This upregulation of LDL-receptor expression is the main physiological mechanism for lowering plasma cholesterol, and is also the mechanism by which statins exert their therapeutic effects.

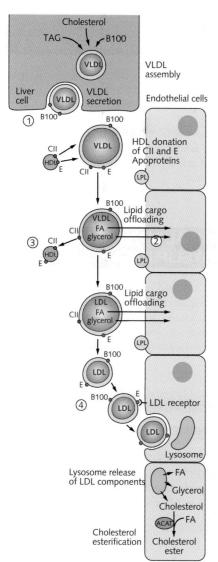

Fig. 7.23 Transport of endogenously synthesized lipids: VLDL, IDL and LDL particles. Square boxed numbers refer to the text. VLDL CII acts as a cofactor for endothelial LPL, allowing hydrolysis of the TAG cargo and offloading the products FA and glycerol. *ACAT,* Acyl-coenzyme A: cholesterol acyltransferase; *FA,* fatty acid; *HDL,* high-density lipoprotein; *IDL,* intermediate-density lipoprotein; *LDL,* low-density lipoprotein; *TAG,* triacylglycerol; *VLDL,* very-low-density lipoprotein.

This esterification is mediated by acyl-CoA:cholesterol acyl transferase (ACAT). See stage 4 in Fig. 7.23.

Upregulation of LDL receptors

Remember that intracellular cholesterol, like statins, inhibits HMG-CoA reductase, inhibiting endogenous synthesis and reducing intracellular cholesterol when it is abundant.

HDL metabolism

HDL particles are the smallest, densest lipid transport vehicle. They are assembled in the liver and intestine from apoproteins AI, AII, E and phospholipids. HDL donate apoproteins to passing CMs and VLDL particles they encounter in the circulation. HDLs also play a key role in lipid and cholesterol metabolism homeostasis: these particles are the only transport vehicles that transport cholesterol *from* the tissue *to* the liver, where it may be excreted in bile. HDL thus 'lowers' a person's total amount of cholesterol, and it is sometimes referred to as 'good cholesterol,' because it is going rather than coming, so to speak.

Cholesterol: modification for transport

Cholesterol in HDL, must be esterified. The polar hydroxyl group at C3 (see Fig. 7.19) is hydrophilic, and cholesterol tends to locate itself superficially in lipid phases, such as the phospholipid monolayer. However, molecular 'shielding' of this hydroxyl group allows cholesterol to be packaged in the hydrophobic interior of lipoproteins, allowing for increased transport capacity.

'Shielding' involves covering the –OH group with an FA acyl group. This is an esterification reaction and the reaction product is a cholesterol ester. This may occur intracellularly, in which case it is catalysed by ACAT. It may also be performed by HDL, when it is catalysed by plasma lecithin:cholesterol acyl transferase (LCAT). In the case of HDL, the FA used to modify cholesterol is sourced from the phospholipid phosphatidylcholine, which is present within the HDL shell.

Excess cellular cholesterol elimination

Specific HDL-mediated transport only commences when the HDL apoprotein AI interacts with the ATP-binding cassette transporter 1 (ABCA1), also known as the 'cholesterol efflux regulatory protein'. ABCA1 is a cellular cholesterol efflux pump, ejecting excess cholesterol from cells into circulating blood. This free cholesterol is then esterified by serum LCAT, and internalized to the HDL interior.

Cellular cholesterol clearance

HDL interacts with (and removes cholesterol from) peripheral cells such as macrophages, which may contribute to the well-established association between higher HDL levels and reduced atheromatous disease.

CLINICAL NOTES

ATHEROSCLEROTIC PLAQUES

These represent arterial wall deposits, which may be fibrous or lipid rich. These lipid-rich plaques consist of cells, connective tissue elements, lipids and debris. They are medically significant because they narrow arterial lumen and, if they rupture, promote thrombus formation and rapid occlusion. In the coronary arteries, a complete occlusion results in ischaemia and necrosis of downstream heart muscle – a myocardial infarction.

GENETIC DYSLIPIDAEMIAS

The term 'dyslipidaemia' refers to abnormalities of the serum lipid profile. Dyslipidaemias of genetic origin usually result from an abnormality of lipid metabolism or uptake. This can be secondary to abnormal/absent enzymes (e.g. LPL), apoproteins (e.g. CII, E) or receptors (e.g. the LDL receptor).

Genetic dyslipidaemias share the clinical features of physical signs and premature atherosclerotic disease with acquired dyslipidaemia, but signs are usually more pronounced and disease manifestations tend to occur even earlier.

Often a family history is known to the patient, but because mutations can occur spontaneously with no previous antecedents affected, or a premature death in a close relative may have been misattributed to another cause, this factor is of variable diagnostic utility. Features of the most common genetic dyslipidaemias are summarized in Table 7.4.

ACQUIRED HYPERCHOLESTEROLAEMIA

Hypercholesterolaemia occurs when total serum cholesterol is more than 5.0 mmol/L. It is described as 'acquired' in the absence of an inherited disorder of lipid metabolism. It is typically accompanied by raised serum LDL greater than 3.0 mmol/L. It is partially attributable to a high intake of saturated fat and low intake of unsaturated fat and is partially correctable by diet and lifestyle modification.

CLINICAL MANAGEMENT OF DYSLIPIDAEMIAS

Whether acquired or genetic, elevations in serum lipids have potentially serious consequences. They are also extremely common, so it is important to be aware of their management. In general, specific disease manifestations occur according to the location of atherosclerosis.

CLINICAL NOTES

LIPID NOMENCLATURE

The term 'triglycerides' is used synonymously with 'triacylglycerol'; however, as 'triglycerides' is used in clinical biochemistry and medicine, this term will be used in this section.

Table 7.4 Lipid derangements in genetic dyslipidaemias

Genetic condition	Mechanism	UK incidence	Lipid profile derangements
Familial hypertriglyceridaemia, also known as 'familial chylomicronaemia' or 'familial lipoprotein lipase deficiency'	LPL deficiency	1 in 1,000,000	Cholesterol normal HDL ↓ or ↔ TG ↑↑ Chylomicrons ↑↑
Familial hypercholesterolaemia	LDL receptor absence/deficiency (95%) Apolipoprotein B100 defect (5%)	1–2 in 500	TG normal Cholesterol ↑ LDL ↑
Familial combined hyperlipidaemia	Impaired fatty acid oxidation, excessive hepatic TG synthesis Impaired fatty acid esterification in adipose tissue Decreased LPL activity	1 in 100 Associated with obesity and insulin resistance	TG ↑ VLDL ↑↑ Cholesterol ↑ HDL ↓

HDL, High-density lipoprotein; LDL, low-density lipoprotein; LPL, lipoprotein lipase; TG, triglyceride; VLDL, very-low-density lipoprotein.

CLINICAL NOTES

MYOCARDIAL INFARCTION

This is the end result of atherosclerosis in coronary arteries. Distal perfusion of the territory of muscle supplied by the artery is impaired by progressive obstruction of the arterial lumen. Myocardial death occurs due to ischaemia. Loss of myocytes impairs subsequent cardiac contractility and function. If extensive, myocardial infarction may be fatal or may result in chronic cardiac failure.

CLINICAL NOTES

ISCHAEMIC STROKE

Cerebral artery atherosclerosis narrows lumens, impairing distal perfusion of brain tissue supplied by the vessel. Embolic thrombi or atherosclerotic plaque rupture usually precipitates complete obstruction and leads to ischaemic death of brain tissue. This manifests with neurological symptoms and signs specific to the area of infarcted brain.

CLINICAL NOTES

PERIPHERAL VASCULAR DISEASE

Atherosclerosis in peripheral arteries compromises distal perfusion, resulting in muscular pain due to ischaemia. This initially occurs on exertion when the muscle oxygen demand is elevated (intermittent claudication), but may progress to cause pain even at rest if arterial perfusion is excessively compromised by critical ischaemia. Rest pain in a poorly perfused limb either requires vascular surgical intervention or amputation.

Clinical signs: the 'dyslipidaemia' phenotype

Excessive lipid deposition in multiple locations, including the skin, connective tissue, corneal limbus and arterial walls, results in development of palmar and tendon xanthomata, periorbital xanthelasma, corneal arcus and atheromata, respectively. These features comprise the clinical phenotype of dyslipidaemia. Recurrent pancreatitis is a dangerous and potentially fatal complication of dyslipidaemias associated

Table 7.5 Desirable fasting lipid parameters (serum 'lipid profile')

Parameter	Normal range
Total cholesterol	<5.1 mmol/L
High-density lipoprotein (HDL)	>1.2 mmol/L (females) >1.0 mmol/L (males)
Total cholesterol:HDL ratio	<5
Low-density lipoprotein	<3 mmol/L
Triglycerides	<1.7 mmol/L

with very high triglyceride concentrations. Identifying these very obvious signs should prompt a request for serum lipid profile.

Serum lipid profile

This is performed on a blood sample drawn from a fasted patient. Normal parameters are given in Table 7.5. Note that the measurement of cholesterol only does not require a fasting sample.

Genetic testing

Particular mutations responsible for the various genetic dyslipidaemias may be identified by specialist, targeted genetic investigations. Positive identification also enables testing and identification of mutations and disease risk in blood relatives. Referral to a geneticist would be indicated in the following contexts:

- A known familial history of genetic dyslipidaemia
- Grossly abnormal lipid profile
- End-organ atherosclerotic damage in a young patient

Clinical management of dyslipidaemia

Disordered lipid profiles, particularly hypercholesterolaemia, can have catastrophic long-term effects on cardiovascular health. This effect is due to atherosclerosis, which is a direct pathological consequence of significant chronic hypercholesterolaemia. Management of dyslipidaemia is threefold and encompasses dietary modification, lifestyle changes and drug treatment.

Dietary modification

Reduction of saturated fat intake and increase in unsaturated fat intake are the mainstays of dietary management of dyslipidaemia. Oily fish contain omega-3 FA, which are thought to reduce endogenous VLDL synthesis in the liver and are sometimes advocated.

Lifestyle advice

Increasing aerobic exercise is the most effective lifestyle modification for decreasing the risk for atherosclerotic

Table 7.6 Lipid-lowering drugs

Drug	Mechanism of action
Statins (e.g. simvastatin)	HMG-CoA-reductase (see the 'Statins' section). Decrease endogenous cholesterol synthesis. Lower both serum cholesterol and LDL. Rather than using particular numerical parameters, statins are usually commenced according to an individual's personal cardiovascular risk.
Fibrates (e.g. fenofibrate)	Potentiation of hepatocyte PPAR-α signalling, enhancing hepatic β-oxidation of fatty acids and HDL synthesis. Useful for lowering both triglycerides and cholesterol. Cholesterol lowering is less effective than by using statins.
Bile acid sequestrants (resins; e.g. colesevelam)	Sequester GI luminal bile acids, impairing bile acid-mediated absorption of dietary lipids and cholesterol. Rarely used now.
Cholesterol absorption inhibitors (e.g. ezetimibe)	Inhibits dietary cholesterol absorption, upregulating LDL-receptor expression, which enhances LDL internalization, lowering serum LDL and cholesterol. Again, cholesterol lowereing is less effective than by statins.
PCSK9 inhibitors (proprotein convertase subtilisin/kexin type 9 inhibitors)	Fortnightly injection of PCSK9 inhibitor. PCSK9 is a hepatocyte protein that downregulates hepatic LDL-R expression. When inhibited, more LDL can be removed from the blood by the liver, substantially lowering serum LDL.

GI, Gastrointestinal; HDL, high-density lipoprotein; HMG-CoA, 3-hydroxy-3-methylglutaryl-coenzyme A; LDL, low-density lipoprotein; PPAR-α, peroxisome proliferator-activated receptor alpha. PCSK9, proprotein convertase subtilisin/kexin type 9

cardiovascular disease irrespective of plasma lipid levels. The lifestyle advice also includes weight reduction, reduction of alcohol intake and smoking cessation.

Lipid-lowering drugs

Because hypercholesterolaemia has such serious implications for cardiovascular health, a number of therapeutic drugs have been developed to manage this risk. These are summarized in Table 7.6.

KETONES AND KETOGENESIS

In biochemistry, the term 'ketones' (also called 'ketone bodies') refers to three particular molecules. They are all derived from acetyl-CoA, and function as substrates for ATP generation. The three biologically significant ketones are:

- Acetoacetate
- 3-Hydroxybutyrate
- Acetone

Ketone synthesis

Ketone synthesis (ketogenesis) occurs in the mitochondrial matrix of hepatocytes and requires $NADH + H^+$ as a redox partner. Acetyl-CoA is the substrate of the synthesis pathway. Acetyl-CoA may be derived from:

- FA catabolism (β-oxidation)
- Ketogenic amino acid catabolism (leucine, isoleucine, lysine, tyrosine, phenylalanine and tryptophan)
- Oxidative decarboxylation of pyruvate mediated by pyruvate dehydrogenase; see Chapter 5)

The pathway is illustrated in Fig. 7.24.

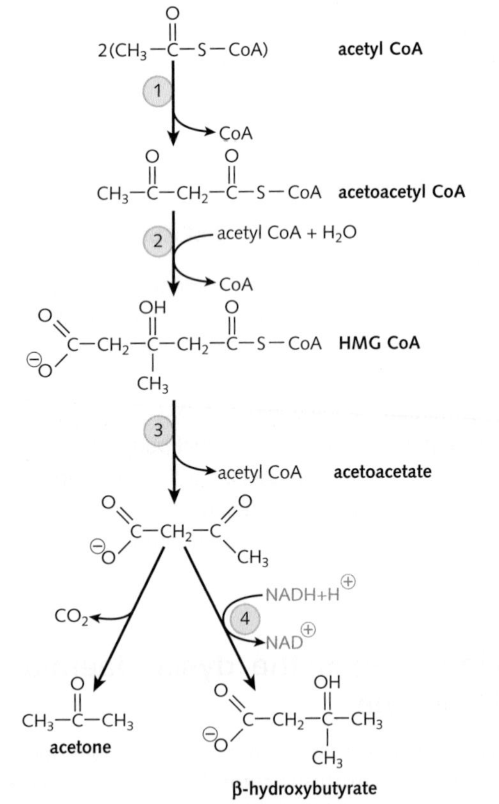

Fig. 7.24 Ketone synthesis. *1,* β-Ketothiolase; *2,* HMG-CoA synthase; *3,* HMG-CoA lyase; *4,* β-hydroxybutyrate-dehydrogenase; *CoA,* coenzyme A; *HMG-CoA,* 3-hydroxy-2-methylglutaryl-CoA; *NAD+,* nicotinamide adenine dinucleotide.

Formation of acetoacetate

Three acetyl-CoA molecules condense to form HMG-CoA, just as in the cholesterol synthesis pathway (Fig. 7.20). Although the reaction is identical, ketone synthesis occurs in the mitochondria, whilst cholesterol synthesis occurs in the cytoplasm. HMG-CoA then releases acetyl-CoA (mediated by HMG-CoA lyase), forming *acetoacetate*.

Acetoacetate conversion to acetone or 3-hydroxybutyrate

Note that catabolism of the amino acids tyrosine, phenylalanine, tryptophan, leucine and lysine generates acetoacetate (Table 9.3). Acetoacetate may spontaneously decarboxylate, forming *acetone*, or may be reduced by 3-hydroxybutyrate dehydrogenase to *3-hydroxybutyrate*. This latter reaction, representing the main fate of acetoacetate, oxidizes $NADH + H^+$ to NAD^+.

Regulation of ketone synthesis

Regulation of ketone synthesis is primarily by substrate (acetyl-CoA) availability. There are two main metabolic contexts in which ketogenesis is particularly active: high rate of lipid catabolism and high rate of gluconeogenesis.

High rate of gluconeogenesis

When gluconeogenesis is increased, oxaloacetate becomes diverted towards gluconeogenesis, instead of participating in the TCA cycle. Reduced TCA cycle activity increases acetyl-CoA availability for ketogenesis. This increases ketogenesis.

High lipid catabolism activity

In the context of lipid catabolism, serum FA is elevated. This provides abundant substrate for β-oxidation by numerous tissues. In the liver, increased β-oxidation increases mitochondrial acetyl-CoA concentration, allowing for greater diversion of acetyl-CoA to ketogenesis in addition to the TCA cycle.

Important clinical examples of metabolic states promoting ketone synthesis

Starvation

During prolonged fasting, once glycogen reserves have been exhausted, hepatic gluconeogenesis is upregulated, because plasma glucose levels must be maintained. In addition, lipid catabolism increases. Therefore, in starvation, both metabolic scenarios promoting ketone synthesis are present. This explains the observed rise in plasma ketones in starvation (see Chapter 9).

Ketoacidosis

Ketoacidosis results from serum accumulation of ketones. Chemically, acetoacetate and 3-hydroxybutyrate are carboxylic acids; at physiological pH they are anions dissociated from their H^+ ions. If ketones production is excessive and sustained, these H^+ ions cause a metabolic acidosis (plasma pH < 7.35, or H^+ > 45 nmol/L) when normal physiological buffering systems are overwhelmed. This scenario is known as 'ketoacidosis' – acidosis due to pathological ketone elevation. See Chapter 6 for discussion of diabetic ketoacidosis.

CLINICAL NOTES

KETOSIS VERSUS KETOACIDOSIS

It is important to understand the difference between these two terms. Ketosis describes an elevated level of ketones in the blood and might be a normal consequence of ketone synthesis. Ketoacidosis is a pathological state occurring when ketones accumulate to the extent they cause significant metabolic acidosis. Ketoacidosis is a feature of decompensated diabetes mellitus (nearly always type 1: see Chapter 6).

Ketone catabolism

Ketones are oxidized in mitochondria, generating acetyl-CoA. In this way, ketones may be thought of as 'alternatives' to glucose, because their oxidation generates acetyl-CoA. This can then enter the TCA cycle, generating $NADH + H^+$ and $FADH_2$ and thus fuelling oxidative phosphorylation to drive ATP synthesis to meet the cell's energy requirements.

In starvation, once glycogen reserves are exhausted, plasma glucose is maintained at the expense of muscle protein breakdown. This provides amino acids to sustain hepatic gluconeogenesis, but with the unhelpful side effect of further weakening the starving individual. Ketone availability as a 'back-up' oxidation substrate reduces the demand placed on gluconeogenesis to produce glucose for cellular oxidation. In starvation, the brain upregulates its ketone catabolism, reducing its usual reliance on glucose as a catabolic substrate.

Ketone catabolism can occur in all mitochondria-containing cells (except hepatocytes, because 3-ketoacyl-CoA transferase is absent in the liver) and results in release of two molecules of acetyl-CoA (and ultimately 20 ATP; 10 per acetyl-CoA molecule). The pathway is shown in Fig. 7.25. The $NADH + H^+$ generation seen here is counterbalanced by the consumption of $NADH + H^+$ during the ketone synthesis process, so there is no *net* generation of $NADH + H^+$.

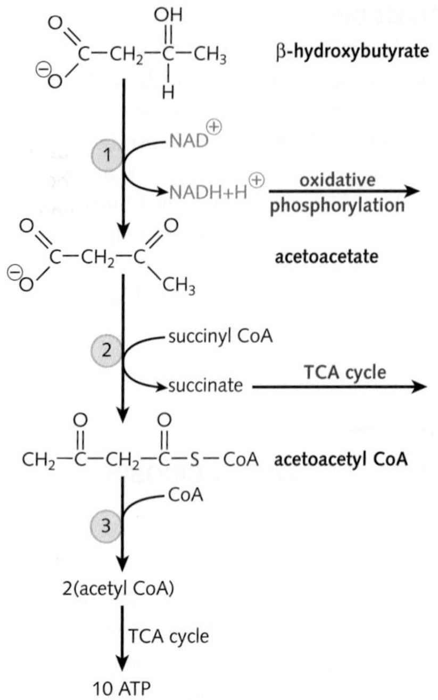

Fig. 7.25 Ketone catabolism. *1*, β-Hydroxybutyrate dehydrogenase; *2*, β-ketoacyl-CoA transferase; *3*, β-ketothiolase; *ATP*, adenosine triphosphate; *CoA*, coenzyme A; *NAD⁺*, nicotinamide adenine dinucleotide; *TCA*, tricarboxylic acid.

Ketone utilization in the central nervous system

When glucose availability decreases, the central nervous system (CNS) is forced to partially switch from glycolysis to ketone oxidation for acetyl-CoA production and thus TCA cycle activity. TCA cycle activity is necessary to supply reduced intermediates needed for ATP generation via oxidative phosphorylation. FA cannot cross the blood–brain barrier and thus are inaccessible to the CNS. Thus the CNS relies on glucose and ketones (which can traverse the blood–brain barrier) as substrates to meet its metabolic demands. CNS usage of ketones gradually increases during sustained hypoglycaemia, but it is unable to make a full transition, so there is a persistent reliance on glucose. This is one very important reason for the necessity of blood glucose level maintenance.

Ketone utilization in cardiac myocytes

Surprisingly, cardiac myocytes preferentially catabolize FA in all metabolic states except starvation. This means that these cells utilize β-oxidation of FA (rather than glycolysis) to generate acetyl-CoA for TCA cycle oxidation and energy generation. In starvation, when plasma FA gradually diminishes, cardiac myocytes are able to switch to ketone catabolism to meet their energy requirements.

● Chapter Summary

- Nomenclature of lipid molecules is based on the number of carbon atoms, double bonds and their positions within the molecule. Triglycerides consist of fatty acid 'tails' bound to glycerol 'heads'.
- The citrate shuttle exports acetyl-coenzyme A (acetyl-CoA) from the mitochondrial matrix to the cytoplasm where the necessary enzymes for fatty acid synthesis reside. β-Oxidation of fatty acids is a sequential four-stage catabolic pathway releasing acetyl-CoA. It is repeated a number of times that is determined by the number of carbons in the fatty acid.
- Diagnosis and management of the various dyslipidaemias (of which the most common by far is acquired hypercholesterolaemia) follow standardized criteria.
- Different lipoprotein particles, which function as lipid transport vehicles, have specific roles and compositions.
- Ketogenesis is physiologically upregulated in the context of low blood glucose and abnormally upregulated in type 1 diabetes mellitus. Ketone catabolism is important for maintenance of substrate provision for the CNS in the starvation state, and the myocardium in the nonstarvation state.

BODY COMPOSITION

The human body is conventionally divided into components of fat and 'lean body mass' (LBM). For simplicity we will use a tall man (2.0 m) who weighs 100 kg (a body mass index (BMI) of 25 kg/m^2) to illustrate the proportions of the various components. If of average body composition, he would be composed of 15 kg of fat (adipose tissue) and 85 kg of LBM (Fig. 8.1).

Lean body mass

LBM refers to a theoretical body compartment composed of water, protein (muscle tissue and structural/enzymatic proteins) and bone mass (i.e. everything except fat). The relative proportions are shown in Fig. 8.1. In our example for the 100-kg man, 7 kg represents bone, 17 kg represents protein, 61 kg represents water and 15 kg represents fat.

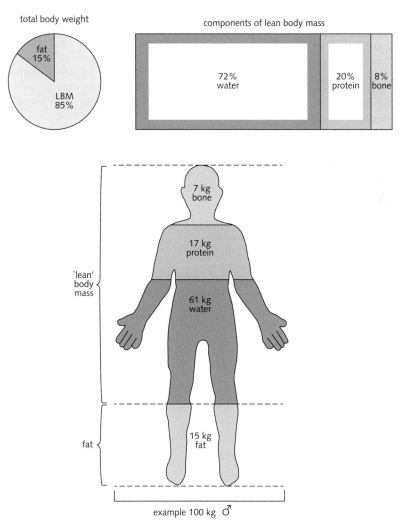

Fig. 8.1 Body composition. *LBM,* Lean body mass.

ENERGY BALANCE

Energy balance refers to the difference between energy intake and energy expenditure.

Energy intake

The total energy content of food, usually stated in kilocalories (kcal) or kilojoules (kJ), represents the chemical potential energy (CPE) intrinsic to the food. This is measured experimentally by bomb calorimetry (i.e. the heat liberated by complete combustion in air).

Different types of macromolecules have different CPE (Table 8.1) as determined by bomb calorimetry, due to their different relative proportions of C, H and N. However, the proportion of an ingested food's CPE that is physiologically liberated by cellular respiration varies according to its macromolecular nature. Proteins, for example, have a greater CPE per gram than carbohydrates, but are incompletely oxidized and consume more adenosine triphosphate (ATP) during their catabolism (due to the energetically costly but necessary generation of urea), so a smaller percentage of their CPE is assimilated than carbohydrates, which are completely oxidized and consume less ATP during their catabolism.

Within a macronutrient group (e.g. carbohydrates) the proportion of ingested nutrient that can access the circulation and is therefore available for cellular metabolism signifies the amount that is 'bioavailable'. Various factors affect the proportion of CPE that can be physiologically assimilated from particular foods.

Consider table sugar, sucrose, a glucose and fructose disaccharide. Enzymes that digest (separate) the two saccharides are abundant, and gastrointestinal (GI) uptake is essentially unlimited. Sugar has maximum bioavailability, and thus cellular metabolism is the only factor limiting the CPE that is assimilated by the body from sugar. Contrast this with leafy greens: the human GI tract lacks enzymes to break down plant cellulose (representing the bulk of carbohydrate making up leaves). Virtually none of the available

CPE of cellulose can be assimilated, so the carbohydrate polymer cannot be digested or absorbed and is therefore lost via faeces.

Energy expenditure

Once assimilated, energy substrates are oxidized by cellular catabolism. This liberates energy. Approximately 50% is unavoidably 'lost' as heat. Around 10% is diverted towards diet-induced thermogenesis (DIT). Only the remaining 40% is available for endergonic physiological processes underlying the basal metabolic rate (BMR), and physical activity (Fig. 8.2). If not directed towards physical activity, energy within this 40% that is not required to drive energy-consuming processes (the BMR) will be incorporated into energy-dense lipid storage molecules (i.e. fat) within adipocytes.

Basal metabolic rate

The BMR is the energy required for organ activity, normal cellular function and involuntary life-sustaining physiological processes. Examples of these processes include bowel motility, neuronal activity and respiratory muscle contraction. BMR is proportional to a person's LBM.

Numerous other factors in addition to the individual's LBM:fat ratio may alter an individual's BMR. It approximately correlates with overall oxygen demand. Usual diet, growth/developmental phase, hormone levels, pregnancy, body composition, body surface area, age, sex and individual genetics all influence BMR. The Harris–Benedict formula is used to calculate an adult individual's BMR based on gender, age (in years), weight (kg) and

Table 8.1 Chemical potential energy versus metabolically liberated energy for different macronutrients

Macronutrient	Actual chemical potential energy per gram (kcal) as determined by complete combustion in oxygen	Metabolically liberated energy per gram (kcal)
Fat	9.3	9.0
Carbohydrate	4.1	4.0
Protein	5.4	4.0

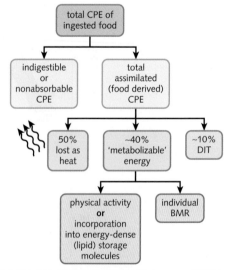

Fig. 8.2 The fate of chemical potential energy (CPE) in ingested food. *BMR*, Basal metabolic rate; *DIT*, diet-induced thermogenesis.

Table 8.2 Multipliers of BMR for various activities

Activity	Physical activity ratio (BMR multiplier)
Sitting	×1.2
Standing	×1.7
Walking on flat, dressing/undressing	×2.0
Household chores	2.5–4.5
Gentle cycling or swimming	×5.0
Walking uphill with a load, jogging, tennis, football	×6.0–8.0

BMR, Basal metabolic rate.

height (cm):
> Men: BMR (in kJ/kg/h) = 66 + (13.7 × weight in kg) +
> (5 × height in cm) – (6.8 × age in years)
> Women: BMR (in kJ/kg/h) = 65 + (9.6 × weight) +
> (1.8 × height) – (4.7 × age)

Diet-induced thermogenesis

Consumption of food increases heat production (thermogenesis). DIT (also known as 'specific dynamic action' and 'thermic effect of food') refers to obligatory energy expenditure (in addition to the BMR) during the process of digesting, absorbing, distributing, metabolizing and storing nutrients derived from ingested food. The energy is ultimately lost as heat, hence 'thermogenesis'.

The main determinants of DIT are the energy (calorie) content and macronutrient composition of ingested food. Proteins (then carbohydrates, then fats) produce the greatest DIT.

Physical activity

Exercise (muscle contraction) ultimately requires energy in the form of ATP. This energy is derived from oxidation of macronutrients. Increasing exercise intensity or duration increases energy consumption. Because we have only limited control over DIT and biological reaction exergonics, altering physical activity is by far the most modifiable component of total energy expenditure.

The intensity of a particular physical activity (physical activity ratio) is expressed in multiples of the BMR (Table 8.2), even though physical activity represents an energy requirement *over and above* the background energy consumption represented by the BMR.

Measurement of total energy expenditure

Given the multiple factors that can influence any of the three major components of energy expenditure (BMR, DIT and physical activity), it should be clear that energy expenditure is highly variable. To measure an individual's energy expenditure (and thus infer their energy requirement), a technique of indirect calorimetry is utilized.

Indirect calorimetry

The equipment used to perform indirect calorimetry is called a 'metabolic cart'. Oxygen consumption and carbon dioxide production are measured noninvasively. The rate of gas exchange is proportional to body consumption of chemical energy derived from food and storage molecules. In other words, oxygen consumption and CO_2 generation correlate with total energy expenditure. Physiological energy requirements under different experimental or disease conditions can therefore be indirectly quantified. The metabolic energy requirement is also related to the rate of catabolism.

Energy intake = energy expenditure

When the CPE of ingested food is *equal* to the energy requirements imposed by BMR, DIT and exercise combined, body weight will remain constant. Assuming the person is a healthy weight, this is the ideal scenario.

Energy intake > energy expenditure

Where the CPE of ingested food *exceeds* the energy requirements imposed on the body by BMR, DIT and exercise combined, the body weight will increase. This is due to the accumulation of storage molecules, primarily triacylglycerols in adipocytes, and thus an increase in the amount of subcutaneous and intraabdominal fat.

Bodybuilding

An alternative scenario where excess energy intake leads to increased body weight that is *not* in the form of fat deposits is that of bodybuilding. Bodybuilders deliberately ingest calories in excess of their requirement, but by regular intense and focussed exercise strategies cause muscle hypertrophy. In this situation, muscle mass rather than fat deposits account for the increase in weight. However, because excess muscle tissue is not a permanent physiological storage strategy, if not regularly exercised, the muscle will soon atrophy with degradation of component proteins. This will also occur if the net increase in energy is not sustained.

Energy intake < energy expenditure

Where the CPE of ingested food *is less than* the energy requirements presented by BMR, DIT and exercise combined, the body weight will decrease. Initially, this occurs as fat deposits are used. However, once these are exhausted, the scenario shifts from weight loss to starvation as functional proteins are utilized and their component amino acids diverted towards gluconeogenesis.

APPETITE REGULATION: HUNGER AND SATIETY

The nature of subjective sensation of hunger is a complex, evolving field of study. Hormones or central neuronal factors that stimulate appetite and hunger are termed 'orexigenic'. An increase in appetite drives the person to increase their energy intake, that is, eat. Appetite suppression has the converse effect, and is described as 'satiety', where the person feels 'full' and their appetite is low or absent.

It is the balance between appetite stimulation and suppression that ultimately determines whether the person is hungry and seeks to eat or feels full and lacks the desire to eat.

Appetite-stimulating signals

Appetite stimulation drives a person to seek food and eat it. Orexigenic signals can be divided into neurohormonal and GI.

Neurohormonal appetite stimulation

Activation of specific orexigenic hypothalamic neurons releases peptide hormones. These stimulate a population of local second-order orexigenic neurons, which then increase sensation of hunger via complex integration of central signals.

Two important orexigenic peptide hormones are neuropeptide Y (NPY) and agouti-related peptide (AGRP). They are potent appetite stimulators. Release of these neurohormones is stimulated by ghrelin (see below). By contrast, NPY and AGRP release is inhibited by appetite-suppressive hormones, for example, leptin, insulin, peptide YY and glucagon-like peptide (GLP-1, see discussion later). Appetite stimulation is much reduced postprandially. This limits excessive energy intake.

Gastrointestinal hormones

Ghrelin

Ghrelin is an orexigenic hormone that has both central and GI effects. Ghrelin is secreted from gastric P/D1 cells. Gastric stretch (as after a meal) inhibits its secretion, whilst it is released in proportion to the emptiness of the stomach. Levels (and appetite) are therefore highest after fasting, and lowest after eating.

Ghrelin modifies hypothalamic regulation of appetite by influencing the arcuate first-order neurons in two ways:

- Enhances appetite-stimulating signals (e.g. NPY and AGRP release)
- Suppresses appetite-suppression signals (e.g. cocaine/amphetamine-regulated transcript (CART) and AGRP)

These signals then stimulate the orexigenic population of second-order neurons to elicit hunger and inhibit the anorexigenic population of second-order neurons, also promoting hunger and suppressing the sensation of satiety. Ghrelin also attenuates pancreatic glucose-induced insulin secretion (indirectly, via promoting somatostatin release).

Appetite-suppressing signals

Neurohormonal appetite suppression

Appetite suppression is promoted by a population of second-order *an*orexigenic neurons that respond to *an*orexigenic peptide hormones released by first-order hypothalamic neurons. The sensation of hunger is then reduced via complex integrations of central signals. Two anorexigenic peptides are CART and melanocyte-stimulating hormone (MSH). As well as opposing their effects, CART and MSH release is inhibited by the orexigenic NPY and AGRP. Leptin, insulin and peptide YY and glucagon-like peptide (GLP-1; see discussion later), are, peripheral hormones associated with the appetite suppression.

Gastrointestinal appetite-suppressing hormones

Cholecystokinin

Cholecystokinin (CCK) is synthesized and secreted in the duodenum in response to gastric stretch and nutrients within the GI lumen. Aside from important roles in digestion, CCK promotes appetite suppression.

The underlying mechanism is CCK stimulation of vagal afferents, which communicate with brainstem nucleus tractus solitarius neurons. These neurons then promote hypothalamic anorexigenic activity (i.e. CART and MSH release) and suppress orexigenic neurohormones (i.e. NPY and AGRP release). Thus orexigenic hypothalamic activity is suppressed and anorexigenic activity is promoted. The overall outcome is that the second-order anorexigenic neuron activity predominates over the second-order orexigenic neuron activity.

Peptide YY

Neuroendocrine L-cells within the mucosa of the GI tract release peptide YY in response to gastric stretch and passage of food through the intestine. Peptide YY induces appetite suppression, as well as slowing GI motility, which increases the time available for digestion and nutrient absorption. Peptide YY is also released from a group of neurons in the medulla. Interestingly, obese individuals are known to release less peptide YY in response to the same stimulus (i.e. eating).

Glucagon-like peptide and gastric inhibitory peptide

GLP-1 and gastric inhibitory polypeptide (GIP) are incretin hormones, that is, hormones released postprandially that provoke a decrease in blood glucose. They are released by the gut and both potentiate glucose-induced insulin release and suppress glucose-induced glucagon release. These effects lead to lowering of blood glucose. They reduce appetite by inhibiting NPY and AGRP release in the hypothalamus.

Pancreatic hormones

Insulin

Insulin, synthesized by β-cells of the pancreas, suppresses appetite. This makes sense, because insulin release is elevated by food ingestion, which means that less energy intake is necessary for a while.

Adipocyte appetite-suppressing hormones

Leptin

Leptin is the most powerful known appetite-suppressing hormone. It is synthesized and released by adipocytes and belongs to the adipokine family. The greater the adipocyte mass, the greater the amount of leptin released. Rather than the dynamic peaks and troughs of the other hormones that respond acutely to fasting or postprandial status, leptin secretion is a tonic background influence that reflects the overall energy status of the person.

Normally, this means that the greater lipid stores present, the less the overall appetite. This is appropriate, because high fat mass reflects a decreased requirement for calorie intake. In chronic obesity, however, the effect of leptin is pathologically reduced, which explains why there is rarely a noticeable suppression of appetite.

CLINICAL ASPECTS OF OBESITY

Weight gain

As outlined earlier, weight gain occurs when dietary energy intake exceeds energy expended by BMR, DIT and exercise. Weight gain is usually in the form of adipose tissue (fat).

Obesity: definition

A person's body weight can be considered excessive once it begins to negatively affect general health and physiology. This is termed 'obesity'. It is usually visibly apparent on cursory inspection as obvious excess fat. Various parameters are available to identify and stratify obesity.

Body mass index

The BMI calculation integrates height and weight into a value that is easy to stratify into the following categories (Fig. 8.3):

- Underweight (BMI < 18.5 kg/m^2)
- Normal (BMI 18.6–24.9 kg/m^2)
- Overweight (BMI 25.0–29.9 kg/m^2)
- Obese (BMI ≥ 30 kg/m^2)

CLINICAL NOTES

CALCULATION OF BODY MASS INDEX (BMI)

To determine BMI, the height *in metres* and the weight *in kilograms* must be known. Weight is divided by the square of the height:
BMI = weight/(height^2)

Obesity may be further subclassified. Class 1 is BMI in the range 30.0–34.9 kg/m^2, Class 2 is BMI between 35 kg/m^2 and 39.9 kg/m^2 and class 3 is BMI of 40.0 kg/m^2 or more. The term 'morbidly obese' is used to describe any patient with class 3 obesity, or in class 2 obese patients suffering from complications directly attributable to the obesity.

Clinical significance

Obesity causes a wide array of health complications. As it also very common, and incidence and prevalence are increasing. It represents a gigantic public health burden. Worldwide, 2.7 billion adults are overweight or obese. In the UK, nearly 1 in 4 adults are obese (24.9%)! This figure has trebled in the last 30 years and is estimated to double to ~50% by 2050. Obesity is a leading cause of mortality, morbidity, disability and healthcare costs.

Causes of obesity

The specific causes underlying the development and persistence of excessive fat deposits are complex and multifactorial, although energy intake outweighing energy expenditure is the universal causative mechanism. In the vast majority of cases, food intake is excessive relative to energy expenditure. In extremely simplistic behavioural

weight lbs	100	105	110	115	120	125	130	135	140	145	150	155	160	165	170	175	180	185	190	195	200	205	210	215
kgs	45.5	47.7	50.0	52.3	54.5	56.8	59.1	61.4	63.6	65.9	68.2	70.5	72.7	75.0	77.3	79.5	81.8	84.1	86.4	88.6	90.9	93.2	95.5	97.7
height in/cm	underweight					healthy						overweight					obese					extremely obese		
5'0" – 152.4	19	20	21	22	23	24	25	26	27	28	29	30	31	32	33	34	35	36	37	38	39	40	41	42
5'1" – 154.9	18	19	20	21	22	23	24	25	26	27	28	29	30	31	32	33	34	35	36	36	37	38	39	40
5'2" – 157.4	18	19	20	21	22	22	23	24	25	26	27	28	29	30	31	32	33	33	34	35	36	37	38	39
5'3" – 160.0	17	18	19	20	21	22	23	24	24	25	26	27	28	29	30	31	32	32	33	34	35	36	37	38
5'4" – 162.5	17	18	18	19	20	21	22	23	24	24	25	26	27	28	29	30	31	31	32	33	34	35	36	37
5'5" – 165.1	16	17	18	19	20	20	21	22	23	24	25	25	26	27	28	29	30	30	31	32	33	34	35	35
5'6" – 167.6	16	17	17	18	19	20	21	21	22	23	24	25	25	26	27	28	29	29	30	31	32	33	34	34
5'7" – 170.1	15	16	17	18	18	19	20	21	22	22	23	24	25	25	26	27	28	29	29	30	31	32	33	33
5'8" – 172.7	15	16	16	17	18	19	19	20	21	22	22	23	24	25	25	26	27	28	28	29	30	31	32	32
5'9" – 175.2	14	15	16	17	17	18	19	20	20	21	22	22	23	24	25	25	26	27	28	28	29	30	31	31
5'10" – 177.8	14	15	15	16	17	18	18	19	20	20	21	22	23	23	24	25	25	26	27	28	28	29	30	30
5'11" – 180.3	14	14	15	16	16	17	18	18	19	20	21	21	22	23	23	24	25	25	26	27	28	28	29	30
6'0" – 182.8	13	14	14	15	16	17	17	18	19	19	20	21	21	22	23	23	24	25	25	26	27	27	28	29
6'1" – 185.4	13	13	14	15	15	16	17	17	18	19	19	20	21	21	22	23	23	24	25	25	26	27	27	28
6'2" – 187.9	12	13	14	14	15	16	16	17	18	18	19	19	20	21	21	22	23	23	24	25	25	26	27	27
6'3" – 190.5	12	13	13	14	15	15	16	16	17	18	18	19	20	20	21	21	22	23	23	24	25	25	26	26
6'4" – 193.0	12	12	13	14	14	15	15	16	17	17	18	18	19	20	20	21	22	22	23	23	24	25	25	26

Fig. 8.3 Body mass index chart.

terms: persistently eating too much, exercising too little, or a combination of both, ultimately leads to obesity.

Factors associated with obesity

Several social and demographic factors are associated with increased likelihood of obesity:

- Financial status
- Psychological stress
- Education level
- Ethnicity

It is extremely important not to confuse *association* with *causality*. Whilst lower earners may be seen to be at greater risk for obesity due to factors themselves associated with greater socioeconomic deprivation, it is not acceptable or accurate to attribute obesity to low financial status.

Rare causes of obesity

In a small minority of people, obesity may develop secondary to a specific disease process. In a case of rapid weight gain without clear predisposing cause (e.g. excessive calorie intake (eating!) or insufficient exercise), it may be clinically relevant to exclude these causes. These include:

- Hypothyroidism (decrease in BMR → reducing total energy expenditure)
- Cushing disease (related to excessive glucocorticoid levels)
- Insulinoma (increased fat storage secondary to anabolic action of insulin)
- Polycystic ovary syndrome (hyperandrogenism and dysregulated insulin homeostasis)
- Hypothalamic disease or injury (impaired satiety sensation or increased hunger)
- Growth hormone deficiencies

Drug-induced obesity

Certain drugs are known to cause weight gain by a variety of mechanisms.

CLINICAL NOTES

DRUGS WHICH MAY CAUSE WEIGHT GAIN

This group includes steroids, diabetes medications (insulin, sulphonylureas, thiazolidinediones), psychiatric medications (most antipsychotics, tricyclic antidepressants, lithium, some selective serotonin reuptake inhibitors), antiepileptic drugs (carbamazepine, valproate, gabapentin), hormonal contraception, β-blockers and antihistamines.

Genetic factors

Some very rare genetic syndromes cause multisystem disturbances of which obesity, almost always developing in early childhood, is a prominent feature. These include:

- Prader–Willi syndrome (a genetic disorder characterized by uncontrolled appetite amongst other diagnostic features)
- Bardet–Biedl syndrome (a genetic multisystem disorder characterized by marked obesity)

- Turner syndrome (females entirely or partially lacking a second X chromosome, i.e. genotype XO rather than XX)

Susceptibility genes

There is ongoing intense research attempting to identify specific genetic features that render individuals more susceptible to weight gain and obesity. Most of the areas under investigation understandably relate to homeostasis of hormones underpinning hunger and satiety.

CLINICAL CONSEQUENCES OF OBESITY

All doctors (surgeons, general practitioners, medics, etc.) should be well-informed of the clinical consequences of obesity because it is so commonplace. The constellation of negative physiological consequences is wide ranging and impairs numerous systems, which are discussed in brief as follows.

Medical complications

Cardiovascular complications

Cardiovascular diseases that may develop or be exacerbated as a direct consequence of obesity include:

- Systemic hypertension
- Atherosclerotic cardiovascular disease (including coronary heart disease, peripheral vascular disease and cerebrovascular disease)
- Obesity-related cardiomyopathy → left ventricular failure → congestive cardiac failure
- Pulmonary hypertension → right heart failure (cor pulmonale)

Electrocardiogram abnormalities associated with obesity are shown below.

CLINICAL NOTES

ELECTROCARDIOGRAM ABNORMALITIES ASSOCIATED WITH OBESITY

Low voltage complexes, ↑ QT interval, inferolateral T wave abnormalities, right axis deviation, right bundle-branch block, left-ventricular hypertrophy or strain criteria and P-pulmonale.

Diabetes

Obesity is one of the leading risk factors for type 2 diabetes mellitus (T2DM; see Chapter 6). With all the potential complications that can arise secondary to poorly controlled diabetes, this is perhaps the most devastating and disabling consequence of obesity.

Respiratory complications

Obesity has an enormous impact on respiratory function. The greater the obesity, the more profound the impact. Spirometric and lung volume abnormalities seen in obese patients are shown in Table 8.3; most are primarily due to reduced chest wall compliance, but reduced lung compliance also contributes. A restrictive defect may also be present. There is also a significant increase in the work of breathing. The integrated outcome of these abnormalities is that obese patients have greater ventilation:perfusion mismatch, increased tendency to hypoxia and collapse of peripheral lung segments.

Obesity-related hypoventilation is also an important cause of type 2 respiratory failure (↓ partial pressure of oxygen in arterial blood (PaO_2), ↑ partial pressure of carbon dioxide in arterial blood ($PaCO_2$)) due to alveolar hypoventilation. Obesity also causes increased collapsibility of the upper airway, which may lead to obstructive sleep apnoea.

Hepatic complications

Chronic obesity leads to development of fatty liver (nonalcoholic steatohepatitis). The physiological impact of these disorders ranges from asymptomatic to catastrophic liver failure.

Gastrointestinal complications

Increased intra-abdominal pressure due to heavy layers of centripetal adipose tissue increases the risk for hiatus hernia and gastro-oesophageal reflux disease (GORD).

Musculoskeletal/rheumatological

The significant impact of obesity on the musculoskeletal system is mainly related to increased mechanical load-bearing, but other factors such as the abnormal systemic inflammatory state also contribute. Both degenerative and inflammatory diseases of bone and soft tissue are common in the obese.

Table 8.3 Respiratory consequences of increasing BMI

Parameter	Effect of increasing BMI
Functional residual capacity	↓
Expiratory reserve volume	↓
Forced expiratory volume in 1 second	↓
Closing capacity	↑

BMI, Body mass index.

Psychiatric/psychological consequences

The psychological consequences of obesity and the negative impact on the individual's body image are strongly related to low self-esteem. Incidence of mental health problems (particularly depression) is greater in the obese. Stigmatization and discrimination are common, both in society in general but also unfortunately among healthcare professionals. An attitude exists that overweight people have brought the obesity-related health problems upon themselves; this is highly detrimental to the patient–doctor interaction.

ETHICS

MANAGING OBESE PATIENTS

Obesity is a clinical entity, and patients deserve our empathy and understanding without prejudice, regardless of any personally-held negative opinions that we may harbour. Even among the medical profession there are those feel that obesity is a self-inflicted problem and that obese patients deserve the associated medical problems. It is therefore even more important not to make the patients' experience any more arduous by communicating blame that increases and complicates our workload. While being well-informed about the medical complexity and being informed about the consequences of obesity, it is very important not to make the patients' journey any harder with an attitude of blame.

Operative risk

In addition to the outlined medical impacts of obesity on normal physiology, obesity presents a special risk in the context of obese patients requiring surgery.

Surgical risk

The following technical and physiological factors contribute to increased surgical risk:

- Organ access difficulty due to increased subcutaneous adipose tissue
- Equipment difficulties (instruments, e.g. too short for the depth of the fat layer)
- Prolonged operating times and increased technical difficulty of operation
- Requirement for specialist equipment (e.g. reinforced operating tables, hover mattresses, hoists)
- ↑ staff manpower necessary for transfer of the anaesthetized patient
- Delayed postoperative mobilization and increased postoperative monitoring requirements (e.g. level 2 care)

Anaesthetic risk

Notwithstanding the high probability of multiple obesity-related comorbidities and their impact on an obese individual's ability to tolerate general anaesthesia, the following factors also greatly increase the challenges and risks of anaesthesia:

- ↑ difficulty of vascular access
- ↑ airway difficulty
- ↑ challenges of effective ventilation
- Pharmacokinetic alterations of drug metabolism
- Enhanced technical difficulties of regional techniques due to adipose distortion of anatomy
- ↑ risk for aspiration at induction and intraoperatively (↑ incidence of hiatus hernia and GORD)
- ↑ risk for postoperative lower respiratory tract infection due to obesity-related respiratory impairment

Thromboembolic risk

Obesity is a significant risk factor for thromboembolism in hospital as well as the community. This risk is additional to the immobility of the very obese. Venous thromboembolism prophylaxis is particularly important, and therapeutic doses are either greater or more frequent in the obese compared with those of normal weight.

Obstetric risk

Obesity significantly impairs fertility, but if a pregnancy is successful, it is far more perilous in an obese woman. Obesity is a significant risk factor for multiple, serious, adverse fetomaternal outcomes.

Antenatally, the probability of developing gestational diabetes or diabetes mellitus in pregnancy (see Chapter 6) and preeclampsia or other hypertensive disorders of pregnancy is dramatically enhanced, along with all the separate risks that these conditions entail in pregnancy. Intrauterine growth retardation and fetal macrosomia are both more likely in obese women.

The chance of needing an induction of labour is greater in obese parturients, but the likelihood of success of induction is reduced, conferring a greater likelihood of an unplanned caesarean section.

For vaginal birth, the risk for obstetric perineal tears is greater, and they are more likely to be more severe. Instrumental assistance and birth trauma for the baby are also more likely, shoulder dystocia in particular being more common in obese women.

For caesarean deliveries, anaesthetic or surgical intervention is needed and the risks are far greater for the obese parturient (as outlined earlier). Epidural and spinal (regional) anaesthesia is far more challenging and likely to fail in an obese woman, meaning the much greater dangers of a general anaesthesia in an obese and pregnant patient must be risked.

OBESITY TREATMENT STRATEGIES

Management of obesity is challenging and often unsuccessful. Weight loss attenuates or reverses the physiological complications of obesity. To maximize the chance of achieving successful and permanent weight loss, an appropriately multifactorial approach is necessary for this condition of multifactorial aetiology. The strategies include lifestyle modification (specifically diet and exercise), drug treatment and surgery.

Diet

Unfortunately, obesity usually develops in individuals who enjoy eating excessive amounts of unhealthy food options. Motivating an individual to make healthy changes to their diet in the long term is extremely challenging. Basic nutritional education will at least empower the patient to make healthier choices for their diet if they choose to. Dietician input is invaluable in this regard. Reduction of calorie intake reduces the intake of CPE intrinsic to food. This can be achieved by counselling reduction of portion sizes *in addition to* calorie restriction.

Exercise

Regular exercise maintained long term has a large evidence base in testament to its efficacy in achieving weight loss and subsequently maintaining a healthy weight. Exercise is synergistic to calorie restriction. However, as with diet modification, obese individuals have often become that way due to dislike of exercise, and motivating someone to start a successful lifelong programme of exercise is perhaps even more challenging than persuading them to make healthier changes to their diet.

Pharmaceutical

Drug treatment for weight loss should be accompanied by diet change and exercise. In the UK, a BMI $\geq 28\,kg/m^2$ in presence of associated risk factors (e.g. T2DM, hypertension, dyslipidaemia) or a BMI $\geq 30\,kg/m^2$ is an indication for drug treatment *as an adjunct* to lifestyle (diet and exercise) interventions. Orlistat is the only weight loss drug currently available in the UK. Certain drugs prescribed for other conditions may cause weight loss as an additional clinical benefit (e.g. liraglutide in T2DM)

but are not prescribed solely for weight loss in the absence of the primary condition. Other centrally acting appetite suppressant drugs are available in the USA, which typically act by modification of central noradrenergic or serotoninergic axes.

Orlistat

Orlistat is a pancreatic lipase inhibitor. It impairs GI lipid degradation, resulting in fat malabsorption. This decreases the proportion of CPE that can be derived from ingested food, overall reducing energy intake and promoting an energetic expenditure > intake weight-loss scenario.

However, the side effect of fat malabsorption, steatorrhoea, is unpleasant and surprise faecal incontinence can occur if too much fat is eaten whilst taking the drug. In some patients, this reduces drug compliance, whilst in others it may actually improve dietary compliance due to the fear of side effects.

Surgical

Bariatric (weight loss) surgery is proposed if diet, exercise and pharmaceutical interventions have failed to achieve lasting weight loss in patients with BMI exceeding $40\,kg/m^2$. It is also indicated for people with BMI > $35\,kg/m^2$ in the presence of severe reversible obesity-related complications. It is a first-line approach if BMI > $50\,kg/m^2$. Essentially, as soon as the risks of obesity outweigh the perils of the surgery and anaesthesia in this patient population, operating is in the patient's best interests. However, a healthy diet and exercise should be promoted both before and after surgery for the best possible outcome.

Bariatric procedures

Gastric bands constrict the access lumen of the stomach and can be performed laparoscopically, avoiding a laparotomy (i.e. major abdominal surgery). Bariatric procedures that require a full laparotomy include reduction of the stomach's volume, removing the 'holding bay' function of the stomach or bypassing it entirely, which dramatically reduces the amount of food that be eaten in one go. These include:

- Gastric bypass (Roux-en-Y procedure), which bypasses the stomach entirely
- Sleeve gastrectomies that reduce the volume of the stomach

All of these procedures limit the amount of food a person is able to physically consume as well as dramatically reducing appetite. This restricts calorie intake, promoting a favourable expenditure > intake energetic weight-loss scenario, which reliably leads to weight loss in the majority of cases.

● Chapter Summary

- The human body composition is conventionally divided into fat and lean body mass (LBM). LBM is composed of water, protein and bone. Proportions of fat versus LBM vary according to individual habitus, whilst LBM composition is more consistent between individuals.
- Total energy expenditure is determined by the sum of energy consumed by the basal metabolic rate, diet-induced thermogenesis and physical activity.
- Different macronutrients have differing chemical potential energies. In addition, the proportion of assimilated chemical potential energy in ingested food is affected by various factors.
- Weight gain or weight loss is almost always due to an imbalance of energy expenditure against energy intake. In normal health, when intake equals expenditure, body weight usually remains constant.
- Obesity has multiple consequences for the main organ systems, as well as significantly increasing surgical, anaesthetic, thromboembolic and obstetric risks.
- There are several treatment strategies used in obesity including diet, exercise, drug and surgical management.

AMINO ACIDS

Proteins are composed of amino acids. Amino acids all share a common structural skeleton (Fig. 9.1) which includes:

- A central carbon atom (the α-carbon)
- An amino (NH₂) group attached to the α-carbon
- A carboxyl group (COOH)
- A side chain (usually designated 'R')

Individual amino acids have different R-groups or side chains. Different R-groups confer the amino acid with differing biochemical properties, summarized in Table 9.1. They may confer the following characteristics upon their parent amino acid:

- Charged or uncharged
- Hydrophobic or hydrophilic
- Acidic or basic

Amino acids link with each other via peptide bonds between the carboxyl and amino groups (Fig. 9.2). Chemically, this reaction is a condensation reaction and the peptide bond formed is covalent in nature. Amino acids are chiral; however, only the L-stereoisomer occurs in humans.

PROTEIN STRUCTURE

A string of amino acids linked end-to-end with each other via peptide bonds forms a polypeptide. The name 'protein' is reserved for polypeptides containing 50+ amino acids. A protein can consist of a single polypeptide or multiple associated polypeptides.

Primary structure

The linear order of the amino acid sequence in a polypeptide (protein) is termed the 'primary structure'. The sequence order is determined by the base sequence in DNA. By convention, the free amino group is considered the start (N terminus) of a polypeptide sequence and the free carboxyl group its end (C terminus).

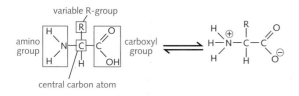

Fig. 9.1 Molecular structure of an amino acid.

Secondary structure

Amino acids also interact with each other by hydrogen bonds. These form between the oxygen atom of the C = O component of the carboxyl group of one amino acid and the amino N atom of another. These hydrogen bonds impose 'secondary structure' – ubiquitous architectural features, such as α-helices and β-pleated sheets.

Tertiary structure

The term 'tertiary structure' describes the three-dimensional structure adopted by a polypeptide (in addition to the secondary structure features). Tertiary structure is determined by the characteristics and intermolecular/interatomic interactions of component amino acid side chains.

Quaternary structure

The quaternary structure of a protein is determined by interactions between two or more different polypeptide subunits. The types of structural bonds forming quaternary structure are the same as those forming tertiary structure; the difference in this instance is that they link different polypeptides rather than different segments within the same polypeptide.

INTERMOLECULAR/INTERATOMIC FORCES THAT SHAPE PROTEINS

The correct 'folded shape' of a protein is determined by the primary, secondary, tertiary and quaternary structural characteristics. These in turn are determined by intermolecular/interatomic forces, which include various types of bonds/interactions.

Covalent bonds

Covalent bonds arise through sharing of electron pairs between atoms. They are extremely strong, and resistant to heat, pH extremes and detergents (Fig. 9.1). A peptide bond is a covalent bond.

Ionic bonds

Ionic interactions, also very strong, are bonds arising via electrostatic attraction between positively and negatively charged atoms.

Table 9.1 Amino acid reference table

One-letter code	Three-letter code	Amino acid	Essential, semiessential or nonessential	Side chain	Additional information
R	ARG	Arginine	Semi-essential	$-CH_2-CH_2-CH_2-C\begin{smallmatrix}NH_2\\+\\NH_2\end{smallmatrix}$	Precursor of nitric oxide. Role in the urea cycle. (Chapter 9, Fig. 9.16) Basic R-group
H	HIS	Histidine	Semi-essential	$-CH_2-$ imidazole N–H	Basic R-group
I	ILE	Isoleucine	Essential	$-CH\begin{smallmatrix}CH_3\\CH_2-CH_3\end{smallmatrix}$	Hydrophobic R-group; hence normally located in the interior of protein structures
L	LEU	Leucine	Essential	$-CH_2-CH\begin{smallmatrix}CH_3\\CH_3\end{smallmatrix}$	Like isoleucine, leucine has a hydrophobic R-group; hence normally located in the interior of protein structures
K	LYS	Lysine	Essential	$-CH_2-CH_2-CH_2-CH_2-NH_3^+$	Basic R-group
M	MET	Methionine	Semiessential	$-CH_2-CH_2-S-CH_3$	Cysteine precursor (see Chapter 9, Fig. 9.9)
T	THR	Threonine	Essential	$-CH\begin{smallmatrix}OH\\CH_3\end{smallmatrix}$	–OH group in the R-group is a site for posttranslational modification such as O-linked glycosylation (see Chapter 9)
W	TRP	Tryptophan	Essential	$-CH_2-$ indole	Precursor of serotonin (see Chapter 9, Fig. 9.13)
F	PHE	Phenylalanine	Semiessential	$-CH_2-$ phenyl	Precursor of catecholamine hormones noradrenaline, adrenaline and dopamine (see Chapter 9, Fig. 9.13), and also the pigment melanin. Precursor of tyrosine (see Chapter 9, Fig. 9.10)
V	VAL	Valine	Essential	$-CH\begin{smallmatrix}CH_3\\CH_3\end{smallmatrix}$	Hydrophobic R-group; hence normally located in the interior of protein structures
A	ALA	Alanine	Nonessential	$-CH_3$	In muscle, via the glucose–alanine cycle, alanine fulfils the role glutamine performs in all other tissues (i.e. transport of nitrogen to the liver for urea synthesis)
N	ASN	Asparagine	Nonessential	$-CH_2-C\begin{smallmatrix}NH_2\\O\end{smallmatrix}$	Few metabolic roles aside from acting as a component of proteins
D	ASP	Aspartate	Nonessential	$-CH_2-C\begin{smallmatrix}O^-\\O\end{smallmatrix}$	Amino group donor of the urea cycle (Chapter 9, Fig. 9.16). Role in purine and pyrimidine synthesis (see Chapter 10). Acidic R-group. Precursor of threonine.

Table 9.1 Amino acid reference table—cont'd

One-letter code	Three-letter code	Amino acid	Essential, semiessential or nonessential	Side chain	Additional information
C	CYS	Cysteine	Nonessential	—CH$_2$—SH	Sulphur-containing R-group allows important structural role in proteins (formation of disulphide bridges). Component of glutathione (see Chapter 5)
E	GLU	Glutamate	Nonessential	—CH$_2$—CH$_2$—C$\lesssim_{\:O}^{\:O^-}$	Operates as an intermediate linking nitrogen metabolism with carbon metabolism. Central neurotransmitter. Acidic R-group
Q	GLU	Glutamine	Nonessential	—CH$_2$—CH$_2$—C$\lesssim_{\:O}^{\:NH_2}$	Able to cross the blood–brain barrier. Functions to transport nitrogen from most tissues to the liver for urea synthesis (see Chapter 9)
G	GLY	Glycine	Nonessential	—H	'Imino' acid. Central neurotransmitter. Important structural component of collagen. Role in synthesis of purines (Chapter 10), haem (see Chapter 10) and creatine. creatine (see Chapter 4) creatine. Participation in drug metabolism. Component of glutathione see Chapter 5
P	PRO	Proline	Nonessential	(pyrrolidine ring structure) —COOH	Also an 'imino' acid. This is the only amino acid where the side chain incorporates the α-amino acid group of the amino acid skeleton
S	SER	Serine	Nonessential	CH$_2$—OH	Contribution of activated one-carbon units required for tetrahydrofolate coenzymes. Required for biosynthesis of cysteine (Chapter 9, Fig. 9.9) and phospholipids
Y	TYR	Tyrosine	Nonessential	—CH$_2$—(benzene ring)—OH	Precursor in synthesis of catecholamines (see Chapter 9, Fig. 9.13). Thyroglobulin tyrosine residues vital for thyroxine synthesis (see Chapter 11).

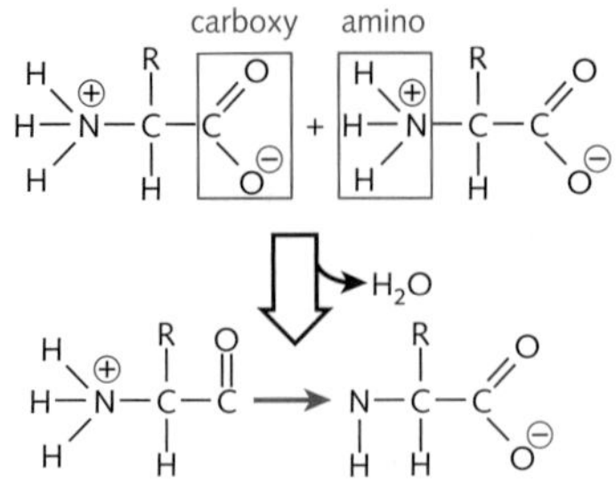

Fig. 9.2 Formation of a peptide bond between the carboxyl and amino groups of two separate amino acids.

Hydrogen bonds

Hydrogen bonds occur between a peptide bond component atom and a polar R-group. A hydrogen atom becomes 'shared' by two electronegative atoms. These bonds are intermediate strength and are important in determining secondary structural features.

Hydrophobic interactions

Amino acids with hydrophobic R-groups (i.e. valine, alanine, leucine and phenylalanine) form nonpolar interactions, rather than true bonds, where they cluster close to one another. These are of weak strength.

van der Waals forces

van der Waals forces are weak attractions between two atoms with nearby electron orbitals. These are the weakest interactions.

Side chain interactions

Four types of bond may occur between different amino acid R-groups. These are:

- Disulphide bridges (covalent)
- Salt bridges (ionic)
- Hydrogen bonds
- Hydrophobic interactions

KEY REACTIONS IN AMINO ACID METABOLISM

There are two types of reaction that one must appreciate before understanding amino acid metabolism. These are transamination and oxidative deamination. Both perform the same function: removal of the amino group ($-NH_2$) from the carbon skeleton of an amino acid.

Transamination: conversion of any amino acid into alanine, glutamate or aspartate

Transamination involves deamination of the amino acid (transfer of the amino group to α-ketoglutarate, converting α-ketoglutarate to glutamate). The remaining (deaminated) molecule is now structurally a keto acid. This is catalysed by the aminotransferases (Fig. 9.3), all of which use pyridoxal phosphate (PLP) as a cofactor.

The amino group of the newly formed glutamate can then be transferred to another ketoacid, forming alanine, aspartate or glutamate, depending on which intermediate of the tricarboxylic acid (TCA) cycle the glutamate is incorporated into:

Pyruvate→alanine
Aspartate→oxaloacetate
Glutamate→α-ketoglutarate

The transaminase catalysing this second reaction is named according to the end product; for example, alanine transaminase or aspartate transaminase (AST).

Oxidative deamination: removal of the amino group

In these reactions, the amino group of an amino acid is removed (resulting in the formation of α-ketoglutarate) and released as ammonia (NH_3). This enters the urea cycle for excretion. The redox partner for this oxidation is nicotinamide adenine dinucleotide (NAD^+; Fig. 9.4). The main substrate for oxidative deamination is glutamate, because most amino acids are degraded (as described previously) by the transamination generating glutamate.

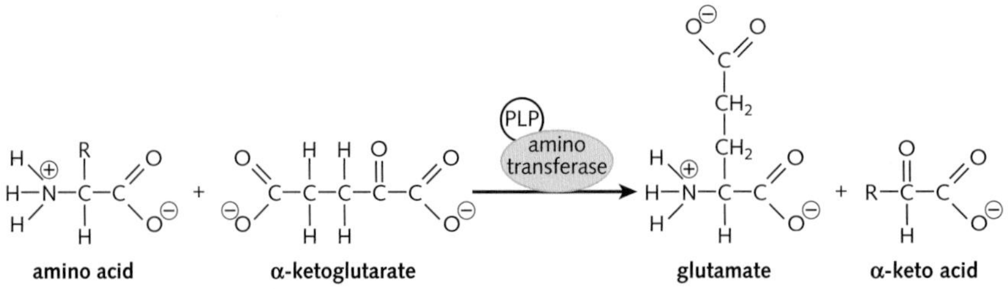

Fig. 9.3 Transamination reactions. The example illustrates the glutamate → α-ketoglutarate transamination. *PLP,* Pyridoxal phosphate.

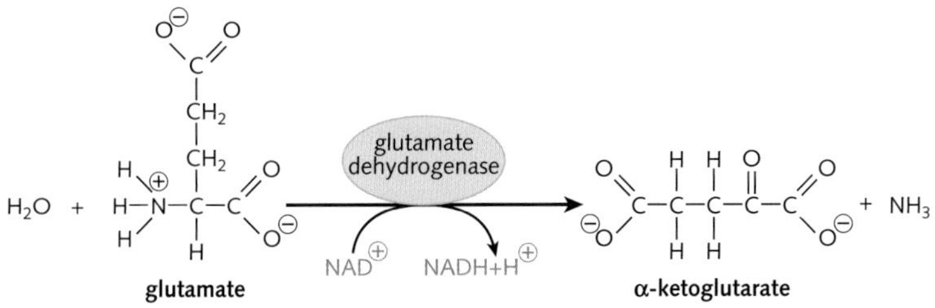

Fig. 9.4 Oxidative deamination of glutamate. *NAD⁺*, Nicotinamide adenine dinucleotide.

Amino acid transport

Because amino acids are present at much higher concentrations intracellularly than extracellularly, amino acid import requires energy. Transporters exist that couple adenosine triphosphate (ATP) hydrolysis (directly or indirectly) to amino acid import. Transporters are grouped by specificity for R-group properties (Table 9.2).

γ-Glutamyl cycle

This cycle imports a wide range of amino acids into cells. It is active transport, requiring three ATP molecules per amino acid imported, it is rapid and has high capacity. It utilizes the peptide glutathione (see Chapter 5).

- Glutathione donates γ-glutamyl residue to the transmembrane enzyme γ-glutamyl transpeptidase (GGT), which transfers γ-glutamyl to the exterior face of the membrane. The glutathione Cys–Gly 'remnant' remains intracellular.
- At the exterior surface of the cell membrane, the γ-glutamyl is attached to the awaiting amino acid, also catalysed by GGT. This modification allows the γ-glutamyl amino acid to be imported by GGT.

- Once imported, the γ-glutamyl component releases the amino acid intracellularly. The γ-glutamate is converted to 5′ oxoproline. Both these functions are performed by intracellular γ-glutamyl cyclotransferase.
- 5′ Oxoproline is then converted to glutamate by oxoprolinase, utilizing 1 ATP.
- Glutamate recombines with Cys forming γ-Glu–Cys, again utilizing 1 ATP. This is catalysed by γ-Glu–Cys synthetase.
- γ-Glu–Cys then reacts with Gly, re-forming glutathione. This is catalysed by glutathione synthetase, again utilizing 1 ATP (Fig. 9.5).

AMINO ACID SYNTHESIS

Essential and nonessential amino acids

There are six essential, four semi-essential and ten non-essential amino acids in human biochemistry (Table 9.1).

- Essential amino acids cannot be endogenously synthesized de novo *at all* and are thus required from dietary protein intake. These include tryptophan, lysine, threonine, valine, leucine and isoleucine.

Table 9.2 Amino acid transporter characteristics

Type of aminoacids transported	Specific amino acids transported	Inheritance and pathology of specific transport system deficiency
Small and neutral	ALA, SER, THR	–
Large and neutral/aromatic	ILE, LEU, VAL, TYR, TRY, PHE	Hartnup disease: autosomal recessive absence of this carrier system. These amino acids cannot be absorbed across the gut or reabsorbed from renal ultrafiltrate, leading to deficiency of these particular amino acids
Basic (positively charged) plus cysteine	ARG, LYS, HIS, CYS	Cystinuria: autosomal recessive condition resulting from absence of this carrier system. This causes inability to reabsorb cysteine from renal ultrafiltrate, leading to crystallization of cysteine and stone formation in the renal tract
Acidic (negatively charged)	GLU, ASP	–
Neutral large/neutral small	ALA, SER, THR, GLY, CYS, GLN, ASN	–
'Imino' acids: proline and glycine	PRO, GLY	Iminoglycinuria: autosomal recessive illness resulting from the carrier deficiency, causing failure of absorption from renal ultrafiltrate.

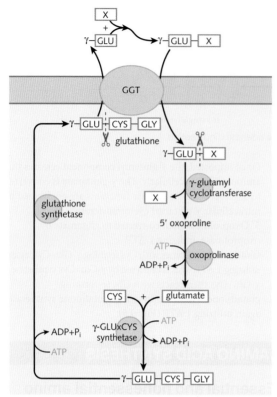

Fig. 9.5 General amino acid intracellular import: the γ-glutamyl cycle. *ADP,* Adenosine diphosphate; *ATP,* adenosine triphosphate; *CYS,* cysteine; *GLU,* glutamate; *GLY,* glycine; *P$_i$,* inorganic phosphate.

- Nonessential amino acids can be synthesized in the human body, so their dietary intake is not mandatory. These include alanine, asparagine, aspartate, cysteine, glutamate, glutamine, glycine, proline, serine and tyrosine.
- Semi essential amino acids *can* be synthesized endogenously, so are not technically 'essential'; however, they are considered essential as maximum biosynthesis cannot meet physiological demands. These include arginine, histidine, phenylalanine and methionine.

Nonessential amino acid biosynthesis is described in the following sections.

Glutamate, glutamine, proline and arginine biosynthesis

These are grouped together because glutamate is used as a substrate for synthesis of the other three.

Glutamate biosynthesis

α-Ketoglutarate is converted to glutamate by transamination (Fig. 9.3).

Glutamine biosynthesis

Glutamine is synthesized by amidation of glutamate by glutamine synthetase (Fig. 9.6). This combines NH_3 (ammonia) with glutamate, and requires ATP hydrolysis.

Proline biosynthesis

This is a three-step pathway (Fig. 9.6):

- Reduction of glutamate to glutamate γ-semialdehyde (redox partner is $NADPH + H^+$).
- Glutamate γ-semialdehyde spontaneously undergoes molecular rearrangement to lower-energy pyrroline-5-carboxylate.
- Pyrroline-5-carboxylate is reduced to proline (reaction redox partner is $NADPH + H^+$).

Arginine biosynthesis

Like proline synthesis, glutamate is first reduced to glutamate γ-semialdehyde (redox partner $NADPH + H^+$). This is then transaminated, forming ornithine. Ornithine enters the urea cycle, ultimately forming arginine.

Aspartate and asparagine biosynthesis

Asparagine is a derivative of aspartate.

- Aspartate is formed by transamination of oxaloacetate. This is catalysed by aspartate aminotransferase, and the amino group is helpfully provided by glutamate (which is converted to α-ketoglutarate).
- Aspartate is then converted to asparagine by asparagine synthetase. The amino group is donated by glutamine. This reaction consumes an ATP (Fig. 9.7).

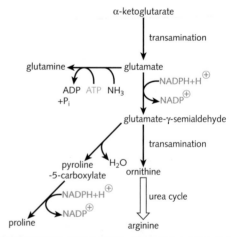

Fig. 9.6 Synthesis of glutamate, glutamine, proline and arginine. *ADP,* Adenosine diphosphate; *ATP,* adenosine triphosphate; *NADP$^+$,* nicotinamide adenine dinucleotide phosphate; *NADPH,* nicotinamide adenine dinucleotide phosphate (reduced form of NADP$^+$).

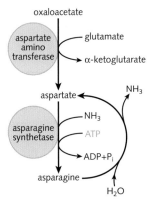

Fig. 9.7 Aspartate and asparagine synthesis. *ADP,* Adenosine diphosphate; *ATP,* adenosine triphosphate; *P_i,* inorganic phosphate.

Serine, glycine and cysteine biosynthesis

Serine biosynthesis

The majority of serine synthesis occurs in the cytoplasm. This utilizes 3-phosphoglycerate (a glycolytic intermediate; see Chapter 4). The pathway involves three steps: oxidation, transamination and hydrolysis (Fig. 9.8).

Glycine biosynthesis

This occurs mitochondrially, via two routes. One is the generation of glycine from serine (by serine hydroxymethyltransferase; Fig. 9.8). The other (not illustrated) is catalysed by glycine synthase, uses $NADH + H^+$ as a redox partner and requires the ammonium ion (NH_4^+), CO_2 and N^5N^{10}-methylene tetrahydrofolate as substrates.

Cysteine biosynthesis

Cysteine is formed from methionine and serine in the cytoplasm. The synthesis pathway is not yet fully identified; however, the main steps are shown in Fig. 9.9. Deficiency of the enzyme cystathionine-β-synthase results in accumulation of the intermediate homocysteine. This causes homocystinuria, a multisystem disorder characterized by elevated serum and urinary homocysteine.

Tyrosine biosynthesis

Tyrosine synthesis is simply hydroxylation of phenylalanine (Fig. 9.10). The reaction is highly exergonic, explaining why phenylalanine cannot be synthesized from tyrosine. The reaction is catalysed by phenylalanine hydroxylase and requires tetrahydrobiopterin as a cofactor. Absent/deficient phenylalanine hydroxylase causes phenylketonuria.

Fig. 9.8 Serine and glycine synthesis. Some of the enzymes in serine synthesis have not yet been identified, so are not illustrated here. *NAD⁺*, nicotinamide adenine dinucleotide; *THF*, tetrahydrofolate.

CLINICAL NOTES

PHENYLKETONURIA

This autosomal recessive disease arises from deficiency/absence of phenylalanine hydroxylase. Tyrosine cannot be synthesized endogenously, making it an essential amino acid. Phenylalanine accumulates, saturating the large-neutral/aromatic amino acid transporter at the blood–brain barrier. This denies other molecules relying on this transporter access to the developing central nervous system. This manifests with progressive brain damage and seizures. Treatment is by dietary exclusion of phenylalanine and tyrosine supplementation.

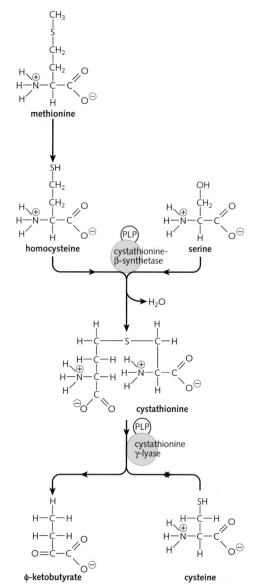

Fig. 9.9 Cysteine synthesis. *PLP*, Pyridoxal phosphate.

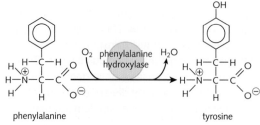

phenylalanine   tyrosine

Fig. 9.10 Tyrosine synthesis.

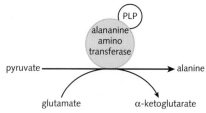

Fig. 9.11 Serotonin synthesis. *PLP*, Pyridoxal phosphate.

Tyrosine is oxidized by the enzyme tyrosinase to produce the pigment melanin. Tyrosinase deficiency results in failure of melanogenesis, leading to oculocutaneous albinism type 1. Ocular complications arising from iris translucency and reduced retinal pigmentation are common.

Alanine biosynthesis

Alanine is synthesized by transamination of pyruvate to alanine (Fig. 9.11). This is catalysed by alanine aminotransferase (cofactor PLP) and requires glutamate to donate the amino group.

BIOLOGICAL DERIVATIVES OF AMINO ACIDS

Amino acids are essential as the building blocks of proteins; however, they also fulfil important functions as individual molecules; for example, the majority of central neurotransmitters are derived from amino acids.

Serotonin synthesis from tryptophan

Serotonin (5-hydroxytryptamine) is synthesized from tryptophan. This is a two-step pathway (Fig. 9.12): tryptophan is hydroxylated to 5-hydroxytryptophan, by tryptophan hydroxylase (cofactor tetrahydrobiopterin). 5-OH-tryptophan is then decarboxylated by amino acid decarboxylase (cofactor PLP) to form 5-hydroxytryptamine.

Adrenaline, noradrenaline and dopamine synthesis from tyrosine

These three neurotransmitters (catecholamines) are all derived from tyrosine. The pathway is best shown as a diagram (Fig. 9.13).

Thyroid hormone synthesis from tyrosine

Two tyrosine residues in the same polypeptide (the glycoprotein thyroglobulin) are iodinated at their R-groups, forming monoiodotyrosine or diiodotyrosine depending

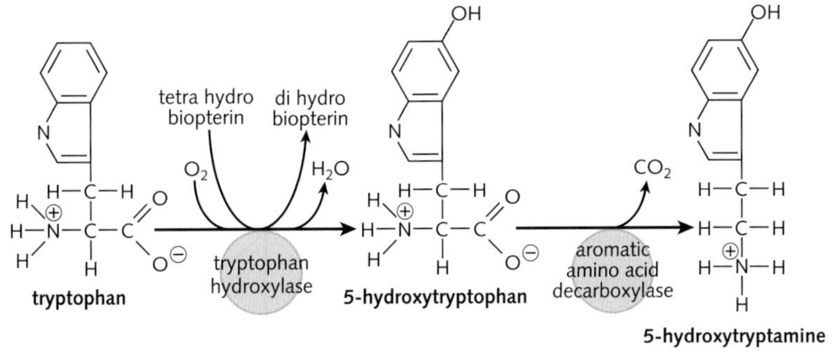

Fig. 9.12 5-hydroxytryptophan (serotonin) synthesis from tryptophan.

on whether iodination occurs at one or two sites. These two iodinated tyrosine residues react with each other. This forms T3 (triiodothyronine) when one diiodotyrosine combines with another monoiodotyrosine, and T4 (thyroxine) if two diiodotyrosines combine with each other. Generation of T3 and T4 (both termed 'thyroid hormones') is catalysed by thyroid peroxidase. The newly formed thyroid hormones are excised from their thyroglobulin scaffold by lysosomal enzymes and are then released in a regulated fashion by the thyroid gland. T3 is much more active than T4; T4 can also be peripherally converted to T3.

NITROGEN BALANCE

As nitrogen breakdown yields toxic products, and biological availability of nitrogen is limited, the balance between synthesis and breakdown of nitrogen-containing (nitrogenous) molecules is closely regulated. Nitrogenous molecules include amino acids and their derivatives, nucleotides, nucleic acids and, of course, proteins. Nitrogen presence in the body is largely accounted for by proteins, and therefore nitrogen balance is primarily determined by the balance between synthesis and degradation of proteins.

Positive nitrogen balance describes the scenario where N intake exceeds N excretion. This is seen during growth, pregnancy and wound healing, all situations where new body tissue (protein) is being generated. Negative nitrogen balance describes the converse scenario – a net loss of N occurs due to excretion exceeding intake. This can be due to:

- Insufficient nitrogen intake: malnutrition, anorexia, dieting
- Excess nitrogen loss: tissue destruction (extensive surgery, trauma, burns, sepsis), muscle wasting
- Combination of both: cachexia (emaciation associated with severe illness)

To excrete nitrogen, proteins are degraded to their constituent amino acids, which are then processed so that the nitrogen they contain can be offloaded. This offloading can be conceptually divided into two stages; removal of the amino group and formation of urea.

AMINO ACID CATABOLISM

There are two components of amino acid catabolism:

- Removal of amino groups and nitrogen elimination
- Catabolism of the carbon skeletons

Removal of the amino group

This may occur via either transamination or deamination. Each route generates different products, but both are able to enter the urea cycle.

Transdeamination: removal of the amino group as NH₃

Amino acids can be converted to their corresponding keto acid (which is further metabolized) and NH_3 is subsequently released, entering the urea cycle. This involves sequential transamination and oxidative deamination:

- Cytoplasmic transamination, where aminotransferases 'convert' the amino acid to glutamate; in reality, the amino group is transferred to α-ketoglutarate, generating glutamate, whereas the amino acid skeleton is released as the corresponding keto acid.
- This is followed by mitochondrial oxidative deamination of glutamate (Fig. 9.4) releasing α-ketoglutarate and NH_3 (Fig. 9.14).

Transamination: incorporation of the amino group into aspartate

Transamination was described earlier in the chapter (Fig. 9.3). In the context of nitrogen excretion, the second transaminase reaction generates aspartate and is mediated by AST. The aspartate is then able to enter the urea cycle (Fig. 9.16).

Catabolism of carbon skeletons

Once the amino group has been removed (from an amino acid), the carbon 'skeleton' remains. This skeleton (the

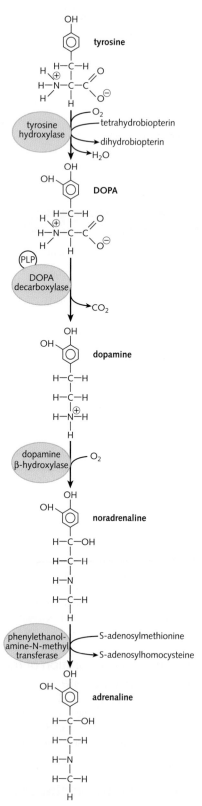

Fig. 9.13 Catecholamine synthesis. *DOPA,* Dihydroxyphenylalanine; *PLP,* pyridoxal phosphate.

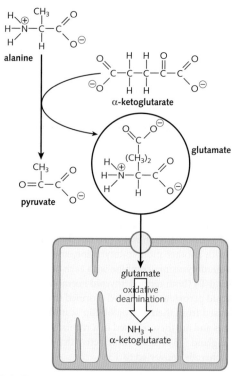

Fig. 9.14 Transdeamination of alanine.

corresponding keto acid) will vary in structure according to the individual amino acid. Each structure is further catabolized to form intermediates of the TCA cycle or ketogenesis. Table 9.3 provides further detail.

The terms 'glucogenic' and 'ketogenic'

Amino acids whose catabolites can enter the gluconeogenesis pathway, ultimately forming glucose, are termed 'glucogenic'. Any amino acids with metabolites that can enter the TCA cycle ultimately form oxaloacetate, which is a gluconeogenic substrate; thus this feature ensures glucogenic status.

Some amino acid catabolism products, however, cannot be converted to TCA cycle or gluconeogenesis intermediates and are instead destined to become intermediates of the ketogenesis pathway (e.g. acetyl-coenzyme A (acetyl-CoA); Chapter 7). These are termed 'ketogenic' amino acids.

Some amino acids are able, depending on their route of catabolism, to generate intermediates of both ketogenesis and the TCA cycle (both 'ketogenic' and 'glucogenic'). Others are only able to ultimately produce intermediates of one or other pathways (Table 9.3):

- Leucine and lysine are purely ketogenic.
- Isoleucine, phenylalanine, tyrosine and tryptophan are both ketogenic and glucogenic.
- All other amino acids are purely glucogenic.

Table 9.3 Catabolism of individual amino acid carbon skeletons.

Amino acid	Tricarboxylic acid/ cycle/ketogenesis pathway intermediate	Processing of deaminated carbon skeleton	Glucogenic	Ketogenic
GLU	α-Ketoglutarate	Undergoes oxidative deamination (Fig. 9.4), forming α-ketoglutarate, NH_3 and $NADH + H^+$	✓	
GLN	α-Ketoglutarate	Hydrolysed by glutaminase to form glutamate	✓	
CYS	Pyruvate	Cysteine aminotransferase converts cysteine into glutamate	✓	
ARG	α-Ketoglutarate	Cleaved to form ornithine and urea in the urea cycle. Ornithine is transaminated to form glutamate γ-semialdehyde, which converts to glutamate	✓	
PRO	α-Ketoglutarate	Proline dehydrogenase and Δ1-pyrroline-5-carboxylate dehydrogenase oxidize proline to glutamate	✓	
HIS	α-Ketoglutarate	Histidine catabolism involves a complex, seven-enzyme pathway culminating in the formation of glutamate. Initial deamination is mediated by histidase: deficiency of this enzyme causes histidinaemia	✓	
ALA	Pyruvate	Transamination of alanine generates pyruvate (and glutamate)	✓	
GLY	Pyruvate	Glycine is converted to serine (which is catabolized ultimately to pyruvate) by serine hydroxymethyltransferase	✓	
SER	Pyruvate	Serine–threonine dehydratase converts serine to pyruvate	✓	
VAL	Succinyl-coenzyme A (succinyl-CoA)	Branched chain amino acid catabolism: see following section	✓	
MET	Succinyl-CoA	Methionine donates its methyl group to various acceptors via the intermediate S-adenosyl-methionine. This generates propionyl-CoA, which is metabolized to succinyl-CoA by the odd-chain fatty acid oxidation pathway	✓	
THR	Succinyl-CoA	Serine–threonine dehydratase converts threonine to α-ketobutyrate, which is converted to propionyl-CoA and CO_2. Propionyl-CoA is metabolized to succinyl-CoA by the odd-chain oxidation pathway	✓	✓
ASP	Fumarate, oxaloacetate	Transaminated by aspartate aminotransferase to produce oxaloacetate	✓	
ASN	Oxaloacetate	Converted first to aspartate by asparaginase	✓	
TYR	Fumarate, acetoacetate	Tyrosine aminotransferase catalyses the first step in this five-step pathway, culminating in fumarate and acetoacetate. Deficiency of homogentisic acid dioxygenase, one of the tyrosine catabolism enzymes, causes alkaptonuria (accumulation of the intermediate homogentisate)	✓	✓
PHE	Fumarate, acetoacetate	Converted first to tyrosine by phenylalanine hydroxylase	✓	✓
ILE	Acetyl-CoA, succinyl-CoA	Branched-chain amino acid catabolism: see the following section. Catabolism yields acetyl-CoA and succinyl-CoA	✓	✓
TRY	Acetyl-CoA	The complex catabolism of tryptophan has not yet been fully elucidated; however, the TRY catabolism pathway culminates with acetyl-CoA	✓	✓
LEU	Acetyl-CoA, Acetoacetate	Branched-chain amino acid catabolism: see the following section		✓
LYS	Acetoacetate	Deaminated lysine undergoes enters a complex pathway which ultimately produces acetoacetate		✓

Branched-chain amino acids

The branched-chain amino acids (BCAAs) are isoleucine, leucine and valine. They are degraded primarily in muscle, because the liver (the usual site for amino acid catabolism) lacks the specific aminotransferase required to cleave off the amino group from BCAA. Their catabolism is as follows: BCAA aminotransferase transfers the amino group from BCAA to α-ketoglutarate. This forms glutamate and a branched-chain α-ketoacid. This α-ketoacid then undergoes oxidative decarboxylation, mediated by mitochondrial branched-chain α-ketoacid dehydrogenase complex (cofactor PLP). This produces branched-chain acyl-CoA derivatives, which are then dehydrogenated by two separate dehydrogenases (Fig. 9.15). Each separate BCAA derivative undergoes oxidation reactions reminiscent of β-oxidation, ultimately producing:

- (Leucine →) acetyl-CoA and acetoacetate
- (Isoleucine →) acetyl-CoA and succinyl-CoA
- (Valine →) succinyl-CoA

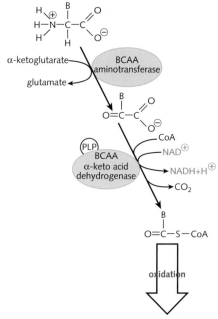

Fig. 9.15 Branched-chain amino acid (BCAA) catabolism. 'B' indicates a branched-chain 'R' group. *CoA*, Coenzyme A; *NAD⁺*, nicotinamide adenine dinucleotide; *PLP*, pyridoxal phosphate.

THE UREA CYCLE

The urea cycle, also known as the 'ornithine cycle', is the process via which ammonia (NH_3) is converted to urea ($NH_2)_2$ C = O in the liver. The cycle also accepts nitrogen in the form of aspartate and integrates it into the urea molecule. The urea cycle operates within hepatocytes across two cellular compartments: the cytoplasm and the mitochondrial matrix. The cycle and relevant enzymes are detailed in Fig. 9.16. In brief:

- Ammonia combines with a bicarbonate ion and two ATP molecules, forming carbamoyl phosphate (catalysed by carbamoyl synthetase-I).
- Carbamoyl phosphate combines with mitochondrial ornithine, forming citrulline.
- Citrulline diffuses out of the mitochondria.

- Citrulline then combines with aspartate, forming arginosuccinate. ATP is hydrolysed.
- Arginosuccinate is cleaved to fumarate and arginine.
- Arginine remains in the urea cycle for the final reaction; hydration of arginine generates urea and regenerates ornithine.
- Ornithine re-enters the mitochondria, completing the cycle.

Fate of urea cycle fumarate

Fumarate produced by cleavage of arginosuccinate is converted by cytoplasmic fumarase to malate. This malate may follow one of two routes:

- Re-enter the mitochondria to participate in the TCA cycle
- Further oxidize to oxaloacetate (catalysed by malate dehydrogenase). This is then transaminated, generating aspartate, by AST. Aspartate can re-enter the urea cycle, as shown in Fig. 9.16.

Sources of urea cycle aspartate

Aspartate may be derived from urea cycle fumarate (as described previously). Alternatively, it may originate from transaminated oxaloacetate. Any amino acid can be transaminated (first via the relevant aminotransferase, and then via AST) to generate aspartate.

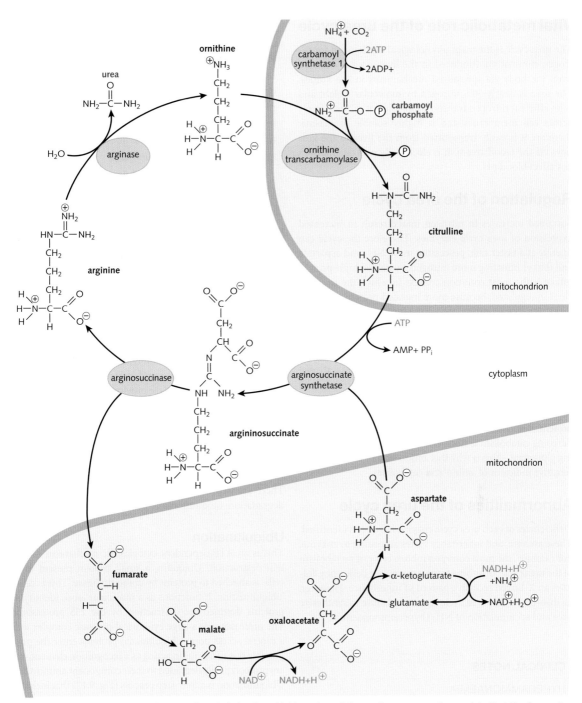

Fig. 9.16 The urea cycle. Note the cytoplasmic/mitochondrial location of the cycle enzymes. Appreciate that the fumarate → malate → oxaloacetate stages are part of the tricarboxylic acid (TCA) cycle; for simplicity most of the enzymes are not shown in this illustration. *ADP,* Adenosine diphosphate; *AMP,* adenosine monophosphate; *ATP,* adenosine triphosphate; *NAD⁺,* nicotinamide adenine dinucleotide; *PPi,* inorganic pyrophosphate.

Vital metabolic role of the urea cycle

The urea cycle is the main physiological mechanism for nitrogen elimination. Produced in the liver, urea is excreted from the body via specialized mechanisms in the kidney. The urea is nearly 50% nitrogen by molecular weight and is an efficient nitrogen transport molecule. It diffuses freely across cell membranes and is highly soluble in plasma; therefore it is easily transported from the liver to the kidneys via the bloodstream. It is electrically neutral and does not affect blood pH.

Regulation of the urea cycle

Sustained increases in nitrogen intake result in increased expression of urea cycle enzymes. Therefore the cycle can operate at a faster rate, processing more NH_3 and aspartate and thus eliminating more nitrogen. Sustained high-protein intake is the most common context in which the urea cycle is upregulated, because more ingested protein results in more nitrogen requiring processing for elimination.

Short-term regulation of the urea cycle is mainly via modulation of mitochondrial carbamoyl-phosphate synthase-I activity, the enzyme that uses ATP, NH_3 and HCO_3^- to form carbamoyl phosphate. This enzyme is allosterically activated by N-acetyl glutamate, itself formed by the combination of acetyl-CoA and glutamate. This is appropriate, because intracellular glutamate will rise following catabolism of ingested protein. Remember that the amino group of amino acids undergoing catabolism is transferred to α-ketoglutarate, forming glutamate – this is why this amino acid in particular is a sensitive indicator of amino acid catabolism.

Abnormalities of the urea cycle

Deficiencies of each urea cycle enzyme have been identified. These are rare, and inheritance varies according to enzyme. For example, the most common inborn error of metabolism of the urea cycle, ornithine transcarbamylase deficiency, follows an X-linked recessive pattern of inheritance. However, all disorders of the urea cycle result in a failure to synthesize urea and accumulation of NH_3 (hyperammonaemia).

PROTEIN SYNTHESIS AND DEGRADATION

Protein turnover

Proteins, both structural and functional, undergo continuous synthesis and degradation. If these processes occur at equal rates, the total protein quantity remains constant. Because proteins are composed of amino acids (nitrogen-containing molecules), protein intake and excretion broadly approximate to nitrogen balance (see previous discussion).

Protein degradation

This section describes enzymatic breakdown of proteins to their constituent amino acids. Enzymes that hydrolyse peptide bonds (between amino acids) are called 'proteases'. There are two major routes of protease-mediated protein degradation: ubiquitination and the lysosomal pathway.

Ubiquitination

This is an ATP-dependent cytoplasmic mechanism of protein destruction. Ubiquitin, a small protein present in all cells, is attached to proteins by ubiquitin ligase. This is called 'ubiquitination'. It functions as a molecular label, identifying proteins destined for destruction by the 25S proteasome. The proteasome is a large cylindrical protease complex with a central access pore. Ubiquitinated proteins enter the pore, possibly due to ubiquitin acting as a recognition element, and are proteolytically degraded to their component amino acids. Ubiquitination is a four-step process (Fig. 9.17) that includes:

- Production of an active adenylated ubiquitin intermediate and covalent binding of activated ubiquitin to enzyme E1 (ubiquitin-activating enzyme).
- Transfer of ubiquitin to enzyme E2 (ubiquitin-conjugating enzyme).
- Association of E2-ubiquitin with substrate-bound E3 (ubiquitin ligase). E3 'reads' the N terminus of a protein.
- If the N terminus is unstable, a peptide bond is generated between ubiquitin and the E3-bound substrate. E2 and E3 then dissociate.

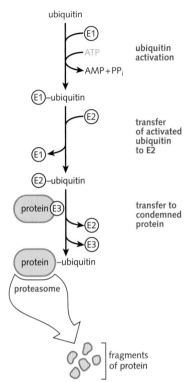

Fig. 9.17 Ubiquitination. *ADP*, Adenosine diphosphate; *AMP*, adenosine monophosphate; *ATP*, adenosine triphosphate; *E1*, Ubiquitin-activating enzyme; *E2*, ubiquitin-conjugating enzyme; *E3*, ubiquitin ligase; *PPi*, inorganic pyrophosphate.

Lysosomal proteolysis

Lysosomes are intracellular organelles. Intralysosomal proteases (cathepsins) mediate lysosomal proteolysis. Proteins gain access to lysosomal interior by either endocytosis (extracellular proteins) or intracellular autophagy. Autophagy is when endoplasmic reticulum wraps around intracellular organelles (e.g. mitochondria), forming an 'autophagosome'.

Intracellular degradation signals

There are various structural features that decrease the lifespan of proteins by conferring susceptibility to various cellular degradation processes. Appreciate that exposure of such features during conformational change also renders a protein vulnerable to degradation.

N-terminus components

High density of the amino acids Met, Gly, Ala and Ser promotes N-terminus stability, because these are not readily ubiquitinated. Thus presence of these amino acids at the N terminus of a protein renders it relatively insensitive to ubiquitin-mediated destruction. Conversely, Phe, Try, Asp, Asn and Lys destabilize the N terminus. These amino acids

are an N-terminal feature of short-lived proteins, because they are readily ubiquitinated by E3.

'PEST' regions

These are features of a protein's primary structure; regions with high density of Pro, Glu, Ser and Thr (P, E, S and T according to the one-letter amino acid code) residues are common in proteins with short lifespans. PEST regions are examples of a 'degradation motif'; their presence condemns a protein to a rapid turnover. The mechanism of PEST-mediated susceptibility is not yet clarified but may be due to caspase or proteasome action.

PROTEIN SYNTHESIS

Introduction

Proteins are fundamental for all cellular functions at every level. Continuous background degradation of senescent and dysfunctional proteins must therefore be balanced by ongoing protein synthesis to maintain protein availability.

Protein biosynthesis at its most simple level can be considered as follows:

Gene expression (messenger RNA (mRNA) synthesis) → ribosomal translation (polypeptide assembly)

Each of these stages is discussed here.

Transcription (mRNA synthesis)

Transcription describes the synthesis of mRNA. mRNA consists of ribonucleotides linked in the order dictated by the original genetic sequence. The DNA sequence that comprises a gene dictates the sequence of ribonucleotide assembly, which directs mRNA synthesis. Transcription occurs in the nucleus and can be broken down into the following steps: initiation, elongation and termination.

Initiation

Transcription kicks off when transcription factors bind to the promoter sequence of a particular gene. The transcription factor–promoter sequence complex recruits RNA polymerase II (POL II).

HINTS AND TIPS

PROMOTER SEQUENCES

Promoter sequences tend to have specific characteristic sequence motifs, for example, TATA 'boxes' which consist of lengths of DNA rich in A and T bases – these features facilitate the initial DNA unwinding.

The RNA POL II enzyme is composed of multiple sub-units and at least six associated transcription factors. It mediates local unwinding of the double helix, exposing the two strands in a 'transcription bubble.' This exposes:

- the coding strand
- the template or noncoding strand

The noncoding strand has a sequence complementary to that of the coding strand. It is the noncoding strand that is used as a template for ribonucleotide binding.

Elongation

The new mRNA strand is formed by POL II-mediated linking of ribonucleotides (A, U, C or G) one at a time, in a 5′ → 3′ direction. The order of ribonucleotide incorporation is determined by the exposed DNA of the template (noncoding) strand within the transcription bubble. G pairs with C, U with A, A with T and C with G (base pairing).

The developing mRNA strand is elongated by POL II-mediated interlinking of assembled ribonucleotides. The new mRNA strand is nearly identical in sequence to the DNA coding strand, because it has used the noncoding complementary DNA strand as a template. However, ribonucleotides lack a T – wherever a T featured in the coding strand, a U is substituted in mRNA.

Termination

RNA POL II continues to transcribe the noncoding strand until it reaches the end of the gene, defined by a terminator sequence of DNA. As this is transcribed, a string of A bases, known as a polyadenylation signal is incorporated at the 3′ end of the developing mRNA. The polyadenylation signal recruits a 5′ exonuclease, which severs and releases the mRNA from RNA POL II.

At this stage, the released mRNA is technically termed a pre-mRNA, because further processing (post-transcriptional modification) is required before the polymer is competent to function as a translation template (a 'mature' mRNA).

Blissfully unaware that its job is done, the POL II continues to transcribe the noncoding strand after this occurs. The mechanism governing the cessation of POL II's transcription is not clear, and the additional RNA is not translated.

Posttranscriptional modifications

Although the following modifications are conceptually post-translational, some actually occur or at least initiate during the transcription process rather than after as the name implies.

Splicing: removal of introns

A gene is composed of a coding strand (i.e. a length of DNA). The coding strand, however, consists of exons and introns. Exons code for the protein, but are disrupted by noncoding introns (sometimes termed 'junk' DNA). The introns do not contribute to the functional code of the gene, and must be clipped out at their start and end, allowing the

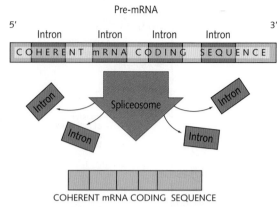

Pre-mRNA

Fig. 9.18 Spliceosome intron excision. Removal of introns allows consecutive exons to link, generating a mature messenger RNA (RNA) coding sequence.

coding exons to run contiguously. This process is known as splicing.

Splicing is performed in the nucleus by a ribonucleoprotein complex called a spliceosome. This assembles itself as soon as the first intron is transcribed. Transcribed introns are manipulated into loop structures (lariats) protruding out from the pre-mRNA transcript, then excised by the spliceosome. These lariats (excised introns) depart, and consecutive exons are left uninterrupted by intervening introns in the mature mRNA (Fig. 9.18).

5′ (Five-prime) capping

The 5′ cap is a 7-methylguanosine molecule, which is added to the 5′ end of the RNA transcript. The cap fulfils several important roles:

- Protecting the mRNA from degradation
- Provides an access point for ribosomes in translation of the mature mRNA transcript

HINTS AND TIPS

IMPORTANT FEATURES OF MESSENGER RNA (MRNA)

The 5′ cap and the poly-A tail can be conceptually considered as analogous to the front and back cover of a book, where the mRNA transcript forms the pages of the book.

3′ Polyadenylate tail addition

A 'tail' of multiple consecutive A ribonucleotides is added to the pre-mRNA at the 3′ end. It is usually about 100–200 A nucleotides in length. The poly-A tail confers molecular stability to the mature mRNA. The length of the tail thus correlates with the mRNA's longevity – typically the longer tails confer greater stability and lifespan to the mature mRNA (Fig. 9.19).

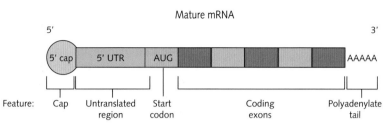

Fig. 9.19 Cartoon representation of a mature messenger RNA (RNA). Note the 5′ cap, 5′ untranslated region (UTR), coding exons and polyadenylate tail at the 3′ end.

Translation (amino acid assembly and interlinking)

Translation is performed by ribosomes in the cytoplasm or at the rough endoplasmic reticulum. Mature mRNA must therefore first be exported from the nucleus before translation can commence.

Translation is the process of assembling amino acids in a sequence dictated by the mRNA codon sequence. Ribosomes act as polypeptide 'factories', using mRNA as the blueprints. The 'workhorses' that shepherd incoming amino acids into the ribosome–mRNA complex for incorporation in the growing polypeptide are the transfer RNAs (tRNA).

Amino acid assembly order

Every trio of consecutive ribonucleotides (every three bases) in a mature mRNA transcript codes for an amino acid. Three consecutive bases are termed a codon. There are 64 possible combinations (codons); 61 codons code for amino acids, and the remaining three are 'stop' codons, which terminate translation.

HINTS AND TIPS

CODONS

There are 61 amino acid coding codons, but only 20 amino acids that are commonly used in polypeptide synthesis. A large proportion of codons are thus considered 'degenerate', that is, >1 codon encodes each amino acid. For example, the codons GGU, GGC, GGA and GGG all encode the amino acid glycine.

Codon recognition

Each codon is recognized by a specific individual tRNA molecule. The specificity is conferred by the tRNA's individual anticodon – a three-ribonucleotide sequence complementary to a particular mRNA codon. This anticodon also defines the particular amino acid carried by the tRNA. In this way, the coded amino acid is recruited to the relevant mRNA codon.

Initiation

During eukaryotic translation the two accepted mechanisms of initiation are:

- The 5′ cap-dependent mechanism
- An 'internal ribosome entry site' (IRES)

Cap-dependent initiation of translation

The 5′ cap acts as a locus for assembly of the small ribosome component, necessary initiation factors (other specialized proteins) and a methionine-bearing tRNA. Once these components interact, scanning occurs. The complex scans the 5′ end of the mRNA, and when the AUG sequence (a start codon) is encountered, the large ribosome component is then recruited and initiation factors are released. Translation is then initiated at that point.

The RNA prior to this start point is known as '5′ untranslated region' or 5′ UTR. The ribosomal/tRNA complex also interacts with the mRNA poly-A tail via a poly-A-binding protein. This forces the mRNA into a large loop with each end within the ribosomal/tRNA complex.

HINTS AND TIPS

RIBOSOMES

Eukaryotic (e.g. human) ribosomes consist of two components (small and large). They are made up of ribosomal RNA which is transcribed from DNA by RNA polymerase (POL) I and III. The large component only unites with the small component to form a functional ribosome at successful initiation of translation.

HINTS AND TIPS

REGULATION OF INITIATION

Initiation is controlled by additional regulatory genes at separate loci, and physiological levels of transcription involve significant external regulation. As the expression of these external regulator genes is tissue specific, gene transcription can be regulated in a similarly tissue-specific fashion.

IRES initiation of translation

Ribosomes/initiation factors commence translation at a start codon in largely the same way as the cap-dependent sequence of events during initiation via an IRES. The key difference is that they incorporate themselves at a start codon present within an 'internal ribosomal entry site' sequence, rather than at the usual 5′ end of the mRNA.

Elongation

The translation elongation cycle adds one amino acid at a time to the growing polypeptide and mediates their interlinking covalent peptide bond formation. The ribosome travels in a 5′ → 3′ direction along the mature mRNA:

1. Recruiting an appropriate amino acid-bearing tRNA
2. Incorporating the tRNA-bound amino acid to the growing polypeptide
3. Releasing the 'empty' tRNA
4. Repeating this sequence

Every new amino acid is incorporated according to the sequential codon on the mRNA strand. Elongation requires the presence eukaryotic elongation factor proteins.

Termination

Three mRNA codons (UAA, UAG and UGA) are unrecognizable to tRNAs, and are termed stop codons. Their presence defines the end of the developing polypeptide, and instructs the ribosome to abort further synthesis. Any of the three stop codons recruits eukaryotic releasing factor proteins when reached by the progressing ribosome synthetic complex. When the eukaryotic releasing factor binds to a stop codon, the mRNA is released from the ribosome. The ribosome then dissociates into its constituent subunits.

Protein synthesis: posttranslational modification

Depending on the ultimate destination of the newly synthesized protein, specific structural motifs act to direct the protein to its appropriate cellular location. These structural motifs may be determined by particular (conserved) amino acid sequences or other posttranslational modifications.

Posttranslational modifications are also vital for the physiological activity of the newly translated polypeptide. Several are discussed as follows.

Glycosylation

Glycosylation occurs in the endoplasmic reticulum lumen or in the Golgi apparatus. An oligosaccharide is covalently bound to specific amino acids. There are two types of glycosylation: N-linked and O-linked.

N-linked glycosylation

An oligosaccharide is incorporated in the polypeptide (via a β-N-glycosidic bond) at an aspartate residue. N-linked glycosylation is significant for directing acid hydrolases to their lysosomal destination, and also in antibody production.

O-linked glycosylation

An oligosaccharide is attached to serine or threonine residues (via an α-O-glycosidic bond). This is an important step in synthesis of cell surface-expressed red cell antigens; these glycoproteins define a person's blood group.

Phosphorylation

This occurs frequently at serine, threonine or tyrosine residues within a polypeptide. Kinases transfer phosphate groups from ATP onto the target residue. Key features concerning the importance of phosphorylation are discussed in Chapter 2.

Sulphation

Frequently, sulphate moieties link at tyrosine residues within a polypeptide. Sulphation plays an important molecular signposting role and facilitates appropriate cellular compartmentalization.

Hydroxylation

The addition of an '–OH' group often occurs at lysine and proline residues. Hydroxylation is particularly structurally significant in collagen synthesis, where it is mandatory for structural integrity.

DIETARY PROTEIN

A protein is composed of at least one polypeptide containing its constituent amino acids. They are an essential part of all organisms, as structural and functional components.

Protein: a macronutrient

Proteins are macronutrients. Along with the other macronutrients, carbohydrates and lipids, proteins are required in relatively large quantities in the diet to permit normal physiological processes including:

- Growth (childhood, adolescence, pregnancy)
- Tissue repair (trauma, surgery, infection, inflammation)
- Energy production (oxidation of 1 g protein provides 17 kJ or 4 kcal)

The reference nutrient intake (RNI) for protein is 0.75 g/kg/day (i.e. ~56 g daily for a 70-kg adult). The RNI for protein is increased in children/adolescents, pregnant or lactating females and the sick.

Protein digestion

Protein digestion is commenced in the stomach. Denaturation is promoted by the low pH, due to HCl secretion by the parietal cells. The enzyme pepsin (secreted by chief cells as pepsinogen) hydrolyses peptide bonds at the low pH values in the stomach. Subsequently, pancreatic proteolytic enzymes (trypsin, chymotrypsin, proelastase and carboxypolypeptidase) further hydrolyse proteins and protein fragments, ultimately degrading them to their constituent amino acids. Enterocytes lining the surface of the small bowel possess surface-bound peptidases that further hydrolyse any remaining dipeptides or tripeptides. Amino acids are absorbed across the enterocyte barrier and extruded into the portal circulation, ultimately reaching the systemic circulation via the liver.

Net dietary protein as % of energy intake

The concept of NDDPE% (net dietary protein as a percentage of energy intake) quantifies the contribution of dietary protein to the total energy intake. Different types of diets can thus be compared with each other. Ideally, a child's diet will provide at least 8% of the caloric intake in the form of protein, whereas in adults 5% suffices.

> **RED FLAG**
>
> Exclusively cereal-based diets. This type of exclusion diet cannot provide >6% NDPPE, thus for children this type of diet does not contribute enough protein-derived calories to avoid protein deficiency, even in the context of satisfactory calorie intake.

Protein 'quality'

The quality of a protein is defined by its essential amino acid components and the bioavailability and digestibility of these amino acids. Various parameters are used to quantify different aspects of proteins.

> **HINTS AND TIPS**
>
> REFERENCE PROTEINS
>
> A 'reference protein' contains all the amino acids in the exact proportions needed for optimal protein synthesis in humans. Albumin (found in egg white) and casein (milk) are closest to the ideal. Other proteins are compared with these reference proteins.

> **HINTS AND TIPS**
>
> LIMITING AMINO ACIDS
>
> The 'limiting' amino acid in a protein is defined as the essential amino acid present in a protein in the lowest amount relative to its requirement for protein synthesis. Examples of protein-containing foods and their limiting amino acids are:
> * Wheat, limited by lysine
> * Meat and fish, limited by methionine and cysteine
> * Maize, limited by tryptophan
>
> Combining different protein sources ensures an adequate intake of all the amino acids. This is particularly important in wide-ranging exclusion diets such as veganism and vegetarianism.

Protein efficiency ratio

This value quantifies the 'efficiency' of a protein by measuring growth in rats fed the protein. The rat weight gain is determined per gram of the test protein consumed. The outcome value is then compared with 2.7 – the standard value defined using casein as the test protein. For rats fed casein, every gram of casein led to a 2.7-g weight increase. A value greater than 2.7 is considered an excellent protein source, in the context of its effect on growth. This parameter correlates poorly to human growth.

Protein biological value

The biological value describes the fraction of the absorbed nitrogen incorporated into the body following consumption of the protein. This makes the biological value an integrated function of protein absorption and utilization. Whole egg is set as the protein digestibility standard and scores 100, but pure protein isolates can exceed this.

Net protein utilization

This quantifies the percent of ingested amino acids that are eventually converted into body proteins.

High net protein utilization values are attained by proteins with both high digestibility and an optimal ratio of essential to nonessential amino acids. This is similar to the biological value parameter but is usually measured indirectly by comparing protein intake against resulting nitrogen excretion.

Protein digestibility-corrected amino acid score

The protein digestibility-corrected amino acid score (PDCAAS) rates a protein as high quality when it is highly absorbed and its composition correlates well with human essential amino acid requirements. Score is from 0 to 1. Pure protein isolates score 1.0. Meat and soy score 0.9, vegetables and legumes 0.7 and grains 0.4. PDCAAS is considered the most reliable protein quality parameter in the context of human nutrition.

PROTEIN–ENERGY MALNUTRITION

The World Health Organization (WHO) defines protein–energy malnutrition (PEM) as a nutritional deficiency resulting in marasmus or kwashiorkor and developing due to (either/or):

- Inadequate calorie intake
- Inadequate protein intake

Causes of PEM

It is primarily a problem in developing countries, where 5 million children die every year from PEM. It is, however, relevant in the UK within populations at risk for general malnutrition, including the following:

- Anyone with severely restricted diet
- Anorexia/bulimia sufferers
- Alcohol-dependent individuals
- Neglected dependants (e.g. children and the elderly)
- Homeless individuals
- Those with severe malabsorption diseases

In hospitals, aside from those listed above, inpatients may be at risk when their protein intake requirement is increased due to disease (e.g. sepsis, inflammation, following major surgery or trauma and critical illness).

Physiological consequences of PEM

There are numerous physiological consequences of extreme starvation.

Weight falls as a consequence first of fat and ultimately muscle loss. Following initial exhaustion of glycogen reserves and subsequent exhaustion of adipose depots, muscle protein catabolism commences to provide amino acid substrates for gluconeogenesis and ketone body synthesis. Eventually, cardiac and respiratory muscles are affected, impairing contractility and respiratory function and leading to death from cardiorespiratory failure.

Metabolically, glycogenolysis initially occurs to maintain serum glucose. Once glycogen reserves are exhausted, lipolysis yields fatty acids which participate in gluconeogenesis and ketogenesis. This shift of primary metabolic substrate from carbohydrate to fat is driven by a fall in insulin and rise in glucagon and catecholamines. The hormonal profile of prolonged starvation is characterised by an elevation of catabolic hormones glucagon, cortisol and adrenaline, and suppression of insulin and thyroxine.

Other derangements include hypoglycaemia, hypokalaemia and hyponatraemia. A metabolic acidosis is seen. Dramatically increased susceptibility to infection and delayed wound healing are likewise hallmarks of extreme starvation. Loss of insulating adipose tissue and impaired calorigenesis place these patients at increased risk for hypothermia.

Specific manifestations of PEM

Classically, two particular clinical syndromes are described in the context of PEM: kwashiorkor and marasmus (Fig. 9.20). The magnitude of weight loss and presence of oedema define each condition. Multiple vitamin and mineral (micronutrient) deficiencies are additional problems in PEM.

Kwashiorkor

Kwashiorkor develops in the context of adequate calorie intake, but inadequate protein intake. Typically, body weight is 60% to 80% of the predicted weight (50th centile) for the measured height, and oedema is present. Muscle wasting is present but may be concealed by the oedema.

Kwashiorkor represents an inappropriate physiological response to protein restriction – subcutaneous fat is conserved whilst muscle catabolism occurs. Widespread flaking dermatitis and hair and skin depigmentation may also be present in kwashiorkor. Hepatomegaly and cardiomegaly with signs of heart failure may be elicited on examination.

Oedema of kwashiorkor

The oedema is secondary to hypoalbuminaemia; decreased plasma oncotic pressure results in inappropriate third-space (e.g. interstitial fluid) expansion. However, the exact causative mechanism of the hypoalbuminaemia of kwashiorkor is not clearly understood. The intravascular hypovolaemia secondary to low serum albumin leads to sodium and water retention, exacerbating the oedema. It is important to note that though these patients are oedematous, due to the hypoalbuminaemia, they are intravascularly hypovolaemic and are extremely vulnerable to hypovolaemic shock with any fluid balance derangement (e.g. diarrhoea).

Marasmus

Marasmus develops in the context of prolonged protein and energy restriction. When body weight is less than 60% of the predicted weight (50th centile) for the measured height, and the oedema is absent, marasmus is diagnosed. If oedema is present, but weight is less than 60% predicted (rather than 60%–80% predicted as in kwashiorkor), the diagnosis is marasmus–kwashiorkor. Extreme emaciation (due to muscle wasting and loss of subcutaneous fat) is striking, and growth retardation in children is more extreme than seen in kwashiorkor. Subcutaneous fat is catabolized, and ultimately muscle protein follows suite. Oedema is not usually a feature.

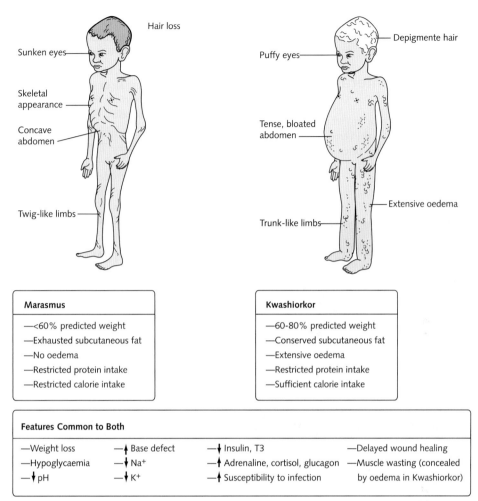

Marasmus

—<60% predicted weight
—Exhausted subcutaneous fat
—No oedema
—Restricted protein intake
—Restricted calorie intake

Kwashiorkor

—60-80% predicted weight
—Conserved subcutaneous fat
—Extensive oedema
—Restricted protein intake
—Sufficient calorie intake

Features Common to Both

—Weight loss   —↑ Base defect   —↓ Insulin, T3   —Delayed wound healing
—Hypoglycaemia   —↓ Na⁺   —↑ Adrenaline, cortisol, glucagon —Muscle wasting (concealed
—↓ pH   —↓ K⁺   —↑ Susceptibility to infection   by oedema in Kwashiorkor)

Fig. 9.20 Comparison of features of marasmus and kwashiorkor. Note that <60% predicted weight where oedema *is* present is termed 'marasmus–kwashiorkor'.

Management of PEM

The immediate priority is treatment of life-threatening complications such as dehydration, electrolyte abnormalities, hypothermia and infection. Then restoration of nutritional status, (typically administering 4 g/kg/day protein and 200 kcal/kg/day) and correction of micronutrient deficiencies can be addressed. Initial refeeding must be done gradually to avoid development of potentially life-treatening refeeding syndrome (see below)

PARENTERAL AND ENTERAL NUTRITION

Enteral nutrition

Enteral nutrition describes delivery of nutritionally complete liquid feed into the gastrointestinal (GI) tract. The enteral route essentially means 'via the enteric system' (i.e. the GI tract). Enteral feed is delivered via a nasogastric (NG) tube, the tip of which sits in the gastric lumen, or a percutaneous gastrostomy/jejunostomy port. The formulation is liquid and may consist of polymeric macronutrients (if digestive enzyme secretion is intact) or elemental macronutrients (no enzymatic digestion required).

Enteral nutrition is employed in situations where the GI tract is capable of absorbing nutrition, but there is a difficulty with eating which has lasted more than 48 hours and is not immediately reversible. This scenario may arise due to:

• Disorders of swallowing (usually patient's swallow will have been deemed 'unsafe')
• Neurological impairment (e.g. stroke) preventing adequate self-feeding
• Conditions causing extreme loss of appetite

If absorptive function is intact, the enteral route for nutrition delivery is always preferred as the intravenous route carries greater risks including infection and mortality.

Enteral feeding maintains GI integrity and function, reduces bacterial translocation, decreases the risk for sepsis and is less expensive.

Complications of enteral feeding

Complications primarily relate to the delivery device. NG tube misplacement (usually in a bronchus) can result in aspiration and death if feed is delivered down the tube. Confused or agitated patients are often poorly tolerant of NG tube, and some people just find the tube's presence particularly upsetting.

> **RED FLAG**
>
> Nasogastric tube placement. As a junior doctor you will regularly be asked to determine that newly placed nasogastric (NG) tubes are safe to use. Essentially, you are being asked 'is the tip in the gastric lumen?' Catastrophic outcomes including death occur when enteral feed is given via a misplaced tube. A combination of visualizing the radiopaque tip well below the diaphragm and an aspirate of fluid with pH < 4 implies the tip is in the gastric lumen, and is a safe and reliable habit to adopt for every NG tube you assess.

Total parenteral nutrition

The parenteral route is any delivery route that excludes the enteric system (i.e. routes other than oral/NG). Total parenteral nutrition (TPN) or intravenous nutrition provides all nutritional requirements including water, macronutrients and micronutrients. It is administered to deliver nutrition when GI digestion, motility and/or absorption are too impaired for sufficient assimilation of dietary nutrients from the GI lumen. Any scenario where chronic GI dysfunction results in failure of digestion or absorption may be an indication for TPN.

TPN components

TPN consists of a carefully balanced formulation of water, carbohydrate, amino acids, fatty acids, vitamins and minerals. Calories are typically added in the form of dextrose. TPN is prescribed by hospital nutrition teams based on individual weight presence of catabolic state and general clinical condition.

TPN administration

Delivery of TPN: requirement for cannulation of a large vein, usually the superior vena cava. This may be via:

- A central line (a large, multilumen cannula) inserted via the internal jugular or subclavian vein
- A peripherally inserted central cannula inserted in the basilic or cephalic vein

In both instances the tip of the cannula must lie in a large-bore vein. This is because TPN preparations are hyperosmolar and therefore highly irritant to vessel walls, and small veins cannot tolerate TPN delivery – painful thrombophlebitis develops if this route is attempted.

Always check whether a TPN formulation is intended for central or peripheral delivery.

Complications of TPN

The most dangerous problems associated with TPN relate to complications of the delivery system: risks of insertion include bleeding, pneumothorax, arrhythmia, malposition and nerve damage. Risks of having a large-bore indwelling invasive venous cannula include infection, discomfort and risk for torrential venous bleeding if pulled out by an agitated or otherwise disgruntled patient. Maintaining strict aseptic procedures during TPN delivery is fundamental.

It is important to appreciate that fluid and electrolyte disturbance is more likely with enteral nutrition, and yet more probable still with parenteral nutrition. Both delivery routes carry the risk for refeeding syndrome; careful monitoring of the patient's serum electrolytes and fluid balance is mandatory.

Pathophysiology of refeeding syndrome

Institution of enteral or parenteral nutrition to malnourished or severely ill patients may cause a constellation of metabolic disturbances collectively referred to as 'refeeding syndrome', particularly if negligible nutrition has been assimilated for 5 days or longer.

Nutrient level rise provokes insulin secretion. This stimulates the synthesis of glycogen, lipid and protein. These intracellular processes require micronutrients such as magnesium, phosphate and B vitamins; these are extracted in large quantities from the serum, lowering their serum concentrations. Na^+/K^+ adenosine triphosphatase (ATPase) stimulation by insulin promotes intracellular diversion of serum potassium, leading to serum hypokalaemia. The clinical features of refeeding syndrome arise due to consequences of the reduction in serum concentration of potassium, magnesium and phosphate.

Chapter Summary

- A typical amino acid molecule consists of a common structural skeleton with a side chain conferring different chemical properties. Amino acids are important functional precursors of many important hormones and neurotransmitters, as well as being components of all proteins.
- Amino acids are categorized according to whether dietary intake is mandatory: these are the 'essential' amino acids where no endogenous synthetic mechanism exists, in contrast to the 'nonessential' amino acids.
- Oxidative deamination and transamination are key amino acid reaction mechanisms. The γ-glutamyl cycle, involving glutathione, is an important mode of amino acid transport across membranes separating intracellular compartments.
- Protein structure is determined by the primary, secondary, tertiary and quaternary structure. Different intermolecular chemical bond types underpin each of these structural components.
- Protein synthesis includes distinct phases: transcription, translation and posttranslational modifications.
- Protein–energy malnutrition has various causes and metabolic consequences. Two important subtypes are marasmus and kwashiorkor.
- Enteral and total parenteral nutrition are therapeutic mechanisms to main energy intake when the usual oral ingestion route is unsafe or compromised. Each has specific indications and associated risks.

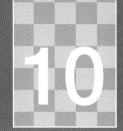

ONE-CARBON TRANSFER

In biochemistry, functional groups containing a single carbon atom (one-carbon 'units'; e.g. a methyl (–CH$_3$) group) are extremely reactive. However, numerous metabolic pathways rely on their transfer between molecules. This transfer of one-carbon units is described as 'one-carbon transfer'. One-carbon units depend on association with specific carrier molecules to 'shepherd' them between reactant molecules as part of biochemical reaction. These one-carbon carriers 'accept' or temporarily incorporate the one-carbon unit into their own molecular structure, and then 'donate' the one-carbon unit to a recipient molecule. The most important biochemical examples of one-carbon carrier molecules are folate (vitamin B9) and S-adenosyl methionine (SAM).

Key one-carbon transfer molecules: folate

Folate is converted to 5,6,7,8-tetrahydrofolate (THF) by two consecutive reduction reactions, which are both catalysed by dihydrofolate reductase (DHFR). THF is the bioactive derivative, which is pivotal in one-carbon transfer.

THF accepts and donates one-carbon units. These bind to its nitrogen atoms at position N^5, N^{10} or both positions, to form the compounds listed in Table 10.1. The one-carbon units transferred from other molecules are then donated on to other metabolic intermediates.

All the one-carbon/THF compounds are interconvertible, except N^5-methyl-THF (starred). Once this compound has sequestered (or 'trapped') THF, the only release mechanism to free up the THF (for further participation in one-carbon transfers) is known as the methionine salvage pathway. It 'salvages' (regenerates) THF from the otherwise unconvertible N^5-methyl-THF (also known as 'methylfolate').

Table 10.1 Compounds formed by combinations of tetrahydrofolate with various one-carbon-units

One-carbon unit	Compound
–CH=NH	N^5-formimino-THF
–CHO	N^5-formyl-THF
–CHO	N^{10}-formyl-THF
=CH–	N^5-N^{10}-methenyl-THF
–CH$_2$–	N^5-N^{10}-methylene-THF
–CH$_3$–	N^5-methyl-THF also known as 'methylfolate'

THF, Tetrahydrofolate.

The responsible enzyme is methionine synthase (MS). Methionine is synthesized from homocysteine during THF regeneration, hence the 'methionine' part of the name 'methionine salvage pathway'. This enzyme requires vitamin B12 (in the form of methylcobalamin) as a cofactor. Release of THF from the 'methylfolate trap' is therefore ultimately dependent on the availability of vitamin B12.

Folate role in nucleotide synthesis

The methylation of deoxyuridylate (an important step in thymidine synthesis) requires THF. Any physiological process involving high rates of cell division is thus dependent on sufficient folate availability. Examples include:

- Growth (childhood and adolescence)
- Pregnancy
- Fetal development
- Haemopoiesis
- Epithelial surface maintenance

Abnormalities of folate metabolism will often manifest clinically with symptoms related to impairment of these processes.

Methotrexate: a folate antagonist

Methotrexate is a folate analogue that exhibits a 1000-fold greater affinity for DHFR than its normal substrate (folate). It is therefore defined as a DHFR inhibitor. Competitively inhibiting folate's bioactivation results in impaired synthesis of key molecules required for nucleotide synthesis. This has the greatest impact on cell populations undergoing rapid division, that is, those with the greatest requirement for available nucleotides (e.g. neoplastic cells). This mechanism of action does, however, also confer the adverse side effect of impairing normal cell populations typically engaged in rapid division, accounting for many of methotrexate's side effects.

Key one-carbon transfer molecules: vitamin B12

Vitamin B12 plays an equally crucial role in nucleotide synthesis via its role in THF regeneration (a vital aspect of folate metabolism). As methylcobalamin, B12 is necessary for regeneration of THF from the inactive form (methylfolate), frequently formed during one-carbon transfer.

Methionine synthase

MS is a critical methyltransferase within the methionine salvage pathway (Fig. 10.1). MS activity relies on presence of vitamin B12 (in the form of methylcobalamin) as a cofactor. MS/B12 mediates transfer of the methyl group from 5-methyl-THF to homocysteine, regenerating THF and synthesizing methionine. This reaction (and thus both THF regeneration and methionine synthesis) is inhibited during vitamin B12 deficiency (see Chapter 12).

Key one-carbon transfer molecules: S-adenosyl methionine

SAM is a methyl group donor necessary for methylation of RNA, DNA, proteins and catecholamines (see Fig. 9.13). SAM is synthesized by a condensation reaction between methionine and adenosine triphosphate (ATP).

PURINES AND PYRIMIDINES: AN OVERVIEW

Purines and pyrimidines comprise the two main groups of nitrogenous bases. These bases are the molecular building blocks of nucleic acids and are thus essential for normal transcription (RNA synthesis) and maintenance of genomic integrity (DNA replication and repair).

Purines consist of a six-atom 'pyrimidine' component fused to a five-atom imidazole ring. Pyrimidines are heterocyclic aromatic compounds (similar to benzene) that contain two nitrogen atoms at positions 1 and 3 of the six-atom ring.

The amino acids glutamine, glycine and aspartate are all required for purine and pyrimidine synthesis. Purines are also obtained directly from the diet, featuring in particularly high concentrations in meat and offal. Plant-based diets are typically low in purines.

PURINE METABOLISM

Purine structure

Purines include the nitrogenous bases *adenine, guanine* and *hypoxanthine* (Fig. 10.2). Purines can exist as these 'free bases' or with an associated pentose sugar (ribose or deoxyribose) attached at the N^9 position. When associated with the pentose, the purine is referred to as a nucleoside as follows:

- adenine + ribose = adenosine
- guanine + ribose = guanosine
- hypoxanthine + ribose = inosine

Phosphorylation of the ribose at the C5 position converts the nucleoside to a nucleotide. The number of phosphate groups defines whether this is a 'mono', 'di' or 'tri' nucleotide (e.g. adenosine + 3 inorganic phosphate (P_i) = ATP, a trinucleotide).

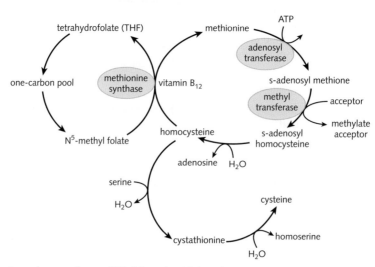

Fig. 10.1 The methionine salvage pathway. *ATP,* Adenosine triphosphate.

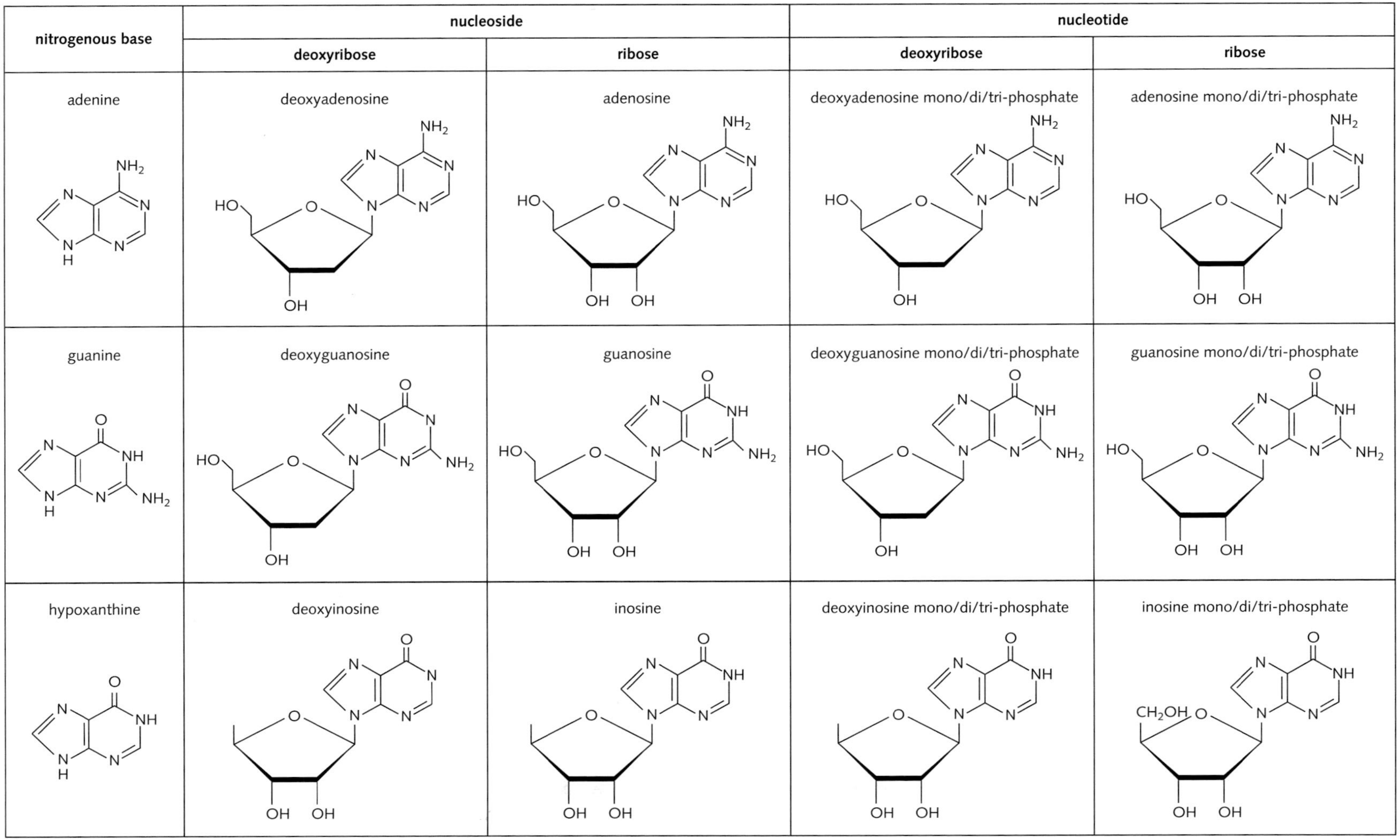

Fig. 10.2 Purines: adenine, guanine and hypoxanthine. Each is pictured with its corresponding nucleoside and nucleotide.

Purines: physiological function

Purines are required for DNA and RNA synthesis (as key components of nucleotides). They are also important in enzyme regulation and cell signalling.

Purine de novo synthesis

Purines are synthesized as mononucleotides rather than free bases. This occurs in hepatocyte cytoplasm in two stages:

1. Formation of inosine monophosphate (IMP)
2. Conversion of IMP to adenosine monophosphate (AMP) or guanosine monophosphate (GMP)

Formation of inosine monophosphate

Adenine, guanine and hypoxanthine are derived from the nucleotide IMP. IMP is the first compound in the pathway to possess a fully formed purine ring.

IMP synthesis requires ribose phosphate (derived from the pentose phosphate pathway) as the primary substrate. This is progressively transformed in a complex pathway (Fig. 10.3) consisting of multiple reactions:

- First, ribose phosphate pyrophosphokinase catalyses the phosphorylation of ribose-5-phosphate at the C1 position, forming 5-phosphoribosyl-1-pyrophosphate (PRPP).
- Second, PRPP amidotransferase catalyses conversion of PRPP to 5-phosphoribosylamine. This is the irreversible rate-limiting step of the pathway.
- Remaining reactions construct the purine ring by incorporation of five carbon and four nitrogen atoms (in total). Please see Fig. 10.3 for the details.

Note that the incorporated C and N atoms are derived from various sources including glycine, glutamine, N^{10}-formyl THF and carbon dioxide.

Conversion of IMP to AMP or GMP

Inosine 5′-monophosphate (IMP) represents a metabolic juncture in purine synthesis as it can be diverted towards formation of either AMP or GMP (Fig 10.4).

Conversion of IMP to GMP first entails an oxidation (employing nicotinamide adenine dinucleotide (NAD^+) as a redox partner) to xanthosine monophosphate. This is followed by an ATP-dependent incorporation of an amino group derived from glutamine. This synthesis is inhibited by GMP, the pathway product.

Conversion of IMP to AMP is guanosine triphosphate dependent, and occurs via formation of adenylosuccinate. Aspartate is converted to fumarate during AMP formation. AMP, the pathway product, inhibits the pathway. Similarly, conversion of IMP to GMP is ATP dependent, with xanthine monophosphate as an intermediate.

Purine synthesis via the salvage pathway

When nucleic acids or nucleotides are catabolized, free bases are released. The salvage pathways recycle these free bases. A ribose-5′-phosphate is derived from PRPP (Fig. 10.5). This reaction is essentially irreversible (highly exergonic), because pyrophosphate is released. Two enzymes are responsible:

- Adenine phosphoribosyl transferase, which salvages adenine, yielding AMP
- Hypoxanthine guanine phosphoribosyl transferase (HGPRT), which salvages guanine, xanthine and hypoxanthine yielding GMP, IMP and IMP, respectively

Each enzyme is starred in Figs 10.3 or 10.4. Salvage of bases is more energy efficient than de novo synthesis, and over 90% purines are synthesized via salvage. Genetic deficiency/absence of the HGPRT enzyme results in failure of purine salvage and manifests with Lesch–Nyhan syndrome. Note that PRPP participates in de novo purine synthesis, purine salvage and the pyrimidine synthesis pathways.

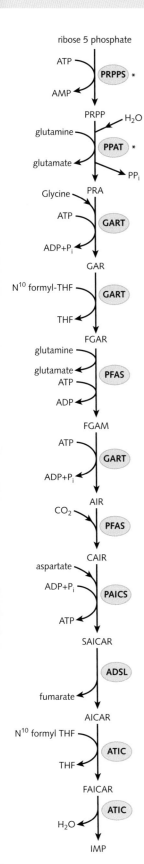

Fig. 10.3 De novo purine synthesis. This commences with ribose phosphate (derived from the pentose phosphate pathway) and ends with IMP. *Starred* enzymes represent regulation points. *ADP,* Adenosine diphosphate; *AMP,* adenosine monophosphate; *ADP,* adenosine monophosphate; *ATP,* adenosine triphosphate; *P$_i$,* inorganic phosphate; *PP$_i$,* inorganic pyrophosphate; *THF,* tetrahydrofolate. Intermediates: *AICAR,* 5-aminoimidazole-4-carboxamide ribonucleotide; *AIR,* aminoimidazole ribotide; *CAIR,* 5′-phosphoribosyl-4-carboxy-5-aminoimidazole; *FAICAR,* 5-formamidoimidazole-4-carboxamide ribotide; *FGAM,* 5′-phosphoribosylformylglycinamidine; *FGAR,* phosphoribosyl-N-formylglycineamide; *GAR,* glycinamide ribonucleotide; *IMP,* inosine monophosphate; *PRA,* 5′ phosphoribosylamine; *PRPP,* phosphoribosyl pyrophosphate; *SAICAR,* phosphoribosyl aminoimidazole succinocarboxamide. For molecular structure of IMP, please see Fig. 10.2. Enzymes: *ADSL,* Adenylosuccinate lyase; *ATIC,* 5-amino 4-carboxy amide ribonucleotide formyl transferase; *GART,* phosphoribosyl glycinamide synthetase; *PAICS,* phosphoribosyl-aminoimidazole carboxylase; *PFAS,* phosphoribosylformylglycinamide synthase; *PPAT,* phosphoribosylpyrophosphate amidotransferase; *PRPPS,* PRPP synthetase.

LESCH–NYAN SYNDROME

This is a rare genetic disease (X-linked disorder) arising from deficient/absent hypoxanthine guanine phosphoribosyl transferase (HGPRT), the purine 'salvage' enzyme responsible for purine recycling. This leads to:

- Hyperuricaemia (secondary to elevated guanine and hypoxanthine), clinically manifesting with symptoms and signs of gout.
- Increased (5-phosphoribosyl-1-pyrophosphate), which is inappropriately diverted towards de novo overproduction of purines. Excess purines cause severe neuropsychiatric disturbances.

Symptoms typically become apparent at ~3 months of age, often heralded by orange urate precipitates seen in the infant's nappies. Hyperuricaemia accompanied by low cellular HGPRT supports the diagnosis. Affected individuals are male due to the heredity pattern – females typically act as silent carriers, though may experience gout in adulthood. Sadly, the prognosis is poor with death usually due to renal failure in the first to second decade of life.

Regulation of purine synthesis

Purine synthesis is regulated at four points in the pathway:

1. PRPP synthetase: inhibited by GMP and AMP
2. PRPP amidotransferase: inhibited by IMP, AMP and GMP
3. Adenylosuccinate lyase: inhibited by AMP
4. IMP dehydrogenase: inhibited by GMP

Dysregulation of purine synthesis arising secondary to deficiency/absence of any of these four regulatory enzymes results in overproduction of the pathway products AMP and GMP.

Purine catabolism

Purines are initially interconverted to either xanthine or hypoxanthine (Fig. 10.6). These intermediates are further metabolized by xanthine oxidase (XO).

Catabolism of hypoxanthine and xanthine to urate

XO mediates catabolism of hypoxanthine to xanthine, followed by xanthine conversion to urate. XO is an unusual flavoprotein, containing both molybdenum and iron ions. It uses molecular oxygen as an oxidizing agent, generating hydrogen peroxide:

1. Hypoxanthine + H_2O + O_2 → xanthine + H_2O_2
2. Xanthine + H_2O + O_2 → uric acid + H_2O_2

Urate

In humans, urate travels in the bloodstream, and is excreted in urine. The acidic pH of urine allows it to precipitate out at high concentrations as sodium urate. Hyperuricaemia (high serum urate) may lead to gout.

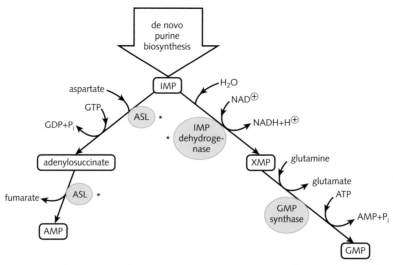

Fig. 10.4 Conversion of inosine monophosphate (IMP) to adenosine monophosphate (AMP) or guanosine monophosphate (GMP). For molecular structure of IMP, AMP, GMP and xanthosine monophosphate (XMP), please see Fig. 10.2. *Starred enzymes represent regulation points. ASL,* Adenylosuccinate lyase; *GDP,* guanosine diphosphate; *GTP,* guanosine triphosphate; *NAD+,* nicotinamide adenine dinucleotide; P_i, inorganic phosphate.

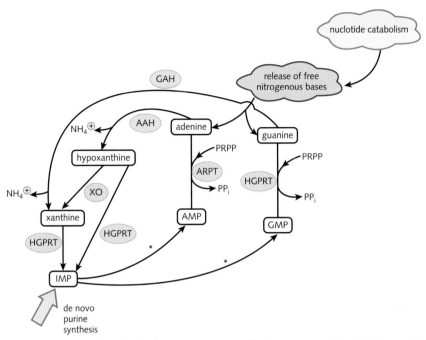

Fig. 10.5 Purine salvage pathways. For details of de novo purine synthesis, please see Fig. 10.3. For details of the reaction sequences IMP → AMP and IMP → GMP (indicated by *starred arrows*), please see Fig. 10.4. *AAH*, Adenine aminohydrolase; *AMP*, adenosine monophosphate; *ARPT*, adenine phosphoribosyltransferase; *GAH*, guanine aminohydrolase; *GMP*, guanosine monophosphate; *HGPRT*, hypoxanthine/guanine phosphoribosyl transferase; *IMP*, inosine monophosphate; *PP$_i$*, inorganic pyrophosphate; *PRPP*, 5′-phosphoribosyl-1-pyrophosphate, *XO*, xanthine oxidase.

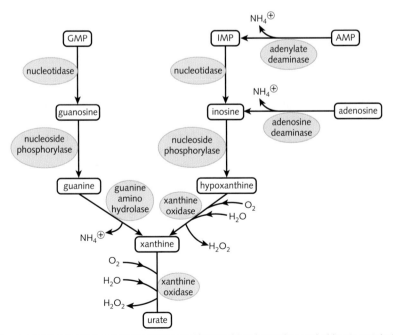

Fig. 10.6 Purine interconversion leading to hypoxanthine and/or xanthine formation and ultimate catabolism to urate. *AMP*, Adenosine monophosphate; *GMP*, guanosine monophosphate; *IMP*, inosine monophosphate.

GOUT

Gout describes the clinical manifestations of sodium urate crystals deposition in soft tissues, joints and the kidney. It arises in the context of hyperuricaemia; however, many people have asymptomatic hyperuricemia: no crystals are deposited, so no symptoms of gout develop.

Hyperuricaemia

Pathological sodium urate deposition occurs in the context of extreme or prolonged elevation of serum urate (hyperuricaemia). Elevated serum urate arises via one of two basic mechanisms discussed in the following sections.

Inadequate urate excretion

This mechanism accounts for the bulk of symptomatic hyperuricaemia (i.e. symptoms of gout). Renal insufficiency, of any cause, results in hyperuricaemia. Metabolic syndrome also consists of multiple pathological conditions that predispose to inadequate urate excretion. Drugs too are common culprits. Acute precipitants of renal impairment include acidosis, ketosis, starvation and dehydration. Finally, lead and alcohol directly impair renal urate excretion.

> **CLINICAL NOTES**
>
> METABOLIC SYNDROME
>
> This syndrome consists of different combinations of obesity, insulin resistance, dyslipidaemia, hypertension, hyperuricaemia and places individuals at high risk for atherosclerotic events.

> **HINTS AND TIPS**
>
> DRUGS CAUSING IMPAIRED RENAL URATE EXCRETION
>
> This includes thiazide and loop diuretics, low-dose aspirin, cyclosporine, pyrazinamide and L-DOPA.

Excessive urate production

Various diverse factors may cause an increase in urate production to pathological levels. All operate via one of the following mechanism:

- High dietary purine intake leads to physiological hyperuricaemia.
- Rapid cell turnover (e.g. haemolysis, lymph/myeloproliferative disease)
- High rates of cell death (e.g. shock, extensive injury/burns/surgery, rhabdomyolysis)

> **HINTS AND TIPS**
>
> PURINE-RICH FOODS
>
> These include meat (red meat > poultry), high-fructose food, seafood, beer and distilled spirits.

Rare genetic enzyme abnormalities

Genetic causes are only responsible for a tiny minority of cases of hyperuricaemia. Excessive de novo purine synthesis leads to increased purine catabolism. This generates high levels of urate. Excessive purine synthesis may arise secondary to various enzyme abnormalities including:

- PRPP synthetase (excessive activity)
- PRPP amidotransferase (resistant to inhibition → overactive)
- HGPRT (underactivity that may be extreme (e.g. Lesch–Nyhan syndrome) or mild)

Clinical manifestations

Crystal arthropathy

Within joints, urate deposition represents a 'crystal arthropathy'. A single joint, most often the first metatarsophalangeal joint, becomes acutely red, hot and swollen secondary to the acute inflammatory response to crystal deposits. It is extremely painful. Chronic recurrent gouty arthritis causes permanent structural damage to joints.

Soft tissue urate deposition

Red, hot, swollen and painful inflammatory masses develop acutely at sites of tissue deposition. Chronically, tophus formation occurs (Fig. 10.7). Whiteish-yellow crystals may be visible within these focal, intradermal nodular masses.

Kidney and urinary tract

In the kidney urate precipitation in renal tubules causes urate nephropathy, which can lead to acute and chronic renal impairment. Conversely, renal impairment may also *cause* hyperuricaemia. Urinary tract formation of urate stones is also a feature of hyperuricaemia.

Gout treatment

Treatment must incorporate both symptomatic relief of pain and inflammation (usually short-term nonsteroidal antiinflammatory drugs and/or colchicine) and management of raised serum urate.

Weight loss, alcohol intake reduction, low-purine diet and cessation of contributory medications are likely to be effective. The main drugs used are allopurinol and probenecid (which impairs tubular urate reabsorption, promoting urinary urate loss).

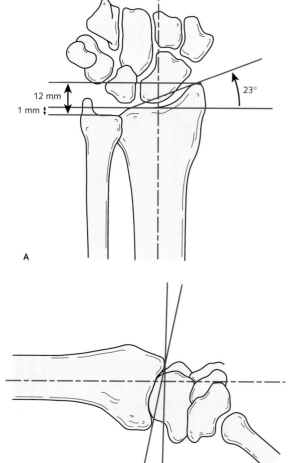

12 mm

1 mm

23°

A

11°

B

Fig. 10.7 Gouty tophi. Note the erythematous overlying skin, which in some areas has broken down to reveal the yellow underlying crystal deposits.

Allopurinol

Treatment with XO inhibitors decreases urate formation, consequently increasing levels of the soluble precursors hypoxanthine and xanthine, which are easily excreted in the urine. Allopurinol, a hypoxanthine analogue, is the most commonly used, with multiple mechanisms of action:

- It competitively inhibits XO by posing as a substrate analogue. Allopurinol ribonucleotide is formed by XO-mediated addition of ribose-5-phosphate.
- Allopurinol ribonucleotide inhibits PRPP amidotransferase, decreasing de novo purine synthesis.
- Allopurinol can be metabolized by XO to oxypurinol, a more potent XO inhibitor.

PYRIMIDINES

Pyrimidine structure

There are three important pyrimidines: *thymine, cytosine* and *uracil* (Fig. 10.8). Note that these are the names of the free bases. When associated with an N1-linked five-carbon sugar, they are referred to as the nucleosides thymidine, cytidine and uridine. When phosphorylated, nucleosides are referred to as nucleotides (uridine triphosphate (UTP), cytidine triphosphate (CTP) and thymidine triphosphate (TTP)).

Pyrimidine function

Pyrimidines, in combination with purines, are vital components of nucleotides and thus mandatory for RNA and DNA synthesis. Thymidine does not feature in RNA; in RNA the adenine pairs with the uracil. Pyrimidine nucleotide derivatives also function as activated intermediates in numerous synthetic reactions. A typical example is the uridine diphosphate (UDP) component of UDP–glucose (see Chapter 5).

Pyrimidines: de novo synthesis

There are three main stages in pyrimidine biosynthesis:

1. Assembly of the pyrimidine ring during UMP synthesis
2. Conversion of UMP to UTP or CTP Deoxyribonucleotide formation (deoxycytidine triphosphate (dCTP) and deoxythymidine triphosphate (dTTP)) follows

Assembly of the pyrimidine ring (UMP formation)

Unlike purine synthesis, the pyrimidine ring is assembled prior to attachment of ribose-5-phosphate. Pyrimidines are synthesised form as free bases, derived from bicarbonate, glutamine, aspartate and CO_2. There are six steps in the reaction sequence (Fig. 10.9).

1. Carbamoyl phosphate synthase II catalyses formation of carbamoyl phosphate from CO_2, ATP and glutamine.
2. Carbamoyl phosphate is conjugated to aspartate, producing N-carbamoylaspartate.
3. The ring structure is 'closed', forming dihydroorotate. Dihydroorotate contains a six-membered ring, with nitrogen and carbon atoms located in their final positions in the mature pyrimidine ring.
4. Oxidation of the dihydroorotate ring, forming a C=C double bond and creating an orotate ring. This reaction is catalysed by dihydroorotate dehydrogenase, which is a mitochondrial enzyme tethered to the inner mitochondrial membrane. This is, however, the only reaction that occurs away from the cytoplasm.

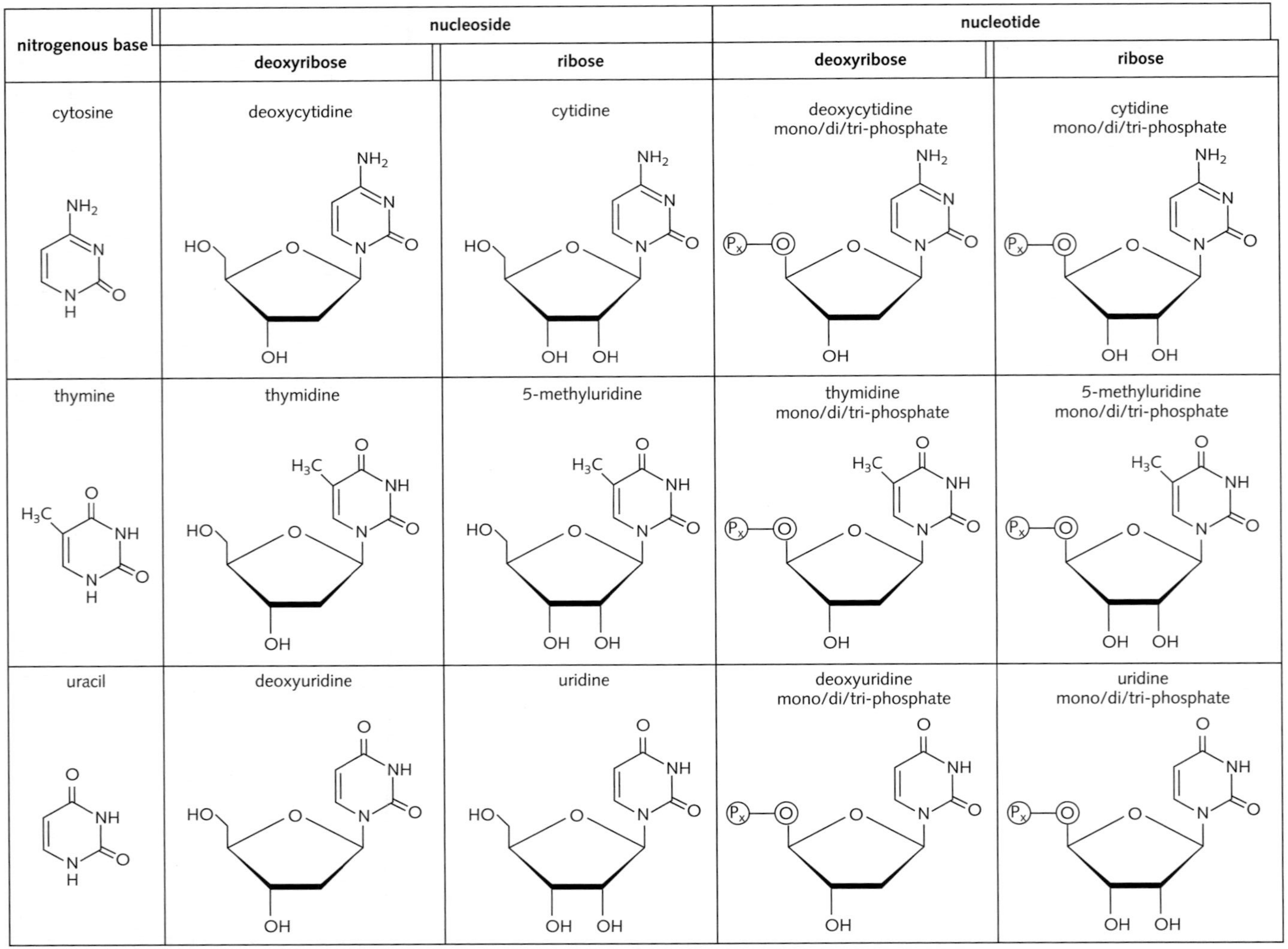

Fig. 10.8 Pyrimidine bases. Each is pictured with its corresponding nucleoside and nucleotide. P_x represents a single phosphate group (monophosphate), a pair of phosphate groups (diphosphate) or three phosphate groups (triphospate).

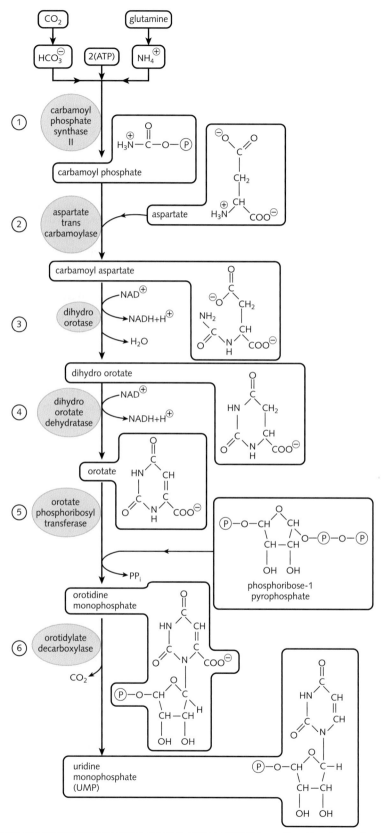

Fig. 10.9 De novo synthesis of pyrimidines: uridine monophosphate (UMP) formation. Numbers refer to the text (see the 'Assembly of the pyrimidine ring (UMP formation)' section). *NAD+*, nicotinamide adenine dinucleotide.

5. The orotate ring is transferred to the phosphoribosyl component of PRPP, forming orotidylate.
6. Orotidylate undergoes decarboxylation, yielding UMP.

Conversion of UMP to UTP, dCTP and dTTP

A typical cell contains 5 to 10 times more RNA than DNA. Most nucleotide biosynthesis is therefore ribonucleotide (ribonucleoside triphosphate) rather than deoxyribonucleotide (deoxyribonucleoside triphosphate) production. Fig. 10.10 illustrates conversion of UMP to UTP, and the subsequent conversion of UTP to CTP.

Background DNA repair is continuous, and during proliferation active replication of DNA occurs. A pool of available pyrimidine nucleotides needs to be permanently available (i.e. dTTP and dCTP). Fig. 10.10 illustrates the de novo synthesis of these pyrimidine nucleotides from the initial substrate UMP (UMP generation shown in Fig. 10.9).

Regulation of pyrimidine synthesis

The rate-limiting step of pyrimidine synthesis is the formation of carbamoyl phosphate by carbamoyl phosphate synthase II. This reaction is activated by ATP and PRPP, and conversely inhibited by UDP and UTP. This regula-tion ensures that a balanced supply of purines and pyrimidines exists for RNA synthesis.

Pyrimidine synthesis via the salvage pathway

Salvage pathways allow conservation of energy, because it is more energetically costly to synthesize de novo UMP than it is to obtain UMP via salvage pathways (Fig. 10.11). Pyrimidine salvage is similar to purine salvage in that free bases (pyrimidine in this case, i.e. thymine, cytosine and uracil) are released from the break down of nucleotides and are then converted into dTMP or UMP. These can then convert (as per Fig. 10.11) into dTTP, dCTP, UTP and CTP *without* requiring the energetically expensive de novo synthesis to form UMP (Fig. 10.10).

Pyrimidine catabolism

Unlike purines, the pyrimidine ring may be broken down into soluble components. Uracil and cytosine are broken down to β-alanine, which can be converted to acetyl-coenzyme A (acetyl-CoA). Thymine is reductively degraded to β-aminoisobutyrate (which forms succinyl-CoA) or oxidatively converted to malonate. These 'carbon skeletons' of pyrimidine catabolism (acetyl CoA, succinyl CoA and malonate) can enter the tricarboxylic acid (TCA) cycle (Fig. 10.12).

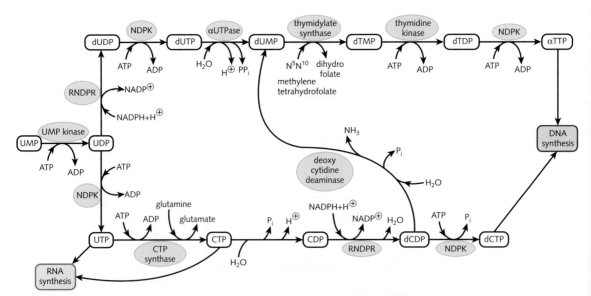

Fig. 10.10 Conversion of uridine monophosphate (UMP) to: uridine triphosphate (UTP), deoxycytidine triphosphate (dCTP) and deoxythymidine triphosphate (dTTP). *ADP*, Adenosine diphosphate; *ATP*, adenosine triphosphate; *CDP*, cytidine diphosphate; *CTP*, cytosine triphosphate; *dCDP*, deoxycytidine diphosphate; *dTDP*, deoxythymidine diphosphate; *dTMP*, deoxythymidine monophosphate; *dUDP*, deoxyuridine diphosphate; *dUMP*, deoxyuridine monophosphate; *NDPK*, nucleoside diphosphate kinase; *PP$_i$*, inorganic pyrophosphate; *RNDPR*, ribonucleoside diphosphate reductase; *UDP*, uridine diphosphate; *UTPase*, uridine triphosphatase. For UMP synthesis, please see Fig. 10.9.

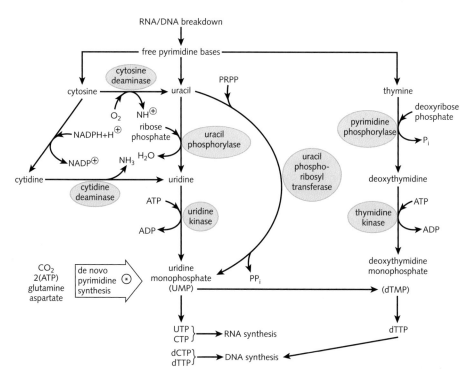

Fig. 10.11 Pyrimidine salvage. For details of de novo pyrimidine synthesis (ringed star), please see Fig. 10.9. For details of conversion of uridine monophosphate (UMP) to UTP, cytosine triphosphate (CTP), deoxycytidine triphosphate (dCTP) and deoxythymidine triphosphate (dTTP; *starred arrows*), please see Fig. 10.10. *ADP,* Adenosine diphosphate; *ATP,* adenosine triphosphate; *NADP⁺,* nicotinamide adenine dinucleotide phosphate; *Pᵢ,* inorganic phosphate; *PRPP,* 5-phosphoribosyl-1-pyrophosphate; *TMP,* thymidine monophosphate.

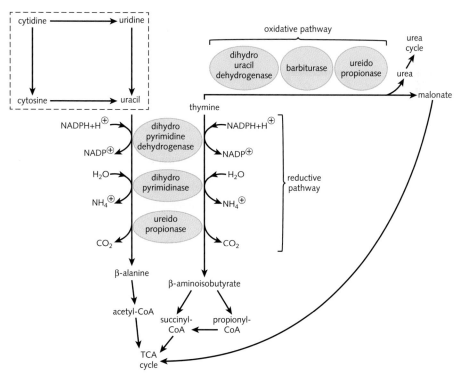

Fig. 10.12 Pyrimidine catabolism. For clarity the intermediate reactions between uracil and β-alanine and thymine and β-aminoisobutyrate are shown as a *single arrow* with their responsible enzymes. For details of the reactions within the *dotted box* please refer to Fig. 10.11. *CoA,* Coenzyme A; *NADP⁺,* nicotinamide adenine dinucleotide phosphate; *TCA,* tricarboxylic acid.

HAEM

Haem is a prosthetic group that functions as a key component of numerous proteins. Haem confers the parent molecule with diverse physiological functions, such as the ability to participate in redox reactions, electron transfer and even diatomic gas transfer. The most well-known haem-containing protein is haemoglobin. The haem component of the component globin chains endows haemoglobin with the ability to reversibly bind molecular oxygen, which is necessary for red cells to fulfil their oxygen transport role.

Structure

Chemically speaking, haem is an iron porphyrin. Haem consists of a ferrous (Fe^{2+}) iron ion located centrally within a protoporphyrin molecule. The protoporphyrin molecule consists of four pyrrole rings, interlinked by methene bridges. This structure is known as a 'tetrapyrrole ring'. The ferrous ion is bonded to each of four N atoms, one from each pyrrole ring. It is also able to bind additional components (e.g. molecular oxygen in the case of haemoglobin) at its fifth and sixth coordination sites (Fig. 10.13).

Haem synthesis

About 40 to 50 mg/day of haem is endogenously synthesized, of which 80% to 85% is incorporated into haemoglobin synthesis during erythropoiesis. Haem biosynthesis occurs partially in the mitochondria and partially in the cytoplasm. The substrates for haem synthesis are glycine and succinyl-CoA. The synthetic pathway (Fig. 10.14) is as follows:

1. δ-Aminolevulinic acid (δ-ALA) synthesis: This is catalysed by δ-ALA synthase and occurs in the mitochondria. Eight molecules of glycine and eight molecules of succinyl-CoA condense to form eight molecules of δ-ALA. This reaction is rate limiting and thus represents a regulation point. Vitamin B6 (pyridoxal phosphate) is required as a cofactor.
2. Porphobilinogen formation: Mitochondrially synthesized δ-ALA is exported to the cytoplasm, where the enzyme ALA dehydratase dimerizes two δ-ALA molecules, forming porphobilinogen.
3. Uroporphyrinogen I formation: Four porphobilinogen molecules are condensed into the linear tetrapyrrole intermediate, uroporphyrinogen I. This is catalysed by uroporphyrinogen I synthase.
4. Uroporphyrinogen III formation: Uroporphyrinogen I is converted to uroporphyrinogen III by uroporphyrinogen III synthase.
5. Coproporphyrinogen III synthesis: The acetate moieties of uroporphyrinogen III are all decarboxylated by uroporphyrinogen decarboxylase. The resultant product (coproporphyrinogen III) therefore features methyl groups in place of acetate.
6. Protoporphyrinogen IX formation: Coproporphyrinogen III is imported into the mitochondrial interior. The oxygen-dependent enzyme coproporphyrinogen III oxidase decarboxylates the two propionate residues, resulting in vinyl moiety incorporation to the two pyrrole rings. The product is protoporphyrinogen IX.
7. Protoporphyrin IX formation: Protoporphyrinogen IX is converted to protoporphyrin IX by protoporphyrinogen IX oxidase. The conjugated ring system is now fully intact.
8. Haem synthesis: The final reaction involves the insertion of the ferrous iron (Fe^{2+}) atom into the ring system. This is catalysed by ferrochelatase, generating haem.

Each number is illustrated in Fig. 10.14.

Regulation of haem metabolism

Although haem is synthesized in virtually all tissues, the principal sites of synthesis are erythroblasts in the bone marrow (~85%) and hepatocytes (~15%). Environmental differences between these two tissues result in different regulatory mechanisms of haem biosynthesis.

Hepatocytes

In hepatocytes, haem is required for incorporation into cytochromes, in particular the P450 superfamily of cytochromes (CYP) that are pivotal in detoxification of assimilated ingested substances and drug metabolism.

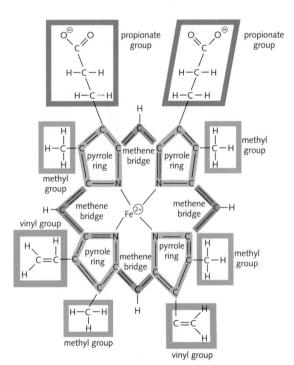

Fig. 10.13 Structure of haem.

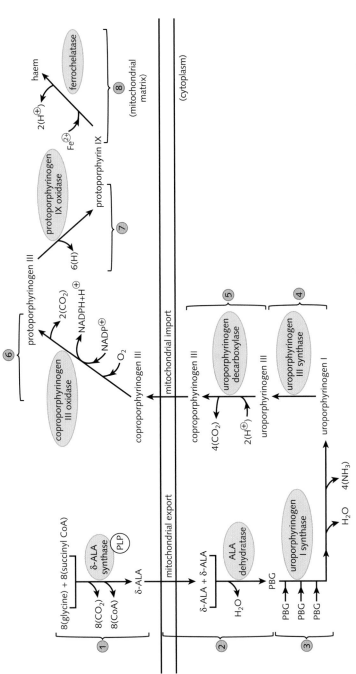

Fig. 10.14 Haem synthesis. The numbers refer to the text. *CoA*, Coenzyme A; *NADP*[+], nicotinamide adenine dinucleotide phosphate; *PBG*, porphobilinogen; *PLP*, pyridoxal phosphate; *δ-ALA*, delta-aminolaevulinic acid.

The rate-limiting step in hepatic haem biosynthesis occurs at δ-ALA synthase (Fig. 10.14). Haem inhibits δ-ALA synthase gene expression. Hemin (haem with a ferric (oxidized, Fe^{3+}) iron ion, rather than a ferrous (Fe^{2+}) iron ion) allosterically inhibits δ-ALA synthase and inhibits mitochondrial import of the enzyme from its site of synthesis in the cytoplasm.

Red blood cells

In developing red blood cells, haem is synthesized exclusively for incorporation into haemoglobin. In contrast to hepatic control of haem biosynthesis, in red cells numerous additional sites are regulation points (in addition to δ-ALA synthase) including ferrochelatase and on uroporphyrinogen I synthase.

Haem catabolism

The largest source of haem in the human body is located within red blood cells as a component of haemoglobin. There is a daily turnover of approximately 6 g of haemoglobin. Breakdown of the protein globin components is straightforward; the peptide bonds are hydrolysed and amino acids in turn are recycled or catabolized as required. The haem moiety, however, presents two challenges:

1. The porphyrin ring is hydrophobic and must be rendered soluble for excretion.
2. The iron must be recycled for further haem synthesis.

Senescent red blood cells are consumed by macrophages of the reticuloendothelial system. Haem is oxidized by haem oxygenase, linearizing the tetrapyrrole ring structure and cleaving one of the methene bridges in a reaction that yields carbon monoxide (Fig. 10.15). This is the only reaction in the body that is known to produce carbon monoxide. The other reaction products are biliverdin (a blue-green pigment) and iron (oxidized to a ferric ion). In the following reaction, a further methene bridge (between rings III and IV) is reduced by biliverdin reductase, producing bilirubin (a yellow-red pigment).

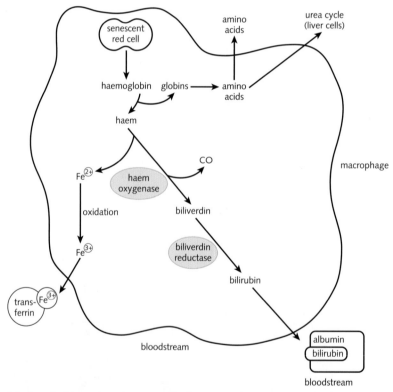

Fig. 10.15 Haem catabolism. In this context, 'senescent' refers to a red blood cell that is either nearing the end of its 120-day life or is damaged in some way and has therefore been engulfed by macrophages of the reticuloendothelial system. Note that one molecule of haemoglobin produces four globins and four haem moieties: only one is shown for clarity. Once released from the haem complex, ferrous iron is oxidized to ferric iron and transported in the bloodstream by transferrin. Amino acids from the dismantled globin molecules may be released into the blood for uptake by other cells and incorporation into new proteins.

Bilirubin

Bilirubin is nonpolar, lipophilic and is only sparingly soluble in aqueous solutions. Bilirubin travels from peripheral sites of catabolism (bound to albumin) to the liver. Here, within hepatocyte endoplasmic reticulum, bilirubin–UDP–glucuronyltransferase conjugates UDP–glucuronate to bilirubin. This produces the water-soluble bilirubin diglucuronide.

Conjugated bilirubin is secreted into the small intestine. Here, bilirubin undergoes bacterial metabolism and is converted to urobilinogen, stercobilinogen and stercobilin. The bulk of urobilinogen is reabsorbed, and renally excreted in urine. Some urobilinogen is converted to urobilin, imparting the yellow colour to urine. Stercobilinogen and stercobilin are excreted in faeces; the latter is a brownish pigment that imparts the characteristic colour to faeces (Fig. 10.16).

PORPHYRIAS

This group of predominantly genetic disorders arise from deficiency/absence of enzymes underpinning stages of haem synthesis (Table 10.2). This has two outcomes:

- Impaired haem synthesis
- Accumulation of upstream precursors

The specific array of precursors that accumulate is determined by the particular enzyme affected. Any failure of haem synthesis has the effect of lifting the negative feedback usually exerted on ALA synthase by haem. As it is the rate-limiting enzyme of haem synthesis, this pathologically *accelerates* pathway activity upstream to the deficient/absent enzyme, exacerbating the precursor accumulation.

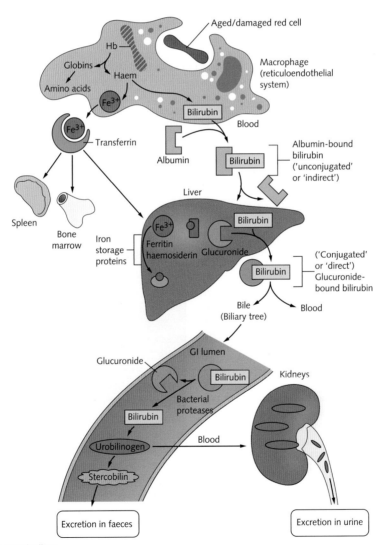

Fig. 10.16 Bilirubin metabolism.

Table 10.2 Clinical features of the porphyrias

Porphyria	Affected enzyme	Elevated parameters	Major symptoms	Inheritance
ALA-dehydratase porphyria	ALA-dehydratase (also known as 'porphobilinogen synthase')	Urinary ALA Urinary PBG	Abdominal pain Neuropsychiatric[a]	Autosomal recessive
Acute intermittent porphyria	Uroporphyrinogen I synthase	Urinary ALA Urinary PBG Red cell PBG deaminase	Abdominal pain Neuropsychiatric[a]	Autosomal dominant
Congenital erythropoietic porphyria	Uroporphyrinogen III cosynthase	Erythrocyte and urinary: uroporphyrin I, coproporphyrin I	Photosensitivity	Autosomal dominant
Porphyria cutanea tarda	Uroporphyrinogen decarboxylase	Faecal isocoproporphyrin Urinary 7-carboxylate, uroporphyrin I	Photosensitivity	Variable
Hereditary coproporphyria	Coproporphyrinogen III oxidase	Urinary ALA Urinary PBG Urinary coproporphyrin III Faecal coproporphyrin III	Abdominal pain Neuropsychiatric[a] Photosensitivity	Autosomal dominant
Variegate porphyria	Protoporphyrinogen IX oxidase	Urinary ALA Urinary PBG Urinary coproporphyrin III Faecal protoporphyrin IX	Abdominal pain Neuropsychiatric[a] Photosensitivity	Autosomal dominant
Erythropoietic protoporphyria (also known as 'protoporphyria')	Ferrochelatase	Urinary ALA Urinary PBG Faecal protoporphyrin IX Red cell protoporphyrin IX	Photosensitivity	Autosomal recessive

Shaded rows indicated the 'acute' porphyrias.
[a] Neuropsychiatric symptoms in this context can include depression, psychosis, anxiety and acute confusion.
ALA, Aminolaevulinic acid; PBG, porphobilinogen.

Clinical relevance of porphyrias

Diagnosis is challenging, because porphyrias are extremely uncommon, as well as typically causing intermittent symptoms interspersed with long symptom-free periods. Although they are genetic, they often arise as spontaneous mutations, in which case family history will be absent, further compounding the difficulty of diagnosis. Porphyrias may be classified as 'acute' or 'cutaneous'.

Acute porphyrias

Sufferers of the 'acute' porphyrias (acute intermittent porphyria, variegate porphyria, hereditary coproporphyria and ALA-dehydratase porphyria (ADP): see Table 10.2) are prone to acute attacks, which are often precipitated by drugs, fasting, stress or alcohol. The causative mechanism of neuropsychiatric symptoms is related to accumulation of neurotoxic porphobilinogen and ALA, in addition to the haem deficiency impairing the availability of haem-containing proteins. Several drugs may provoke an acute attack and must be avoided in known porphyria patients.

RED FLAG

Acute attack of porphyria. These occur in the acute porphyrias only. Severe abdominal pain, nausea, vomiting, constipation, abnormal behaviour, confusion occur commonly; muscular weakness and convulsions may occur rarely. Raised urinary porphobilinogen (at least 5-fold and up to 50-fold increase) and aminolevulinic acid confirm an acute attack. Classically, urine with elevated porphyrins may turn dark red or even purple on standing, fluorescing shows coral-red under ultraviolet light. Intravenous haem arginate addresses the biochemical haem deficit and attenuates precursor accumulation. Analgesia and antiemetics are usually needed for symptomatic relief. Early administration of carbohydrate (oral or intravenous) may attenuate an acute attack.

AVOIDANCE OF DRUGS PRECIPITATING ACUTE ATTACKS OF PORPHYRIAS

Commonplace culprits include alcohol, hormonal contraceptives and barbiturates. A list of drugs safe to prescribe in porphyrias can be accessed at www.drugs-porphyria.org.

Avoidance of hypoglycaemia in porphyria

A diet relatively high in carbohydrate (~60% of calories from carbohydrates) and avoidance of fasting are advised, because hypoglycaemia may provoke an acute attack. This is because hypoglycaemia activates peroxisome proliferator-activated receptor gamma coactivator 1-alpha (PGC-1α), a transcription factor that promotes the expression of various gluconeogenesis enzymes and δ-ALA synthase. In a normal individual, this is of little consequence; however, in porphyria the haem synthesis pathway is arrested at various locations, resulting in accumulation of upstream precursors. Enhanced δ-ALA synthase activity exacerbates this pathological precursor accumulation, increasing the likelihood of exceeding precursor levels above the symptom threshold.

Cutaneous porphyrias

Individuals with the 'cutaneous' porphyrias (congenital erythropoietic porphyria, porphyria cutanea tarda and erythropoietic protoporphyria: see Table 10.2 for abbreviations) experience blistering skin rashes. Photosensitivity is prominent, and these individuals must avoid sun exposure or limit skin exposure to ultraviolet (UV) light with high sun protection factor (SPF) and UVA protection sunblock. Variable extents of photosensitivity can also occur in many of the 'acute' porphyrias. The mechanism of photosensitivity is accumulation of porphyrinogens in skin, where they spontaneously oxidase to porphyrins.

LEAD POISONING

Lead poisoning usually develops gradually with chronic exposure. Children are particularly susceptible to lead poisoning and consequent irreversible neurological damage. It is difficult to diagnose as it may present with any of a wide range of (frequently nonspecific) symptoms.

POSSIBLE SIGNS AND SYMPTOMS OF LEAD POISONING

These are diverse and highly variable in their manifestation.

- Haematological: microcytic, sideroblastic anaemia
- Peripheral neuropathy (motor > sensory): numbness, paraesthesia, weakness
- Cognitive symptoms: memory impairment, fatigue, poor concentration
- Psychiatric symptoms: depression, anxiety
- Gastrointestinal symptoms: intermittent abdominal pain, constipation
- Disrupted bone metabolism
- Disrupted tooth structure: blue line along gum – 'Burton line'

Lead exposure

Skin contact, ingestion and inhalation are the main routes of lead accumulation. This is rare in the UK. Specific occupations carry risk for exposure and likewise soil and water contamination. Lead-based paint (no longer manufactured but still quite common to encounter where it has not been removed) can lead to lead accumulation with sustained skin contact. Lead water pipes are rarely still in use but present a significant risk for lead toxicity where they exist as drinking water conduits.

Pathophysiology

Lead inhibits three key enzymes of haem synthesis, resulting in the accumulation of intermediates:

- ALA dehydratase: ALA accumulation
- Coproporphyrinogen III oxidase: coproporphyrinogen III accumulation
- Ferrochelatase: erythrocyte accumulation of protoporphyrin IX

Impaired haem synthesis manifests clinically with symptoms and signs of anaemia, which is microcytic. Failure of haem synthesis causes impaired iron incorporation into haemoglobin, leading to iron overload of red cell precursors (ring sideroblasts).

Haem precursors are also neurotoxic in excess. In this aspect, lead poisoning shares many features with the porphyrias. Lead also:

- Binds sulphydryl enzyme components, disrupting their structural integrity and function, or displaces other heavy metal ions functioning as enzyme cofactors. Such impairment of the activity of myriad enzymes may in part account for the numerous and diverse symptoms of lead poisoning.

- Disrupts neurotransmitter release and antagonizes neuronal N-methyl-D-aspartate receptors, which probably contributes to the neuropathological effects of lead poisoning.
- Is a source of free radicals, causing oxidative stress to cellular proteins and membranes.

Diagnosis and treatment

Diagnosis is suggested by characteristic blood film features (e.g. 'basophilic stippling' of red cells), elevated red cell protoporphyrins, raised serum lead and X-ray fluorescence bone analysis. Treatment is with lead chelators (e.g. desferrioxamine), calcium edetate or penicillamine. These sequester lead ions in water-soluble complexes, allowing renal lead excretion.

● Chapter Summary

- One-carbon transfer is important for allowing the vital transfer of highly reactive one-carbon units (e.g. methyl groups) between different metabolic pathways. Folate and B12 are key molecules necessary for normal one-carbon transfers.
- Purines and pyrimidines are two classes of nitrogenous bases, which represent the molecular building blocks of nucleic acids. They are therefore essential for normal RNA and DNA synthesis. Synthesis of both purines and pyrimidines relies on glutamine, glycine and aspartate availability.
- Gout may occur in the metabolic context of hyperuricaemia, which may develop due to excessive urate production or impaired urate excretion. Gout has renal, joint and soft tissue manifestations.
- The porphyrias are a group of diseases arising from enzyme deficiencies within haem metabolism pathway. They are subdivided into acute and cutaneous porphyrias, where each type shares several common features.

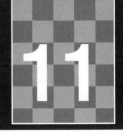

The thyroid gland 11

INTRODUCTION

The thyroid gland secretes both thyroid hormones and calcitonin. Thyroid hormones regulate the transcription of an enormous number of different proteins, in nearly all cell types. Normal thyroid hormone levels are therefore essential for normal metabolism, growth and development. Deficiency or excess of thyroid hormone leads to characteristic clinical features. Calcitonin is important in calcium and phosphate homeostasis (see Chapter 13).

ANATOMY

Ultrastructure

The thyroid gland has a bi-lobed structure, each conical lobe connected by the slender median isthmus. Each lobe lies slightly anterolateral to the anterior trachea (Fig. 11.1). The adult thyroid weighs between 10 g and 20 g. (See Figs. 11.6 and 11.9.)

Histology

Histologically, the thyroid gland consists of multiple spherical follicles, each made up of a monolayer of follicular cell enclosing colloid. These represent the functional units of thyroid parenchyma. Calcitonin-secreting parafollicular cells (C cells) are located in the interstitial regions, between the follicles.

Anatomical relations

The thyroid gland is situated at the C6 vertebral level. The median isthmus is typically a midline structure, whilst overall the gland lies:

- Anterior to the anterior face of the trachea
- Posterior to the sternohyoid and sternothyroid muscles

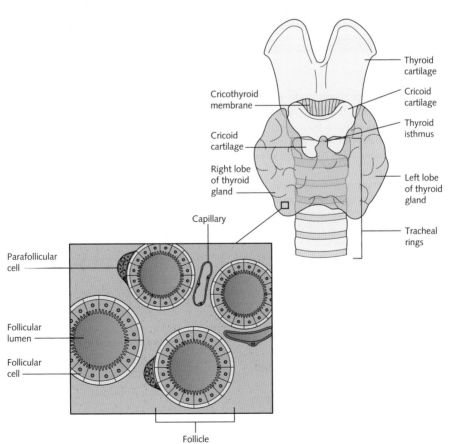

Fig. 11.1 Gross anatomy of the thyroid gland, with magnified area to illustrate the main histological features.

- Superior to the paired inferior thyroid arteries
- Inferior to the anterior portions of the thyroid and cricoid cartilages

Posterolateral to each lobe lies the ipsilateral carotid sheath, containing the carotid artery, vagus nerve and internal jugular vein.

Blood supply

In common with all endocrine organs, the thyroid is highly vascular. Arterial supply is derived from paired inferior and superior thyroid arteries, which anastomose extensively. In approximately 10% of people, additional blood flow is also derived from the thyroid *ima* artery.

Each lobe is drained by the paired superior and middle thyroid veins. These emerge laterally from the ipsilateral lobe and drain into the ipsilateral internal jugular vein. The central isthmus is drained by the paired inferior thyroid veins, which unite to form a venous plexus. This plexus ultimately drains into the left brachiocephalic vein.

Lymphatic drainage

The thyroid has extensive lymphatic drainage. Lymph first flows to periglandular nodes, then to prelaryngeal, pretracheal and paratracheal nodes, following the course of the recurrent laryngeal nerve. Subsequent lymph drainage is then to the mediastinal lymph nodes.

Innervation

Innervation of the thyroid is predominantly autonomic. Parasympathetic fibres originate from the right and left vagus nerves, and sympathetic fibres from cervical ganglia of each ipsilateral sympathetic chain. The innervation is primarily vasomotor, rather than regulating glandular secretion.

Importantly, four important nerves supplying the larynx (the right and superior laryngeal nerves and the right and left recurrent laryngeal nerves) are closely anatomically related to the thyroid gland and are at risk during surgical resection of the gland (thyroidectomy).

HINTS AND TIPS	

REVERSE T3

Reverse T3 (rT3) is a structural T3 isomer. It is synthesized by inner ring deiodination of T4. Approximately 10% of circulating rT3 is secreted by the thyroid gland, whereas the remained is converted by inner ring deiodination of circulating T4 peripherally (in contrast to T3, which is converted from T4 by outer ring deiodination).

THYROID HORMONES

The physiologically significant thyroid hormones are thyroxine (T4) and triiodothyronine (T3). T3 is regarded as the 'active' thyroid hormone, because it is approximately three to four times more potent than T4, in terms of its effects. Reverse triiodothyronine (rT3) is also secreted, but it is metabolically inactive.

Molecular structures

The structures of T4, T3 and rT3 are illustrated in Fig. 11.2. Note that T4 features four covalently bound iodine atoms, whereas T3 features only three. T3 is synthesized by deiodination of the outer ring of T4.

Synthesis

Synthesis of thyroid hormones is illustrated in Fig. 11.3.

Thyroglobulin synthesis

Thyroglobulin is synthesized by follicular cells and secreted into follicle lumens, forming the main component of lumenal colloid. Thyroglobulin functions as a glycoprotein scaffold for the synthesis of thyroid hormone, contributing the required tyrosine residues. Each molecule contains 134 tyrosine residues, but only a few are ultimately incorporated into new thyroid hormone molecules.

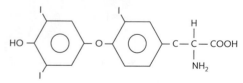

Fig. 11.2 Molecular structure of the thyroid hormones: T4, T3 and reverse triiodothyronine (rT3).

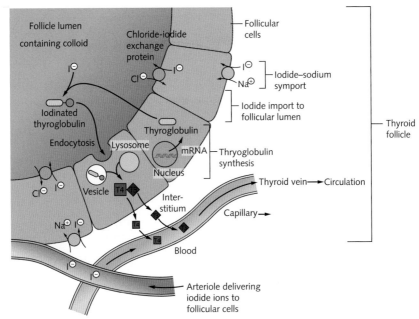

Fig. 11.3 Thyroid hormone synthesis. *mRNA,* Messenger RNA.

Iodine accumulation in follicular cells

The iodine component of T4, T3 and rT3 originates exclusively from the diet. Dietary iodine occurs naturally in coastal soil, where it is assimilated into plants growing in the soil. It is then assimilated into herbivores, and ultimately carnivores and omnivores like ourselves. It can also be artificially incorporated into food at the manufacturing stage. Diets deficient in iodine (e.g. in central African regions) typically manifest clinically with enlarged thyroid glands and/or symptoms of hypothyroidism.

Iodide ions absorbed from the gut are actively transported from the circulation into thyroid follicles via the sodium–iodide symporter (NIS), which is situated at the basolateral membrane of follicular cells.

Iodine import into follicle lumen

Iodide ions (accumulated in high concentration by the follicular cells) are extruded across the apical membrane of follicular cells into the follicle lumen via the chloride-iodide exchange protein pendrin.

Thyroid peroxidase-mediated iodination of thyroglobulin

At the luminal (apical) face of the follicular cell, the enzyme thyroid peroxidase (TPO) catalyses the stages of the formation of iodothyroglobulin:

- Oxidation of iodide ions
- Iodination of tyrosine residues
- Conjugation of iodinated tyrosine residue pairs

The tyrosine residues are components of the primary structure of lumenal thyroglobulin. Incorporation of a single iodine atom to a tyrosine residue (within the thyroglobulin molecule) forms monoiodotyrosine (MIT), whereas the incorporation of a second iodine atom forms diiodotyrosine (DIT; Fig. 11.4). The iodine may incorporate into the carbon ring of the tyrosine R group at position 3, position 5 or both. Note that the MIT and DIT are still part of the thyroglobulin molecule; once iodinated the molecule is known as 'iodothyroglobulin'.

TPO-mediated conjugation of iodinated tyrosine pairs

Two iodinated tyrosine residues are then linked to each other at their benzyl moieties. If two DITs join together, thyroxine (T4) will be synthesized. If DIT and MIT join together, triiodothyronine (T3) will be synthesized. Remember, this pairing is also catalysed by TPO.

Lysosomal proteolysis of iodothyroglobulin

Iodothyroglobulin is imported into follicular cells from the follicle lumens by endocytosis. Intralysosomal proteolysis excises the linked tyrosine components from the iodothyroglobulin scaffold. T4, T3 and rT3 are the final products, depending on:

- Whether the tyrosine pair consisted of two DIT (T4) or a DIT and an MIT (T3 or rT3)
- Whether the MIT component was iodinated at the outer (T3) or inner (rT3) ring

149

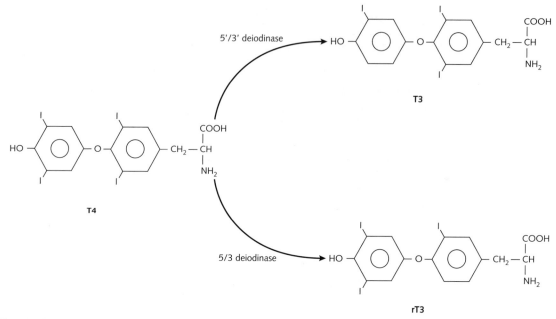

Fig. 11.4 Deiodination of T4. 5′/3′ deiodinase converts T4 to T3 by outer ring deiodination, whereas 5/3 deiodinase converts T4 to reverse triiodothyronine (rT3) by inner ring deiodination. Note that such peripheral intracellular conversion of T4 to T3 is responsible for approximately 75% of the total T3 circulating in the bloodstream.

THYROID HOMEOSTASIS: THE HYPOTHALAMIC–PITUITARY–THYROID AXIS

The hypothalamic–pituitary–thyroid (HPT) axis is a typical hierarchical hormone regulation system. The hypothalamus releases thyrotropin-releasing hormone (TRH) into the hypophyseal portal system. TRH travels to the anterior pituitary, where it binds to TRH receptors on thyrotrophic cells, stimulating them to release thyroid-stimulating hormone (TSH) into the systemic circulation. TSH is 28-kDa glycoprotein with α and β components. TSH (in concert with T3 and T4) exerts negative feedback on hypothalamic TRH secretion.

TSH released by the anterior pituitary subsequently binds to TSH receptors at the basolateral surface of thyroid follicular cells. This binding promotes synthesis and secretion of the thyroid hormones (T4, T3 and rT3) from fol-licular cells, in part by promoting hyperplasia (increase in functional thyroid parenchymal tissue) and in part because of increased expression of TPO. T3, T4 and TSH exert negative feedback on TSH synthesis and release. Somatostatin and dopamine likewise attenuate TSH synthesis and secretion (Fig. 11.5).

SECRETION AND TRANSPORT

Transport in the circulation

Thyroid hormones are hydrophobic, therefore once secreted into the circulation, they immediately bind to plasma proteins, namely, thyroid-binding globulin, transthyretin and albumin.

Secretion from the thyroid gland

The ratio of T4 to T3 secretion *from the thyroid gland* is approximately 10:2. However, the bulk of circulating T3 is in fact derived from peripheral deiodinase conversion of T4. Approximately 75% of plasma T3 originates from converted T4, whereas only approximately 25% of plasma T3 is secreted directly by the thyroid gland.

Peripheral deiodination

The 5/3 deiodinases convert T4 to T3 (Fig. 11.4). Type II deiodinase (D2) is responsible for the vast majority of

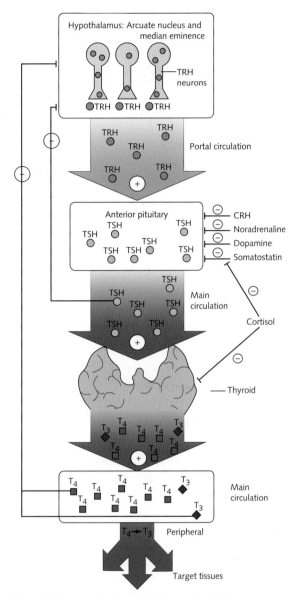

Fig. 11.5 The hypothalamic–pituitary axis. *CRH,*
Corticotropin-releasing hormone; *TRH,* thyrotropin-releasing
hormone; *TSH,* thyroid-stimulating hormone. Note the
relative proportions of T4 and T3 release from the thyroid.
Blue squares represent T4; Red squares represent T3.

T4:T3 ratio

Plasma T4:T3 ratios

The actual ratio of *total plasma* T4 to T3 is approximately
50:1. The physiologically significant fraction, however, is
the 'free' T4 or T3 (i.e. that not bound to plasma proteins).
As a greater proportion of total T4 (compared with T3)
is bound to plasma proteins, three to five times greater
amount of free T4 is present in plasma than the amount
of free T3.

Cytoplasmic T4:T3 ratio

T4 and T3 diffuse across plasma membranes to access cells.
Once T4 has passed into a cell, about 50% is converted
into T3. This equalizes the T4:T3 ratio intracellularly to
approximately 1:1.

CELLULAR EFFECTS OF THYROID HORMONE

Thyroid hormone receptors are intranuclear, associated
with chromatin. They are present in all cell types, accounting in part for the enormous range of physiological
processes influenced by thyroid hormones (represented in
diagram form in Fig. 11.6).

T3 or T4 binds to intranuclear thyroid receptors. T3 has a
10-fold greater affinity for thyroid hormone receptors than
T4. The subsequent receptor–ligand complex then forms a
heterodimer with the retinoid X ligand–receptor complex.
This heterodimer then influences (activates or represses,
depending on the particular gene) the transcription of a
multitude of thyroid-sensitive genes by binding particular
DNA sequences.

Whereas this mechanism of transcriptional regulation
represents the primary mechanism by which thyroid hormones exert their cellular effect, there are now known to
be multiple thyroid hormone-binding sites in the cytoplasm, mitochondria and microsomes, in addition to the
intranuclear receptors. It is thought that the mitochondrial
effects, for example, could contribute to the enhanced oxidative phosphorylation observed in cells exposed to thyroid
hormone.

METABOLIC EFFECTS

Basal metabolic rate

Thyroid hormones increase the basal metabolic rate (see
Chapter 8), which has two very important effects:

- Cellular oxygen and energy requirements increase.
  Tissue perfusion must therefore increase to enhance

peripheral T4→T3 conversion (accounting for ~75% of
plasma T3). Type 3 deiodinase (D3) inactivates T3 and prevents the peripheral T4→T3 conversion.

When humans experience physiological stressors (e.g.
starvation and some instances of depression), 5/3 deiodinase
type I downregulates. This causes a decrease in peripheral
T4→T3 conversion and thus a decrease in total (and free)
plasma T3 levels. Because plasma T3 is a key determinant of
the basal metabolic rate, caloric expenditure is appropriately
decreased in the context of stressors, allowing conservation
of metabolic reserves such as glycogen and lipid stores.

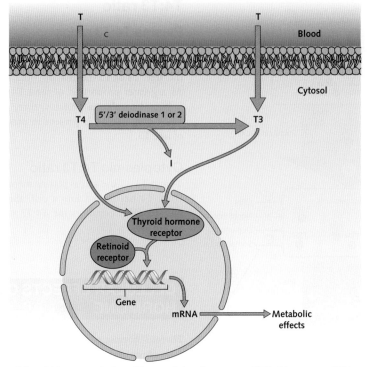

Fig. 11.6 Mechanism of thyroid hormone-induced intracellular changes. *mRNA,* Messenger RNA.

delivery of oxygen and metabolic substrates. An increase in cardiac output contributes to this increase in perfusion (which is partially achieved due to an increase in the heart rate because cardiac output = heart rate × stroke volume).

- Carbon dioxide production increases, mainly due to upregulation of oxidative phosphorylation. Excretion of additional CO_2 requires an increase in pulmonary minute volume (minute volume = respiratory rate × tidal volume). This is observed clinically as an increase in respiratory rate.

Carbohydrate metabolism

Thyroid hormones upregulate hepatic gluconeogenesis, increasing hepatic glucose production. This effect is mediated via induction of gluconeogenic enzymes, including phosphoenolpyruvate carboxykinase, pyruvate carboxylase and glucose-6-phosphatase (see Chapter 5). Glycogenolysis is also stimulated by thyroid hormones.

Lipid metabolism

Upregulation of gluconeogenesis increases the demand for gluconeogenic substrates. One such substrate is glycerol. Thyroid hormones upregulate lipolysis in adipose stores, leading to increased triglyceride hydrolysis. This liberates glycerol and fatty acids (see Chapter 7).

Protein metabolism

Thyroid hormones stimulate proteolysis, most notably within skeletal muscle. The resultant amino acids may then travel to the liver to participate in gluconeogenesis. Protein synthesis is suppressed by T3 and T4.

Thermogenesis

Thyroid hormone uncouple oxidative phosphorylation occurring in brown fat cells by inducing mitochondrial uncoupling protein and thermogenin expression. These proteins uncouple adenosine triphosphate (ATP) synthesis from oxidative phosphorylation, instead causing the energy to be released as heat (see Chapter 4).

PHYSIOLOGICAL EFFECTS

Autonomic (sympathetic) potentiation

Thyroid hormones increase tissue sensitivity to adrenergic β-agonist hormones (e.g. adrenaline, noradrenaline) by upregulation of β-adrenoreceptors. Normal sympathetic tone thus elicits an enhanced response, exemplified by an increased heart rate and thermogenesis for the same magnitude of adrenergic stimulus.

Cardiac function

Thyroid hormones upregulate synthesis of the α-chain subunit of the myosin heavy chain. Presence of this particular subunit in myosin fibres is associated with increased actin and calcium adenosine triphosphatase (ATPase) activity. This translates into increased cardiac contractility, stroke volume and therefore cardiac output.

Na$^+$/K$^+$ ATPase activity

Na$^+$/K$^+$ ATPase activity represents a large fraction of total cellular energy expenditure, because its action is fundamental to maintaining resting membrane potential. Thyroid hormone causes upregulation of Na$^+$/K$^+$ ATPase expression, and increases its membrane insertion. This in part contributes to the increase in ATP and oxygen consumption.

DISORDERS OF THYROID FUNCTION

These can be grouped into hyperthyroidism (excessive secretion of thyroid hormone) and hypothyroidism (inadequate secretion of thyroid hormone).

Hyperthyroidism

Excessive secretion of thyroid hormones leads to elevation of their plasma concentration above the normal physiological range (thyrotoxicosis). The main mechanisms leading to thyrotoxicosis are:

- Graves disease
- Excessive parenchymal mass (hyperplasia of the thyroid gland)
- Neoplasia

Regardless of the underlying mechanism, thyrotoxicosis leads to a common set of clinical features (Fig. 11.7). In addition, due to intact negative feedback, TSH and TRH levels are typically appropriately low in hyperthyroidism. Drug treatments used in hyperthyroidism are known as 'antithyroid drugs'. The two antithyroid drugs in use in the UK are carbimazole and propylthiouracil.

Graves disease

Graves disease is the most common cause of thyrotoxicosis, responsible for approximately 75% of cases. Aetiology is autoimmune: an autoantibody specific for the TSH receptor is produced. This autoantibody binds to, and inappropriately overstimulates the TSH receptor, causing hypersecretion of thyroid hormones and diffuse glandular hyperplasia (goitre).

The autoantibody also affects connective tissue, particularly in the retro-orbital and pretibial locations.

Retro-orbital inflammation and oedema retro-orbitally lead to proptosis and eyelid retraction. These changes can result in eye damage and visual symptoms. In the pretibial region of the lower limb, the striking phenomenon of pretibial myxoedema (an infiltrative dermopathy) may develop (Fig. 11.8).

Thyroid storm

Thyroid storm is a rare but life-threatening complication (mortality ~10%), which usually develops in patients with existing hyperthyroidism. Thyroid storm is usually precipitated by stress, acute illness, infection, pregnancy or therapeutic interventions (e.g. surgery, radioiodine therapy). It is hallmarked by hyperpyrexia, diarrhoea, vomiting, tachycardia, extreme agitation and confusion, and ultimately coma. Treatment is urgent resuscitation, antithyroid drugs, β blockade and supportive therapy in intensive care, whilst the precipitating cause is urgently identified and treated. Thyroidectomy or radioablation is reserved for intractable cases, because these interventions cause lifelong hypothyroidism.

Hypothyroidism

Insufficient secretion of thyroid hormones results in plasma concentrations of T3 and T4 below the normal range. The main mechanisms leading to hypothyroidism are:

- Iodine deficiency
- Autoimmune disease (e.g. Hashimoto thyroiditis)
- Viral infection (de Quervain thyroiditis)
- Loss of functional parenchyma (radioablation, resection, radiotherapy local to anterior neck or infiltrative diseases, e.g. amyloidosis)
- Drugs

Regardless of the underlying cause, hypothyroidism causes a typical set of clinical features (Fig. 11.9). In addition, due to the absence of negative feedback by the low plasma T3 and T4, TSH and TRH levels are *usually* appropriately elevated in hypothyroidism. The exception is when a disturbance of the HPT axis with a consequent insufficient TRH or TSH secretion is the underlying cause of the hypothyroidism.

On a global scale, iodine deficiency is the most common cause of hypothyroidism. It is usually a feature in, for instance, central regions of Africa. In the UK, autoimmunity or iatrogenic destruction of the gland predominates. Treatment is with daily oral levothyroxine replacement.

Congenital hypothyroidism

Congenital hypothyroidism is a condition of neonatal thyroid hormone deficiency, present in approximately 1/4000 newborns. Newborn blood spot screening (see Chapter 14) attempts to identify these babies at birth so that prompt thyroxine replacement can be instigated. Untreated,

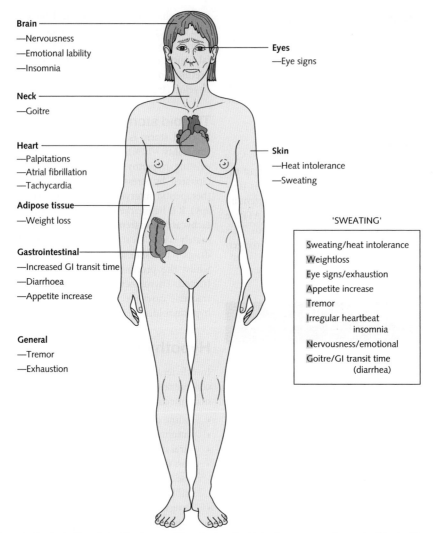

Brain
—Nervousness
—Emotional lability
—Insomnia

Eyes
—Eye signs

Neck
—Goitre

Heart
—Palpitations
—Atrial fibrillation
—Tachycardia

Skin
—Heat intolerance
—Sweating

Adipose tissue
—Weight loss

Gastrointestinal
—Increased GI transit time
—Diarrhoea
—Appetite increase

General
—Tremor
—Exhaustion

'SWEATING'

Sweating/heat intolerance
Weightloss
Eye signs/exhaustion
Appetite increase
Tremor
Irregular heartbeat
          insomnia
Nervousness/emotional
Goitre/GI transit time
          (diarrhea)

Fig. 11.7 Cartoon to illustrate the clinical features of thyrotoxicosis. Note the acronym 'sweating' to facilitate recall of individual symptoms and signs. *GI,* Gastrointestinal.

congenital hypothyroidism leads to impaired growth and development with characteristic deformities and significant cognitive deficiencies, a constellation of symptoms/signs previously known as 'cretinism' (see Chapter 13). Iodine deficiency accounts for most cases of congenital hypothyroidism on a global scale, but in the UK the cause is usually unclear.

Myxoedema coma

Myxoedema coma is a rare, life-threatening state of severe hypothyroidism. It may occur as the first presentation of hypothyroidism, but more commonly develops as an acute phenomenon in individuals with existing hypothyroidism. Precipitating factors include trauma, surgery, burns, non-compliance with oral thyroxine treatment, acute infection and severe illness.

Myxoedema coma is characterized by the following:

- Severe hypothermia
- Reduced respiratory rate and carbon dioxide retention (secondary to hypothermia-induced brainstem insensitivity to arterial partial pressure of oxygen and arterial partial pressure of carbon dioxide)
- Bradycardia and impaired contractility, leading to a reduced cardiac output
- Symptoms and signs of multiple organ dysfunction (due to insufficient cardiac output)
- Hyponatraemia (due to fluid retention)
- Effusions, for example, pleural, pericardial (due to increased vascular permeability)
- Lowered Glasgow Coma Scale (GCS) score: reduced consciousness and coma (due to impaired cerebral perfusion)

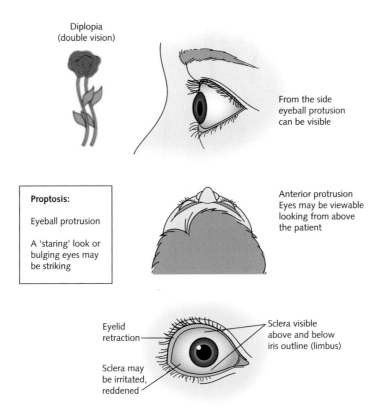

Diplopia
(double vision)

From the side
eyeball protusion
can be visible

Proptosis:

Eyeball protrusion

A 'staring' look or
bulging eyes may
be striking

Anterior protrusion
Eyes may be viewable
looking from above
the patient

Eyelid
retraction

Sclera visible
above and below
iris outline (limbus)

Sclera may
be irritated,
reddened

Fig. 11.8 Clinical features of Graves disease, represented as a cartoon. Note that Graves disease is a specific form of thyrotoxicosis, and the illustrated features are present *in addition* to the symptoms and signs of thyrotoxicosis. The most striking signs relate to the eyes. Proptosis is a combination of lid retraction and anterior displacement of the eyeballs due to oedema in the connective tissue posterior to the eyeball. Pretibial myxoedema, most often present on the shins, is a reddened symmetrical plaque-like swelling with a lumpy texture. It affects up to 5% of patients with Graves disease, and is seen more commonly in females.

Treatment typically involves supportive treatment in intensive care and urgent oral levothyroxine loading, if the oral route remains uncompromised by the low GCS. If the patient is too ill to swallow safely, intravenous liothyronine is the only alternative.

Sick euthyroid syndrome

Sick euthyroid syndrome is defined by low total and free plasma T3 accompanied by a normal or decreased plasma T4, usually normal TSH. Importantly, these derangements are *unaccompanied* by any clinical symptoms of hypothyroidism. Sick euthyroid syndrome is not uncommon in starvation, chronic disease or in critically ill patients, and the biochemical derangement usually resolves when the primary illness resolves. It does not warrant treatment. It is thought to arise due to impaired peripheral deiodination of T4 by deiodinases, secondary to metabolic disturbances induced by the precipitating factor.

INVESTIGATIONS OF THYROID FUNCTION

Clinical examination

A thorough clinical examination of the thyroid gland evaluates potential pathology and guides further investigations. Clinical examination of the thyroid is covered in appropriate detail in dedicated texts and will not be discussed here.

Biochemical investigations of thyroid function

Laboratory tests are necessary for both diagnosis and monitoring of thyroid disease. Most laboratories perform a standard profile of thyroid function (usually consisting of serum TSH and free T4). If either of these are abnormal, further tests may subsequently be requested, for example, free T3, thyroid-binding globulin.

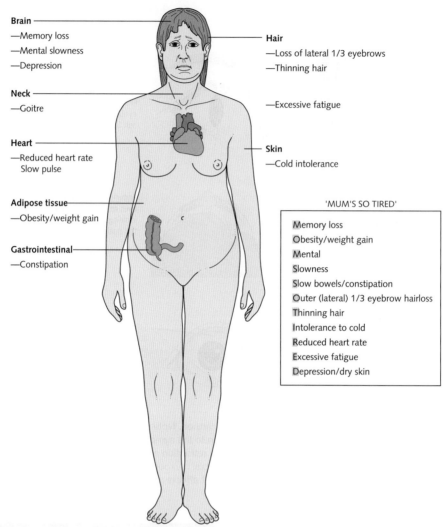

Brain
—Memory loss
—Mental slowness
—Depression

Neck
—Goitre

Heart
—Reduced heart rate
 Slow pulse

Adipose tissue
—Obesity/weight gain

Gastrointestinal
—Constipation

Hair
—Loss of lateral 1/3 eyebrows
—Thinning hair

—Excessive fatigue

Skin
—Cold intolerance

'MUM'S SO TIRED'

Memory loss
Obesity/weight gain
Mental
Slowness
Slow bowels/constipation
Outer (lateral) 1/3 eyebrow hairloss
Thinning hair
Intolerance to cold
Reduced heart rate
Excessive fatigue
Depression/dry skin

Fig. 11.9 Clinical features of hypothyroidism, represented as a cartoon. Note the acronym 'mom's so tired' to facilitate recall.

Imaging of the thyroid gland

Thyroid imaging techniques usually involve ultrasound scans; these permit estimation of parenchymal volume, vascular dynamics and enable image-guided biopsies.

Computed tomography scanning allows visualization of any retrosternal extension of large goitres (lying deep to bone, this compartment is not amenable to ultrasound visualization).

● **Chapter Summary**

- Thyroid hormones (T3 and T4) are synthesized and released from the thyroid gland. They bind to plasma proteins in the bloodstream. T4 is peripherally converted to T3 by deiodinases. T3 is considered the 'active' or more potent hormone.
- Thyroid hormones affect all cells of the body, influencing basal metabolic rate, macronutrient metabolism and thermogenesis. They also potentiate autonomic sympathetic activity and promote an increase in cardiac output.
- Thyroid homeostasis is primarily regulated by the hypothalamic–pituitary–thyroid endocrine axis.
- Disorders of thyroid function are extremely common. Hyperthyroidism describes the constellation of symptoms and signs associated with excessive plasma levels. Antithyroid drugs are used to treat hyperthyroidism. Graves disease is the most common cause for hyperthyroidism.
- Hypothyroidism describes the symptoms and signs associated with a reduced plasma concentration of T3 and T4. Various causative mechanisms may be responsible, but treatment is almost always with oral levothyroxine.

INTRODUCTION

'Vitamin' is the name given to a complex organic substance that must be consumed regularly in small amounts to maintain health. In terms of structure, they are unrelated despite many of them sharing a letter suffix (e.g. B vitamins).

Vitamins are micronutrients, in contrast to macronutrients, which must be consumed in large amounts. As essential micronutrients, their regular intake is mandatory for health and insufficient dietary intake leads to deficiency syndromes. Vitamins are classified according to their solubility (i.e. water soluble and fat soluble).

The exact daily amount of each vitamin that is required to maintain health in the majority of UK adults is given by the 'reference nutrient intake' (RNI). In this context, the 'majority' is defined as the mean population requirement ± two standard deviations; this encompasses 97.5% of the normal population and encompasses interindividual variation. RNIs for vitamins, rich dietary sources and groups at risk for nutritional deficiency are given in Table 12.1; water-soluble vitamins are shaded for clarity.

Certain factors predispose to specific vitamin (and mineral) deficiencies.

CLINICAL NOTES

MALNUTRITION

Malnutrition may be associated with starvation, food deprivation, alcohol dependence, psychiatric disease, bariatric surgery, hyperemesis gravidarum or chronic malabsorption.

CLINICAL NOTES

MALABSORPTION

Malabsorption occurs in inflammatory bowel diseases, chronic gastrointestinal infections (bacterial, viral, protozoal and parasitic), coeliac disease and true lactose intolerance. Malabsorption syndromes predominantly affecting lipid absorption include pancreatic insufficiency, biliary obstruction, bacterial overgrowth, chronic cholestasis and terminal ileal disease. Terminal ileal-specific/predominant diseases include ileal tuberculosis, Whipple disease, tropical sprue, coeliac, exudative enteropathy and terminal ileal resection.

CLINICAL NOTES

VITAMIN DEFICIENCIES IN PREMATURE BABIES

Preterm babies are at high risk for fat-soluble vitamin deficiencies for several reasons: (1) insufficient time *in utero* for accumulation of stores, (2) impaired gastrointestinal fat absorption, limiting absorption from breast milk or formula and (3) reduced circulating lipoproteins, impairing tissue delivery of fat-soluble vitamins.

FAT-SOLUBLE VITAMINS

The fat-soluble vitamins include vitamins A, D, E and K. They share common characteristics in that they are:

- Stored in the liver and adipose tissue, usually for long periods
- Toxic in significant excess (vitamins A and D)
- Not typically degraded by cooking processes
- Reliant on normal gastrointestinal (GI) fat absorption for their absorption
- Share a common mechanism of absorption

Absorption of dietary fat-soluble vitamins

Approximately 80% of ingested fat-soluble vitamins are absorbed via a common mechanism – in the proximal intestine following solubilization into mixed micelles (bile salts and lipolyzed fat). Enterocytes assemble absorbed fat and fat-soluble vitamins into chylomicrons. They are secreted into lymph. Within lymph, chylomicrons access the main circulation via the thoracic duct. From then on, they access the liver and peripheral tissues. In the liver, hepatocytes may:

- Reintegrate vitamins into lipoproteins for export to tissues
- Utilize the vitamin for a specific purpose
- Convert a vitamin into a storage ester for storage in liver parenchyma or stellate cells

Table 12.1 Vitamins: reference nutrient intakes (RNIs), dietary sources and groups at risk for intake deficiency[a]

Vitamin	RNI (or alternative intake parameter if RNI not set)	Rich dietary sources	Risk factors for intake deficiency
A	600 µg	Liver (animal, fish), full-fat dairy products, egg yolk, intensely green/yellow/orange vegetables	Fat malabsorption syndromes Preterm babies Malnutrition Diseases associated with malabsorption Living in geographical zones with high prevalence of vitamin A deficiency
D	10 µg	Oily fish, fish liver oil, fungi irradiated with ultraviolet (UV) light	Fat malabsorption syndromes Preterm babies Malnutrition Diseases associated with malabsorption Chronic renal disease Multiple demographic and behavioural risk factors (see the 'Groups at risk for deficiency' section)
E	(RNI not set) RDA: 15 mg	Plant-derived oils, nuts, spinach, carrots, avocado, apricot, freshwater fish	Fat malabsorption syndromes Preterm babies Malnutrition Diseases associated with malabsorption
K	(RNI not set) AI: 120 µg (♂) 90 µg (♀)	K1: Leafy green vegetables, vegetable oils K2: Animal liver, fermented foods, commensal gut flora	Fat malabsorption syndromes All newborns (preterm > term, exclusively breastfed > formula fed) Malnutrition Diseases associated with malabsorption
B1 (thiamine)	900 µg (♂) 700 µg (♀)	Unprocessed 'wholegrain' cereals, legumes (pulses, beans, groundnuts)	Dietary thiamine antagonists: certain polyphenols (tannins, (e.g. tea), caffeine (e.g. coffee) and flavonoids) Dietary thiaminases: raw shellfish and freshwater/fermented fish Long-term diuretic use Chronic renal replacement (e.g. dialysis) Alcohol dependence Malnutrition Diseases associated with malabsorption
B2 (riboflavin)	1.2 mg (♂) 1.1 mg (♀)	Dairy products, offal, lean meat, eggs, almonds, avocado, dark green vegetables	Oral contraceptive pill use Veganism Pregnancy/lactation Lactose intolerance Malnutrition Diseases associated with malabsorption
B3 (niacin)	15 mg (♂) 12 mg (♀)	Tryptophan-rich foods: meat, fish, dairy products, eggs, yeast, cereals, green vegetables	Staple diet of maize Alcohol dependence B6 antagonists: isoniazid, azathioprine Chronic renal replacement (e.g. dialysis) HIV infection Pathological scenarios of high tryptophan utilization (e.g. carcinoid syndrome) Hartnup disease (impaired tryptophan absorption) Malnutrition Diseases associated with malabsorption
B5 (pantothenic acid)	(RNI not set) AI 5 mg	Offal, fish, shellfish, dairy products, eggs, legumes (pulses, beans, groundnuts), mushrooms, avocado, sweet potato	Malnutrition Diseases associated with malabsorption

Table 12.1 Vitamins: reference nutrient intakes (RNIs), dietary sources and groups at risk for intake deficiencya—cont'd

Vitamin	RNI (or alternative intake parameter if RNI not set)	Rich dietary sources	Risk factors for intake deficiency
B6 (pyridoxine)	1.2 mg (♂) 1.0 mg (♀)	Nuts, seeds, legumes (pulses, beans, groundnuts), fish, meat, avocado, garlic, banana, potato, green vegetables	Isoniazid, chloramphenicol High protein intake (increases B6 requirements) Alcohol dependence Malnutrition Diseases associated with malabsorption
B7 (biotin)	(RNI not set) AI 30 µg	Offal, meat, fish, egg yolk, avocado	Malnutrition Diseases associated with malabsorption Prolonged high consumption of raw egg whites Rare inborn errors of biotin metabolism
B9 (folate)	200 µg	Liver, yeast, dark green leafy vegetables	Increased folate requirement: Childhood, adolescence, pregnancy, lactation, haemolysis Impaired folate absorption: phenytoin Dihydrofolate reductase inhibitors: methotrexate Antifolate drugs: sulphasalazine, trimethoprim, pyrimethamine High therapeutic nonsteroidal antiinflammatory drug dosage Smoking Alcohol dependence Malnutrition Diseases associated with malabsorption
B12 (cobalamin)	1.2 mg	Liver, oily fish, dairy products, eggs, shellfish	Antacids/H1 receptor antagonists/proton pump inhibitors, foscarnet Veganism Increased B12 requirement: Childhood, adolescence, pregnancy, lactation, haemolysis, hyperthyroidism Autoimmunity (pernicious anaemia) Terminal ileal disease B12 annexing by bacteria/parasites: bacterial overgrowth syndrome, tapeworm infestation Genetic defects of cubilin Malnutrition Diseases associated with malabsorption
C (ascorbic acid)	35 mg (nonsmokers) 70 mg (smokers)	Fruit (especially citrus), tomato, berries, green vegetables	Diet poor in plant matter Alcohol dependence Smoking Malnutrition Diseases associated with malabsorption

a RNI values shown here are taken from Department of Health dietary reference values and refer to adults only. Please note that RNI values change often, as nutrition research progresses. Please consult www.BDA.uk.com or other authentic sources for the latest intake recommendations. Where an RNI is not available, alternative parameters such as adequate intake (AI) or recommended daily allowance (RDA) are stated and given.

In peripheral tissues, endothelium-bound lipoprotein lipase facilitates offloading of fat-soluble vitamin cargo from chylomicrons or very-low-density lipoproteins, allowing it access to peripheral cells.

WATER-SOLUBLE VITAMINS

Water-soluble vitamins include the vitamins B1, B2, B3, B5, B6, B7, B9, B12 and vitamin C. Features common to water-soluble vitamins are as follows:

- Minimally toxic in excess (due to effective excretion mechanisms)
- Not stored in the body – regular dietary intake is necessary
- Easily degraded by cooking processes
- Absorption is independent of lipid absorption

VITAMIN A (FAT SOLUBLE)

The term 'vitamin A' refers to both 'formed' retinol (animal derived) and provitamin A carotenoids (plant derived). See Table 12.1 for RNI, deficiency risk factors and vitamin A-rich foods.

Active forms and physiological roles

Vitamin A participates in vision, immunity, erythropoiesis, embryogenesis, growth and development. It is also vital for normal keratinocyte proliferation and differentiation and thus normal epithelialization. The biologically active forms of vitamin A are:

- Retinol: absorbed intact from animal products or derived from conversion of carotenoids. Retinol is converted into retinal and retinoic acid, the active forms of vitamin A.
- 11-*cis* retinal: from plant-derived carotenoids, or retinol oxidation. 11-*cis* Retinal combines with opsin to form rhodopsin, the light-sensitive pigment in retinal cells.
- Retinoic acid: derived from retinal oxidation. Retinoic acid is a signalling molecule that also influences gene transcription.

Vitamin A metabolism

Ingested dietary retinol (animal derived) and retinal (carotenoid derived) are absorbed in the typical manner of fat-soluble vitamins. Incorporation into chylomicrons is as retinyl esters. Retinyl esters may be stored in stellate cells or incorporated into a transthyretin/retinol-binding protein complex for export into the circulation for travel onwards to other tissues (Fig. 12.1). Vitamin A stores last approximately 1–2 years.

Clinical features of vitamin A deficiency

Vitamin A deficiency is predominantly a disease of developing countries, where it is associated with dietary deficiency. Infection susceptibility increases secondary to impaired immunity. Eye and skin symptoms are prominent. In children, defective bone and teeth formation also occur. Deficiency is confirmed by low serum retinol and retinol-binding protein. Treatment is oral/intramuscular retinol palmitate.

Eye symptoms

As the extent of deficiency progresses, so do the clinical symptoms of vitamin A deficiency. Initially dark adaptation failure (night blindness) occurs, progressing to xerophthalmia with Bitot spots and ultimately keratomalacia, corneal ulceration, cataract formation and blindness. These symptoms arise due to failure of both rhodopsin synthesis and corneal epithelialization.

Skin/mucosal surface symptoms

As with the cornea, failure of normal epithelialization at skin and mucosal surfaces leads to drying (xerosis) and follicular hyperkeratosis.

Therapeutic indications

Vitamin A is used therapeutically in treatment of retinitis pigmentosa, promyelocytic leukaemia and various skin diseases. Most commonly encountered is oral/topical isotretinoin, used to treat severe acne and psoriasis.

Teratogenicity

Excessive vitamin A ingestion during pregnancy results in fetal malformations. Vitamin supplements containing vitamin A and foods high in vitamin A must therefore be avoided during pregnancy. Isotretinoin is contraindicated in pregnancy for the same reason.

Clinical features of toxicity: hypervitaminosis A

Hypervitaminosis A is usually a result of excessive supplement intake of retinol or derivatives (excluding carotenoids; reduced bioavailability means that they are less likely to cause toxicity). Acute toxicity from a single, massive (>90,000 mg) exposure manifests with neurological symptoms including drowsiness, irritability and vomiting. Chronic toxicity from sustained excess exposure (>15,000 mg daily) causes exfoliation (skin peeling), hair loss, anorexia, pruritus, hypercalcaemia, hepatomegaly and abnormalities in growing bones (in children). There is no specific treatment other than preventing further excess intake.

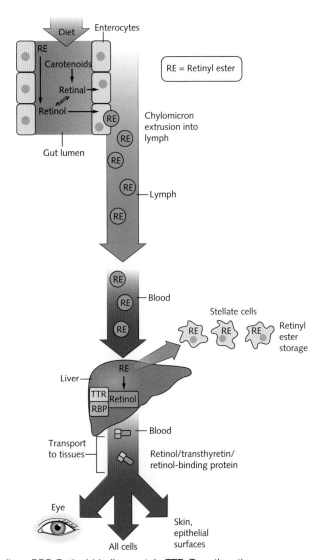

Fig. 12.1 Vitamin A metabolism. *RBP,* Retinol-binding protein *TTR,* Transthyretin.

VITAMIN D (FAT SOLUBLE)

A fat-soluble vitamin that is functionally a steroid hormone, vitamin D occurring in food takes the form of:

- Vitamin D3 (cholecalciferol); naturally low in most foods, unless deliberately fortified. Where present, it is usually in the form of 25-hydroxycholecalciferol, a precursor of the active metabolite.
- Vitamin D2 (ergocalciferol) is present in fungi exposed to UV light.

The majority of vitamin D is endogenously synthesized in most individuals, assuming sufficient sun exposure to uncovered skin. See Table 12.1 for RNI, deficiency risk factors and foods high in vitamin D.

Active forms and physiological roles

The bioactive form of vitamin D is the doubly hydroxylated cholecalciferol metabolite 1,25-dihydroxycholecalciferol. This binds to intranuclear vitamin D receptors, which act as transcription factors. Sufficient vitamin D is essential for normal:

- Regulation of calcium homeostasis
- Bone mineralization

It also participates in:

- Regulation of insulin secretion
- Cellular growth and differentiation
- Vascular tone
- Immune cell differentiation
- Tumour suppression

Effects on calcium and phosphate

1,25-Dihydroxycholecalciferol elevates serum calcium and phosphate via the following mechanisms:

- Increased intestinal absorption of calcium and phosphate
- Potentiated parathyroid hormone-mediated bone resorption
- Reduced renal excretion of calcium and phosphate.

Vitamin D metabolism

This is summarized in Fig. 12.2. Ingested ergocalciferol (D2) and cholecalciferol (D3) are absorbed across enterocytes into the portal circulation in the typical manner of fat-soluble vitamins. Vitamin D is transported in the circulation bound to vitamin D-binding protein.

Activation of vitamin D (by double hydroxylation)

Vitamin D2 and D3 are converted in the liver to 25-hydroxycholecalciferol (also known as 'calcidiol') by hydroxylation at carbon 25. This metabolite may be stored in the liver, or travel in the circulation to the kidney, where it is hydroxylated a second time at carbon 1, forming 1,25-dihydroxycholecalciferol (calcitriol), the bioactive form of vitamin D.

Endogenous synthesis of vitamin D3

The ultraviolet component of sunlight causes keratinocyte (skin cell) conversion of 7-dehydrocholesterol to cholecalciferol (vitamin D3), which joins absorbed dietary

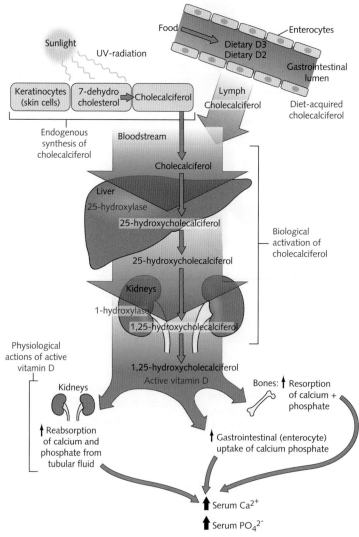

Fig. 12.2 Vitamin D metabolism.

cholecalciferol in the circulation. It undergoes hydroxylation in the liver and then kidney as described earlier.

Groups at risk for deficiency

Because of the sun-exposure aspect of vitamin D synthesis, multiple factors related to geography, behaviour, beliefs, ethnic origin and age influence the risk for deficiency.

CLINICAL NOTES

Risk factors for vitamin D deficiency include:

- Chronic renal disease: impaired renal hydroxylation of 25-hydroxycholecalciferol.
- Living at high latitude or areas with frequent dense cloud cover: reduced incident ultraviolet radiation.
- Pigmented skin: deeper pigmentation impairs cutaneous absorption of ultraviolet light.
- Cultural/religious beliefs regarding modest clothing: the less uncovered/exposed skin, the less potential endogenous cholecalciferol synthesis.
- Elderly/housebound lifestyle: reduced time outside limits sun exposure.
- Vegans, vegetarians: most dietary vitamin D is in food of animal origin.
- Breastfed infants of vitamin D-deficient mothers: milk (vitamin D) is dependent on maternal vitamin D status.
- Infants exclusively breastfed beyond ~6 months: after maternal vitamin D stores are exhausted, breast milk can no longer meet intake requirements of a growing baby.

Clinical features of vitamin D deficiency

Vitamin D deficiency is the most common nutritional deficiency worldwide. Symptoms and signs in part relate to disturbance of calcium and phosphate homeostasis. This manifests in children as rickets and in adults as osteomalacia (see Chapter 13). Generalized muscle pain and weakness are also symptoms of vitamin D deficiency, but in adults the symptoms (aside from osteomalacia-related complications such as fractures) tend to be nonspecific.

Diagnosis is confirmed by low serum 25-hydroxycholecalciferol. Treatment is cholecalciferol supplementation (usually combined with calcium). Note that as the bulk of vitamin D is endogenously synthesized, deficiency is usually attributable to insufficient sun exposure (Table 12.1). However, because sun exposure carries the risk for skin cancer, dietary supplementation is a much safer way of preventing deficiency.

Clinical features of toxicity: hypervitaminosis D

Vitamin D toxicity only results from excessive supplement intake (never from excessive sun exposure). Symptoms are insidious and nonspecific, pathophysiologically due to hypercalcaemia arising as a consequence of excessive vitamin D. There is no specific treatment other than preventing further excessive intake.

VITAMIN E (FAT SOLUBLE)

Vitamin E constitutes the major lipid-soluble antioxidant in the human body. By readily donating a hydrogen ion from the hydroxyl component, tocopherols and tocotrienols neutralize free radicals, limiting oxidative stress. See Table 12.1 for RNI, deficiency risk factors and vitamin E-rich dietary sources.

CLINICAL NOTES

ANTIOXIDANTS

Many important intracellular molecules, including DNA and proteins, are susceptible to oxidation. Endogenous and exogenous free radicals thus impose oxidative damage on these molecules, with consequent functional impairment. There is a complex array of antioxidant 'defences' to prevent this scenario, which is known as 'oxidative stress', as it is highly pathological. Vitamins E and C are the primary human antioxidants.

Active forms and physiological roles

Vitamin E consists of tocopherols (α, β, γ and δ) and tocotrienols (α, β, γ and δ), of which α-tocopherol is the most physiologically active. Biological functions include:

- Antioxidant activity
- Maintenance of normal neuronal function
- Immune cell function
- Antiplatelet activity

Vitamin E metabolism

Dietary tocopherol esters are first hydrolysed. They are then absorbed and transported in the typical manner of fat-soluble vitamins (as esterified tocopherols) but are also transported in the blood by erythrocytes. Storage is in liver parenchymal cells and adipose tissue.

Clinical features of vitamin E deficiency

Adults

Profound vitamin E deficiency in adults can cause haemolytic anaemia, ataxia, profound muscle weakness and retinal damage. If prolonged, it ultimately leads to blindness, cardiac arrhythmias and dementia. It is extremely rare in adults.

Neonates

Vitamin E deficiency is particularly significant in premature infants, where it can cause haemolytic anaemia and neurological damage. The latter is irreversible if not promptly treated with exogenous vitamin E. Low serum α-tocopherol confirms the diagnosis. Treatment is oral supplementation if GI absorption is intact, otherwise parenteral supplementation is used.

Clinical features of toxicity: hypervitaminosis E

This is extremely rare – excessive intake must be sustained long-term for toxicity symptoms to develop; these are primarily due to vitamin E's antiplatelet effects (i.e. bleeding).

VITAMIN K (FAT SOLUBLE)

Dietary vitamin K1 (phylloquinone) is a fat-soluble vitamin. Vitamin K2 (menaquinones) is a group of compounds synthesized by intestinal bacteria – however, menaquinones do not satisfy the vitamin K intake requirement, thus dietary intake is necessary. See Table 12.1 for RNI, deficiency risk factors and vitamin K-rich dietary sources.

Active forms and physiological roles

Vitamin K is an essential cofactor for the enzyme performing γ-carboxylation at specific glutamate residues of coagulation factors II, VII, IX and X, and proteins C and S. This carboxylation step is mandatory for their synthesis, meaning that intact coagulation is dependent on sufficient vitamin K availability.

Vitamin K metabolism

Absorption is typical for fat-soluble vitamins. Vitamin K stores last approximately 1 week in the absence of dietary intake. Effective 'recycling' occurs, lessening the dietary intake requirement. Excretion is via urine and bile.

Clinical features of vitamin K deficiency

Severe vitamin K deficiency manifests with bleeding, which can be severe and even fatal. This may be:

- Internal: into joints (haemarthrosis), muscle (haematomas) and organs, for example, brain (haemorrhage)
- Epithelial: for example, urinary or GI tracts → haematuria, melaena

Unexplained bleeding in the above patterns, in the context of normal platelet levels and function, should lead to measurement of coagulation parameters (see Chapter 14). A prolonged prothrombin time suggests either vitamin K deficiency or warfarin use. In very severe deficiency, a prolonged activated partial thromboplastin time can also be seen. Both warfarin overdose and severe vitamin K deficiency manifesting with haemorrhage are treated with prothrombin concentrate (containing factors II, VII, IX and X, i.e. the vitamin K-dependent factors) and intravenous/oral vitamin K as phytomenadione.

In neonates, vitamin K deficiency manifests as haemorrhagic disease of the newborn.

CLINICAL NOTES

HAEMORRHAGIC DISEASE OF THE NEWBORN

Neonates born with low vitamin K stores (the placenta does not readily transfer vitamin K) and with scarce vitamin K in breast milk are at risk for vitamin K deficiency. A sterile gut means they also cannot benefit from intestinal bacterially synthesized vitamin K2. Neonatal vitamin K deficiency is known as 'haemorrhagic disease of the newborn,' and typically presents with gastrointestinal bleeding. Newborns are given intramuscular phytomenadione at birth as prophylaxis against this potentially fatal manifestation of vitamin K deficiency.

Clinical features of vitamin K toxicity

Unusually for a fat-soluble vitamin, toxicity of vitamin K1 and K2 is low.

THIAMINE: VITAMIN B1 (WATER SOLUBLE)

As is typical for water-soluble vitamins, thiamine is nontoxic in excess. For RNI and thiamine-rich food sources, see Table 12.1.

Table 12.2 Cofactor roles of thiamine pyrophosphate and metabolic consequences of thiamine deficiency

Enzyme	Reaction catalysed	Cellular and physiological consequences of thiamine deficiency
Pyruvate dehydrogenase	Pyruvate → acetyl-CoA conversion	Accumulation of pyruvate, which is then diverted to anaerobic oxidation, forming lactate.
	Tricarboxylic acid (TCA) cycle progression impeded	Decreased acetyl-CoA formation → reduced production of $NADH + H^+$ and $FADH_2$ → impaired adenosine triphosphate (ATP) generation via oxidative phosphorylation (see Chapter 4).
α-Ketoglutarate dehydrogenase	α-Ketoglutarate → succinyl-CoA	Reduced succinyl-CoA generation, leading to substrate depletion for haem and other porphyrin synthesis.
	TCA cycle progression impeded	Decreased acetyl-CoA formation → reduced production of $NADH + H^+$ and $FADH_2$ → impaired ATP generation via oxidative phosphorylation (see Chapter 4).
Branched-chain amino acid α-ketoacid dehydrogenase complex	Branched-chain α-ketoacid → branched-chain acyl-CoA derivatives	Impaired catabolism of branched-chain amino acids → serum and urine elevation of leucine, isoleucine and valine → neurological dysfunction.
Transketolase	Pentose phosphate pathway progression impaired → Reduced $NADPH + H^+$ formation	Impaired fatty acid synthesis → impaired myelination → central and peripheral neural damage.

CoA, Coenzyme A.

Active forms and physiological roles

Thiamine pyrophosphate (TPP) is the bioactive version of thiamine. It is generated by pyrophosphate transfer from adenosine triphosphate (ATP) to thiamine. TPP functions as a cofactor for key metabolic pathway enzymes (Table 12.2). As such, it is vital for normal progression of the tricarboxylic acid (TCA) cycle (see Chapter 3), the pentose phosphate pathway (see Chapter 5) and branched-chain amino acid metabolism (see Chapter 9).

Metabolic consequences of thiamine deficiency

These are summarized in Table 12.2.

Clinical features of thiamine deficiency

This is classically associated with consumption of polished (husked) rice as the staple diet. Husked rice is very low in thiamine; prewashing and then boiling rice leach out the thiamine present into the cooking water.

Traditionally, red cell transketolase activity was used as a surrogate indicator of thiamine status (recall that TPP is an essential cofactor for this enzyme). Now, determination of serum thiamine by high-performance liquid chromatography is more typical. Elevated serum lactate supports the diagnosis. Treatment is thiamine supplementation (intravenous/intramuscular/oral).

Beriberi

There are three 'classic' subtypes of beriberi, delineated in Table 12.3. In reality, adult symptoms and signs usually overlap or combine cardiovascular features of 'wet' beriberi with neurological features of 'dry' beriberi. Infantile beriberi is rapidly fatal if untreated.

Wernicke encephalopathy

This is a triad of (1) acute/subacute mental status change, (2) cerebellar dysfunction and (3) eye signs (nystagmus > sixth nerve palsy > other ophthalmoplegia). It is typically precipitated by acute illness (e.g. infection) in thiamine-deficient individuals (often malnourished alcoholics) and represents a medical emergency.

RED FLAG

Wernicke encephalopathy. This medical emergency is completely reversible *if* promptly treated with thiamine. If untreated, permanent Korsakoff psychosis will develop. Prophylactic vitamin B is given to all alcoholics admitted to hospital to try and prevent the development of Wernicke encephalopathy, most commonly in the form of parenteral Pabrinex (see the 'Parenteral vitamins' section).

Table 12.3 Beriberi: clinical features

Subtype	Symptoms	Signs
'Wet' beriberi: cardiovascular manifestations of thiamine deficiency	Those of end-stage cardiac failure: breathlessness (exertional → rest), orthopnoea, syncope, chest pain, dependent oedema	Elevated jugular venous pressure, tachycardia, hypotension and end-organ hypoperfusion, bibasal crepitations, dependent peripheral pitting oedema, cardiomegaly (→ displaced apex beat)
Dry beriberi: neurological manifestations of thiamine deficiency	Ascending distal paraesthesia, muscle weakness and wasting or paralysis, autonomic neuropathy: postural hypotension, constipation → nausea, vomiting	Peripheral neuropathy (sensory deficits, impaired reflexes and reduced power)
Infantile beriberi	Dyspnoea, constipation, agitation/apathy, vomiting, anorexia, gastrointestinal disturbance	Voice loss (laryngeal oedema), peripheral oedema, grunting, nystagmus, convulsions, oliguria, cyanosis, death

Korsakoff psychosis

This condition is the irreversible neuropsychiatric condition progressing from an untreated Wernicke encephalopathy. Classical hallmarks are confabulation, striking anterograde amnesia (inability to form new memories) and variable retrograde amnesia (memory loss).

COMMON PITFALLS

WERNICKE ENCEPHALOPATHY AND KORSAKOFF PSYCHOSIS DIFFERENTIATION

These are two different diagnoses, but because Korsakoff is usually preceded by Wernicke, the misleading term 'Wernicke–Korsakoff syndrome' is often used.

RIBOFLAVIN: VITAMIN B2 (WATER SOLUBLE)

Dietary riboflavin occurs in the form of flavin adenine dinucleotide (FAD; see Chapter 2, Fig. 2.17). These coenzymes are hydrolysed by intestinal phosphatases before absorption. Riboflavin is approximately 60% absorbed from the diet, and is also synthesized by intestinal bacteria. It is nontoxic in excess, as it is efficiently excreted in urine. Riboflavin is degraded by visible and UV light. Table 12.1 gives the RNI, deficiency risk factors and riboflavin-rich dietary sources.

Active forms and physiological roles

Riboflavin is the precursor of the electron carriers FAD and FMN. These coenzymes act as electron carriers in multiple redox reactions in the TCA cycle (see Chapter 3) and oxidative phosphorylation (see Chapter 4). Importantly, aside from energy generation, the following processes rely on sufficient riboflavin:

- Vitamin B6 conversion to its bioactive form, pyridoxal-5′-phosphate (PLP); this is FMN dependent.
- Nicotinamide adenine dinucleotide (NAD$^+$) and nicotinamide adenine dinucleotide phosphate (NADP$^+$) synthesis (from tryptophan) requires a FAD-dependent enzyme.
- Methionine synthesis and folate metabolism both involve FAD-dependent enzymes.
- Absorption and utilization of iron.

Clinical features of riboflavin deficiency: ariboflavinosis

Isolated ariboflavinosis is rare; it usually manifests accompanied by other water-soluble vitamin deficiencies. Symptoms include glossitis, angular stomatitis (Table 14.6, Fig. 14.6), pruritus, hair loss, seborrheic dermatitis, visual symptoms and degenerative central nervous system changes. Because FAD and FMN deficiency impacts on iron, vitamins B3, B6 and B9 (folate) metabolism, secondary deficiency of these other essential micronutrients may also arise as a consequence of ariboflavinosis. Riboflavin status is assessed by erythrocyte glutathione reductase activity assay. The result is expressed as a ratio of enzyme activity with/without added FAD. A ratio greater than 1.3 indicates functional B2 deficiency. Treatment is with oral riboflavin supplements.

NIACIN: VITAMIN B3 (WATER SOLUBLE)

Table 12.1 provides the niacin RNI, deficiency risk factors and niacin-rich dietary sources.

Active forms and physiological roles

Niacin and its derivative nicotinamide are precursors of NAD$^+$ and NADP$^+$. Both these electron carriers are pivotal in metabolism (see Chapter 2, Fig. 2.17 and 'NADP$^+$' and Fig. 2.20). In addition to these important roles, NAD$^+$ also functions as an adenosine diphosphate (ADP)-ribose donor in deoxyribonucleotide synthesis (see Chapter 10); sufficient niacin is therefore necessary for DNA replication in cell division and DNA repair (i.e. genome stability).

Endogenous synthesis from dietary tryptophan

Synthesis of niacin by tryptophan oxidation (via the kynurenine pathway) can only occur if two requirements are met:

- Sufficient vitamins B1, B2 and B6 are available (to act as cofactors in niacin biosynthesis).
- The physiological requirement for tryptophan in protein synthesis has already been met.

Less than 2% of the body's niacin is obtained by endogenous tryptophan oxidation; this becomes significant only in the context of severe dietary B3 restriction. B6 deficiency in particular can lead to B3 deficiency in this scenario.

HINTS AND TIPS

B3 DEFICIENCY SECONDARY TO B6 DEFICIENCY

The kynurenine pathway, which is responsible for endogenous synthesis of niacin from tryptophan, relies on presence of pyridoxal phosphate to act as a cofactor for kynureninase. By this mechanism, B6 deficiency can lead to B3 deficiency in conditions of inadequate dietary B3 intake.

Clinical features of B3 deficiency: pellagra

Pellagra is rare, but commonly examined. Classically, it is described by the '3Ds' (i.e. diarrhoea, dermatitis and dementia). Diarrhoea may be accompanied by nausea, vomiting and abdominal pain. The 'dermatitis' component refers to a photosensitive symmetrical erythematous scaling rash that can occur anywhere on the body. 'Casal necklace' describes a different rash that can occur: this is a fairly dramatic-looking circumferential necklace-shaped rash that is seen only with niacin deficiency. Onycholysis (Table 14.6, Fig. 14.3), angular stomatitis and glossitis (Table 14.10, Fig. 14.6) may also occur. Diagnosis is made in context of low serum niacin, tryptophan and a combined 24-hour urinary excretion of niacin metabolites less than 1.5 mg. GI and dermatological symptoms are reversible with rescue supplementation, but dementia is progressive and irreversible. Pellagra is fatal if untreated (with oral/parenteral nicotinamide supplementation).

HINTS AND TIPS

There are three 'D' symptoms in vitamin B3 deficiency (diarrhoea, dermatitis and dementia).

Vitamin B3 toxicity

Oral niacin typically causes facial flushing as a side effect; however, *excessive* oral supplementation causes nausea, vomiting and liver toxicity.

PANTOTHENIC ACID: VITAMIN B5 (WATER SOLUBLE)

Table 12.1 gives the RNI, deficiency risk factors and B5-rich food sources.

Active forms and physiological roles

Vitamin B5 is the dietary precursor of coenzyme A (CoA; see Fig. 2.21). CoA is essential to multiple life-sustaining biochemical reactions. In its acetylated version (acetyl-CoA), vitamin B5 is central to metabolism (see Chapter 2). The phosphopantetheinyl moiety of CoA is an essential component of several proteins, for example, acetyl-CoA and malonyl-CoA:ACP transacylase (see Fig. 7.9), a key player in fatty acid synthesis. It uses the same transporter as vitamin B7 for intestinal absorption.

Clinical features of B5 deficiency

Dietary deficiency is extremely rare due to the widespread presence of B5 in food ('pantos' meaning 'everywhere' in Greek). Experimentally induced B5 deficiency with a pantothenic kinase inhibitor/deficient diet combination led participants to complain of headache, fatigue, insomnia, GI disturbance and paraesthesia in the extremities, so theoretically these symptoms could occur in severe deficiency, but B5 deficiency has not been reported outside of this context.

Potential drug interactions

Oral B5 supplementation potentiates cholinesterase inhibitor action, which could be dangerous if such drugs (e.g. donepezil, memantine or rivastigmine) were co-ingested with large amounts of B5 supplements.

PYRIDOXINE: VITAMIN B6 (WATER SOLUBLE)

The RNI, deficiency risk factors and B6-rich dietary sources are given in Table 12.1.

Active forms and physiological roles

There are three forms of nonphosphorylated vitamin B6: pyridoxal, pyridoxine and pyridoxamine. The phosphate ester derivative of pyridoxal, pyridoxal phosphate (PLP), is the bioactive cofactor utilized by the majority of B6-dependent enzymes. Important PLP-dependent enzymes include the following:

- Amino acid decarboxylase (serotonin and dopamine synthesis (see Fig. 9.13))
- Glycogen phosphorylase (glycogenolysis; see Chapter 5)
- Cystathionine synthetase and lyase (see Chapter 9 and Fig. 9.11)
- Kynureninase (involved in endogenous vitamin B3 synthesis)
- 5-Aminolevulinic acid synthase (haem synthesis; see Chapter 10)
- Serine hydroxymethyltransferase (one-carbon metabolism; see Chapter 10)

Clinical features of B6 deficiency

The most clinically relevant scenario of B6 deficiency is secondary to use of specific drugs without co-prescribed B6 supplementation. Neuropsychiatric symptoms include confusion, irritability and depression. Glossitis, aphthous mouth ulcers and angular stomatitis (Table 14.10, Fig. 14.6) may be seen. Low serum PLP confirms the diagnosis, and treatment consists of oral B6 supplements.

CLINICAL NOTES

ISONIAZID AS A CAUSE OF VITAMIN B6 DEFICIENCIES

Isoniazid, along with drugs including cycloserine, penicillamine and L-3,4-dihydroxyphenylalanine (L-DOPA), forms complexes with ingested B6, limiting its bioavailability and resulting in deficiency. Oral B6 supplementation must be co-prescribed prophylactically to prevent iatrogenic B6 deficiency.

BIOTIN: VITAMIN B7 (WATER SOLUBLE)

Biotin intake (from diet or commensal bacterial synthesis) is necessary as an endogenous synthetic mechanism is lacking. Absorption across enterocytes uses the same sodium-dependent transporter as vitamin B5. Biotin is nontoxic in excess.

Active forms and physiological roles

Biotin functions as a cofactor for several key carboxylases, which are necessary for catabolism of branched-chain amino acids, gluconeogenesis and fatty acid synthesis.

Clinical features of B7 deficiency

Clinical features of deficiency range include neurological symptoms (ataxia, depression, lethargy, hallucinations, paraesthesia and convulsions) and epithelial symptoms (dermatitis, glossitis, angular stomatitis, hair loss). B7 deficiency is extremely rare and is only known to occur in the following scenarios:

- Prolonged high consumption of raw egg whites (contain avidin, which binds to biotin, preventing intestinal absorption)
- Prolonged total parenteral nutrition lacking biotin
- Exclusively formula-fed infants where manufacturing error had led to the formula being devoid of biotin
- Rare inborn errors of biotin metabolism (e.g. biotinidase deficiency)

Because deficiency is so rare, biotin status indicators are rarely clinically relevant; however, the most reliable biomarker is the lymphocyte levels of specific biotin-dependent carboxylases.

FOLATE: VITAMIN B9 (WATER SOLUBLE)

See Table 12.1 for RNI, deficiency risk factors and folate-rich foods.

Active forms and physiological roles

5,6,7,8-Tetrahydrofolate (THF) is the bioactive derivative of folate, formed by two sequential reduction reactions catalysed by dihydrofolate reductase. DNA and RNA syntheses require an available pool of THF, as the methylation of deoxyuridylate (an important step in thymidine synthesis) requires THF. Any physiological process involving cell division is thus dependent on sufficient folate availability.

One-carbon transfer

Please see Chapter 10 for details on folate's role in one-carbon transfer.

Role of folate in embryogenesis

The developing fetus requires folate for neural tube closure. Incomplete closure results in anencephaly (incompatible with life) or spina bifida (permanent disability). The developmental stage at which the neural tube closes (24–26 days postconception) is when the developing embryo is most susceptible to the devastating consequences of maternal folate deficiency. For this reason, preconception folate supplements should be taken by women attempting to get pregnant and continued during pregnancy and breastfeeding.

Dietary absorption and storage

Ingested folate is absorbed into duodenal and jejunal enterocytes, via hydrogen-coupled transporter. Some folate is extruded unaltered into the portal circulation, and the remainder first converted within enterocytes to 5-methyl-THF. The liver sequesters some folate, and approximately 15 mg is stored here, with a further approximately 15 mg 'stored' in blood cells and tissues. Folate stores last only a few months, as the storage amount is small relative to daily demand.

Clinical features of folate deficiency

As with B12 deficiency, early symptoms of folate deficiency are related to the macrocytic anaemia ('megaloblastic' according to characteristic blood film appearance) that results (see Chapter 14). In addition, angular stomatitis, glossitis and neuropsychiatric deficits are likely in severe deficiency. Serum folate and red cell folate are used as biomarkers of folate status, the latter being more representative of long-term status. Deficiency is treated with oral folate supplementation, accompanied by B12 supplements.

RED FLAG

Clarification of folate/B12 status in megaloblastic anaemia. This is paramount, because a B12 deficiency will cause a secondary folate deficiency. However, folate supplementation in the absence of B12 supplementation in this context will correct the megaloblastic anaemia, but will allow the B12 deficiency to persist and neurological deficits to progress to permanence.

B12 deficiency: impact on folate metabolism

Reduced activity of methionine synthase (secondary to B12 deficiency) impairs THF availability, as folate becomes 'trapped' as methylfolate. THF is then not available to participate in DNA synthesis and repair, and symptoms of folate deficiency manifest paradoxically, because the body is technically folate replete.

COBALAMIN: VITAMIN B12

Vitamin B12 is a large, complex molecule containing a cobalt ion. GI absorption is complex, with numerous stages. This multistaged process is thus vulnerable to diverse pathologies that have the common outcome of B12 deficiency secondary to failed absorption. As B12 cannot be synthesized endogenously, it is an essential dietary component. See Table 12.1 for RNI, deficiency risk factors and B12-rich dietary sources. B12 is nontoxic in excess.

Active forms and physiological roles

The bioactive vitamin B12 molecules are 5'-deoxyadenosylcobalamin and methylcobalamin. It is a complex tetrapyrrole (known as corrin) ring with an associated cobalt ion. Availability of methylcobalamin is mandatory for maintaining bioavailability of folate and thus maintenance of DNA integrity and genomic stability (see Chapter 10). Vitamin B12 is also essential for normal neuronal myelination, accounting for the neurological symptoms associated with deficiency.

Methylcobalamin

Methylcobalamin is a cofactor for methionine synthase, which:

1. Catalyses the homocysteine → methionine reaction. Methionine is required for S-adenosyl methionine (SAM) synthesis. SAM is important in one-carbon transfer, where it functions as a methyl group recipient and donor in the methylation of RNA, DNA and proteins.
2. Is required for the reaction that releases THF from the 'methylfolate' molecule, allowing it to participate in purine and pyrimidine synthesis, which are necessary for RNA and DNA synthesis and repair.

5'-Deoxyadenosylcobalamin

5'-Deoxyadenosylcobalamin is a cofactor for an enzyme required for succinyl-CoA synthesis from propionyl-CoA (methylmalonyl-CoA mutase). Succinyl-CoA is an important gateway molecule for catabolic metabolites derived from valine, isoleucine, threonine and methionine to access the TCA cycle. Odd-numbered fatty acid catabolism likewise generates propionyl-CoA, which accesses the TCA cycle via conversion to succinyl-CoA. Succinyl-CoA is a substrate for haem synthesis (see Chapter 10).

B12 deficiency-induced loss of methylmalonyl-CoA mutase function results in accumulation of methylmalonyl-CoA. This molecule inhibits fatty acid synthesis. Myelin sheath maintenance requires a continuous turnover of fatty acids, and structural disintegration results from sustained underactivity of fatty acid synthesis. This mechanism most likely accounts for the neurological pathology seen in B12 deficiency.

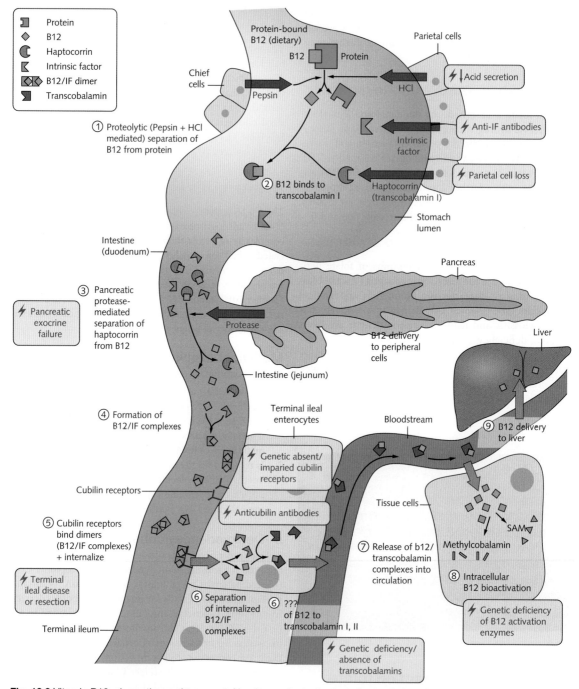

Fig. 12.3 Vitamin B12: absorption and transport. Numbers refer to the text. Anatomic locations are highlighted in blue. Red lightning bolts highlighted in yellow indicate various specific disorders of B12 metabolism which can all contribute to B12 deficiency. *IF,* Intrinsic factor; *SAM,* S-adenosyl methionine.

Vitamin B12 absorption and transport

Numbers refer to Fig. 12.3.

1. Dietary vitamin B12 released from proteins by hydrolysis in gastric lumen

2. Free B12 then binds to R-protein (also known as 'haptocorrin')

3. R-protein/B12 complex is cleaved by a pancreatic protease in the duodenum, releasing B12

4. Intrinsic factor (IF) binds the freed B12 and dimerizes

5. IF-bound B12 dimers bind to specific enterocyte receptors (cubilin) in the terminal ileum and are internalized.
6. Within the enterocyte, B12 binds to transcobalamin proteins 1, 2 or 3
7. B12/transcobalamin complexes are extruded into the portal circulation.
8. B12 may be stored in the liver (total stores last ~2 years) or delivered to peripheral tissues (liver, bone marrow)
9. Intracellular conversion to bioactive forms (deoxyadenosylcobalamin and methylcobalamin)

Pathophysiology of various mechanisms leading to B12 deficiency

Any abnormalities of any of the steps in the aforementioned list will lead to B12 deficiency.

Clinical features of deficiency

Endogenous B12 stores usually last up to 2 years, so symptoms/signs of deficiency may lag up to 2 years after dietary intake becomes inadequate. Onset is usually insidious. Symptoms and signs of anaemia (see Chapter 14: Anaemia) appear early, and later neurological symptoms may include:

- Peripheral paraesthesia and numbness
- Myelopathy: ascending distal motor weakness, gait disturbance
- Progressive cognitive deficit, depression

Non-neurological symptoms include anorexia, glossitis, angular stomatitis and constipation.

Diagnosis and treatment of B12 deficiency

Symptoms/signs consistent with B12 deficiency usually prompt an initial full blood count and serum B12 measurements, which will reveal a macrocytic anaemia with megaloblastic features on the blood film. Elevation of serum homocysteine (which cannot be converted to methionine in B12 deficiency) and methylmalonic acid (a metabolite of methylmalonyl-CoA, which accumulates in B12 deficiency) confirms deficiency and will be elevated even before symptoms manifest. Classically, the Schilling test (see Chapter 14) is used to confirm/refute IF deficiency as the cause of an established B12 deficiency. Treatment is with oral/parenteral B12.

Specific forms of B12 deficiency

Certain pathophysiological mechanisms are popular examination topics.

CLINICAL NOTES

SUBACUTE COMBINED DEGENERATION OF THE CORD

This pattern of neurological signs is seen secondary to deficiency of folate, B12 or a combination of both. A combination of dorsal and lateral spinal columns is impaired. Classically, examination reveals absent distal (ankle) reflexes with relative proximal (knee) hyperreflexia and progressive sensory impairment (proprioception > vibration > light touch > pinprick > temperature).

Pernicious anaemia

Pernicious anaemia is the most common cause of non-dietary B12 deficiency. It arises via autoimmunity: usually secondary to antibody-mediated gastric parietal cell destruction (with failure of IF secretion), but cubilin- or transcobalamin-bound B12 is also a potential auto-antibody targets.

Classically, in addition to anaemia, neurological and mucosal symptoms, premature greying/whitening of the hair is seen when B12 deficiency arises by this mechanism, and a 'lemon-yellow pallor' is used to describe the combination of mild jaundice (ineffective erythropoiesis → increased red cell fragility and haemolysis) and anaemia-induced pallor.

VITAMIN C (WATER SOLUBLE)

Vitamin C is ascorbic acid. Table 12.1 provides the RNI, deficiency risk factors and examples of vitamin C-rich foods.

Active forms and physiological roles

As a powerful reducing agent (electron donor), vitamin C plays a role in multiple intracellular redox reactions. It is the primary water-soluble antioxidant, offering intracellular molecules protection from oxidative stress. Furthermore, vitamin C regenerates oxidized vitamin E, the primary fat-soluble antioxidant. Vitamin C also promotes enterocyte absorption of nonhaem (ferric) iron, by promoting the $Fe^{3+} \rightarrow Fe^{2+}$ reduction. It also plays an important role in normal immune function. Finally, vitamin C functions as cofactor for several key enzymes:

- Dopamine β-hydroxylase, responsible for catecholamine synthesis (see Chapter 9 and Fig. 9.13)
- 4-Hydroxyphenylpyruvate dioxygenase, responsible for tyrosine catabolism
- Three separate hydroxylases required for normal proline and lysine hydroxylation in collagen synthesis

Collagen synthesis, necessary for normal vascular wall integrity and tissue repair, is defective in vitamin C deficiency, leading to many of the observable clinical symptoms/signs.

Dietary vitamin C absorption

Vitamin C is directly absorbed in its dietary form. Multiple absorption mechanisms exist, including active and secondary active sodium-coupled transporters, simple and facilitated diffusion. Up to approximately 90% of ingested vitamin C is absorbed. Pectin, zinc and iron can impair vitamin C absorption if co-ingested in high amounts. When vitamin C status is replete, active absorption is reduced, limiting dietary absorption when not physiologically needed. Vitamin C travels unbound in plasma, or in red cells. Renal conservation or excretion effectively regulates serum vitamin C, so serious side effects of toxicity are rare (although >2 g/day will cause GI upset) with normal renal function. A limited amount is stored, mostly in skeletal muscle.

Clinical features of deficiency

Severe vitamin C deficiency (scurvy) is rare nowadays, although smokers are more vulnerable due to nicotine-induced increase in intake requirement. Historically, scurvy caused great morbidity and mortality among sailors due to extended periods without access to fruit and vegetables.

Deficiency symptoms include lethargy and susceptibility to infection, but relate primarily to defective collagen synthesis (i.e. impaired tissue repair leading to poor wound healing and vascular fragility), resulting in:

- Perifollicular haemorrhages
- Mucosal membrane bleeding (gums, nose)
- Easy bruising
- Joint effusions and joint pain

Serum vitamin C and leucocyte vitamin C are used as biomarkers of vitamin C repletion. The latter gives a better indicator of long-term status. Treatment of deficiency is with oral supplements.

PARENTERAL VITAMINS

Acute admissions can be complicated in alcohol-dependent patients by Wernicke encephalopathy (see the 'Wernicke encephalopathy' section). Parenteral vitamin B1 is administered with intravenous dextrose as prophylaxis against this acute manifestation of thiamine deficiency. The most-used formulation (Pabrinex) also contains vitamins B2, B3, B6 and C in addition to B1, because alcohol dependence is particularly associated with deficiencies of these essential vitamins. Pabrinex is used for emergency treatment of severe vitamin depletion seen in patients with malabsorption, severe malnutrition and certain psychiatric syndromes. It is also used to prevent the development of refeeding syndrome.

● Chapter Summary

- Vitamins, along with minerals (see Chapter 13), represent micronutrients. The discrimination between macronutrients (such as proteins, lipids and carbohydrates) is based on the magnitude of the daily intake requirement.
- Vitamins are classified as either fat soluble (A, D, E and K) or water soluble (the B vitamins and vitamin C).
- There are various parameters used to characterize the various recommended daily intakes of each vitamin. The reference nutrient intake is used in the UK.
- Certain disease conditions (e.g. malnutrition, malabsorption) predispose to multiple vitamin and mineral deficiencies. Other factors may predispose to specific vitamin/mineral deficiencies.
- Deficiencies of each vitamin may arise due to chronic insufficient dietary intake, or other factors specific to the vitamin. Deficiencies can lead to clinical features characteristic of the deficient vitamin. In the case of fat-soluble vitamins, excessive intake can also lead to toxicity.

Minerals and their deficiencies 13

INTRODUCTION

The term 'mineral' refers to inorganic elements that must be consumed regularly in small amounts for growth and maintenance of health. A typical human diet is composed of approximately 5% minerals.

The World Health Organization (WHO) defines a mineral as 'essential' when prolonged insufficient intake impairs physiological processes/function. This is usually because the mineral is an integral component of an important protein, often an enzyme.

Minerals: important definitions

Minerals are 'micronutrients', that is, their intake is required in small amounts (compared with the 'macronutrients'; e.g. carbohydrates). If sustained, insufficient mineral intake results in chronic disease, whereas excessive intake may result in toxicity.

Minerals can be classified as 'major minerals' (also known as 'nontrace' elements) or 'trace elements'. The differentiation is according to daily intake requirements and relative body composition. The major elements are required in more than 100 mg daily and are present in the body in quantities greater than 5 g, whereas trace elements have daily intake requirements under 100 mg and are present in the body in quantities less than 5 g.

Iron, zinc, copper and iodine are the most medically significant essential trace elements and are discussed in this chapter. Reference nutrient intakes (RNIs), dietary sources and patient groups at risk for deficiency for these essential trace elements and major minerals are given in Table 13.1.

SODIUM, POTASSIUM AND CHLORIDE

Total body deficiency or overload of each of these clinically significant ions is rare. However, their concentration in plasma often becomes abnormal due to acute or chronic metabolic disturbances affecting their distribution across body compartments. Because the serum concentration of these ions influences cardiac and neuronal action potentials, fluid distribution and plasma osmolality, their homeostasis is clinically significant. Derangements outside the normal clinical parameters have characteristic clinical effects, addressed in the following section.

Sodium

Na^+ ions are the major determinant of fluid distribution between intracellular, extracellular and intravascular compartments. The differential concentration across cell membranes affects the resting membrane potential in all cells and the threshold potential for action potential generation in electrically excitable cells such as cardiac myocytes and neurons.

Because of the abundance of sodium in all food, dietary deficiency is vanishingly rare. Excessive intake is self-limiting (large intake rapidly causes vomiting). However, derangements of plasma concentration are very common and have a multitude of potential causes (Tables 13.2 and 13.3).

The diagnostic utility of the serum level is that it provides information about a patient's fluid status. Most commonly, a high Na^+ represents intravascular depletion secondary to dehydration, whereas a low Na^+ often represents intravascular fluid overload – but it is often not that simple. It is vital to clinically assess the patient (Table 13.4) and determine the cause rather than making assumptions and restricting/administering fluid inappropriately. Fig. 13.1 provides a sample diagnostic approach.

Management of raised/lowered serum Na^+

Identifying and correcting the cause of the derangement should gradually normalize the plasma Na^+. If this approach does not attain sufficient normalization:

- Euvolaemic hyponatraemia can be treated with mild fluid restriction
- Hypovolaemic hyponatraemia can be treated with isotonic saline
- Hypervolaemic hyponatraemia can be treated with fluid restriction and diuresis
- Hypernatremia can be treated with isotonic glucose (dextrose) solution

Table 13.1 Minerals: RNI, dietary sources and specific groups at risk for deficiency[a,b]

Mineral	RNI (mg)[c]	Particularly rich dietary sources	Dietary factors placing individuals at risk for deficiency
Sodium	1600	Salt, cereals, meat	—
Potassium	3500	Fruit and vegetables, fish, shellfish, poultry, milk	—
Chloride	2500	Salt, salt substitutes, seaweed, rye, tomatoes, olives	—
Calcium	700	Dairy products, leafy green vegetables, Brazil and hazel nuts	Exclusion of dairy products (e.g. veganism).
Phosphate	550	Fish, poultry, red meat	—
Magnesium	300	Unprocessed grains, seeds, nuts, leafy vegetables	—
Iron	6.7 (males) 11.4 (females)	Haem iron: meat, poultry, fish Nonhaem iron: beans, nuts, wholegrain, dark-green leafy vegetables	High consumption of iron absorption inhibitors. Veganism/vegetarianism; despite high nonhaem iron intake, nonhaem iron is relatively poorly absorbed.
Copper	1.2	Offal, shellfish, crustaceans, nuts	—
Zinc	10	Oysters, beef, pork	High phytate consumption (e.g. vegetarian diet). Phytate impairs GI zinc absorption. Oral metal chelator therapy (e.g. penicillamine).
Iodine	0.14	Seafood (marine fish, shellfish), seaweed, sea salt, cow's milk and dairy products	Living in an iodine-deficient area lacking an iodine fortification programme. Exclusion of seafood and dairy (e.g. vegan diet).

[a] *Diseases causing malabsorption, such as inflammatory bowel disease, gastric bypass surgery and generalized malnutrition may cause deficiencies in any/all minerals.*
[b] *Major minerals are bold.*
[c] *RNI values shown here are taken from Department of Health dietary reference values and refer to adults only. Please note that RNI values change often, as nutrition research progresses. Please consult www.BDA.uk.com or other authentic sources for the latest intake recommendations.*
GI, Gastrointestinal; RNI, reference nutrient intake.

Table 13.2 Causes of hyponatraemia. Hyponatraemia is classified according to intravascular volume status[a]

Intravascular volume status	Example causes
Hypovolaemic hyponatraemia	Diuretics Diarrhoea Vomiting Pancreatitis Osmotic diuresis Renal tubular acidosis Burns Cerebral salt wasting Mineralocorticoid deficiency
Normovolaemic hyponatraemia	Hypothyroidism Primary polydipsia Syndrome of inappropriate antidiuretic hormone secretion Glucocorticoid deficiency Drugs
Hypervolaemic hyponatraemia	Congestive cardiac failure Renal failure Nephrotic syndrome Cirrhotic liver disease

[a] *Certain conditions can lead to hyponatraemia or hypernatraemia, depending on whether it is the water or sodium loss that is predominant.*

Table 13.3 Causes of hypernatraemia, classified by underlying mechanism[a]

Mechanism	Examples
Water deficit (insufficient water intake)	Psychiatric illness Debility/excessive frailty Inadequate supply by carers
Water deficit (excessive water loss)	Diabetes insipidus Excessive sweating
Relative water deficit (loss of sodium, but relatively greater loss of water)	Diarrhoea Vomiting Osmotic diuresis[b] Burns Renal disease Polyuric acute tubular necrosis
Excessive sodium	Overenthusiastic administration of intravenous saline Inappropriate administration of intravenous hypertonic saline Mineralocorticoid excess

[a] *Certain conditions can lead to hyponatraemia or hypernatraemia, depending on the whether it is the water or sodium loss that is predominant.*
[b] *Osmotic diuresis occurs with mannitol administration, a very high protein diet, hyperglycaemia or excessive tissue catabolism.*

Table 13.4 Clinical assessment of intravascular fluid status

	Hypovolaemia	Euvolaemia	Hypervolaemia
Mucosal membrane hydration	Reduced	Normal, moist	Moist
Jugular venous pressure level	Absent	<4 cm above sternal angle	>4 cm above sternal angle
Skin turgor	Reduced	Normal	Normal
Capillary refill time	>3 seconds	<3 seconds	<3 seconds
Heart rate	Tachycardia	Normal	Tachycardia
Peripheral oedema	Unlikely[a]	Unlikely[a]	Likely
Basal lung auscultation (pulmonary oedema)	Normal[a]	Normal[a]	Fine, end-inspiratory crepitations
Reported thirst	Yes	Unlikely	Unlikely
Urine output (mL/kg/hour)	<0.5	0.5–1.0	>1.0
Systolic blood pressure (SBP)	<90 mmHg (caution – fall in SBP is a late sign of severe dehydration)	Normal	Normal
Postural drop in SBP	>10 mmHg	<10 mmHg	
Total body weight	Reduced	Normal	Increased

[a] Caution in renal or cardiac failure – peripheral and pulmonary oedema may be present despite intravascular hypovolaemia.

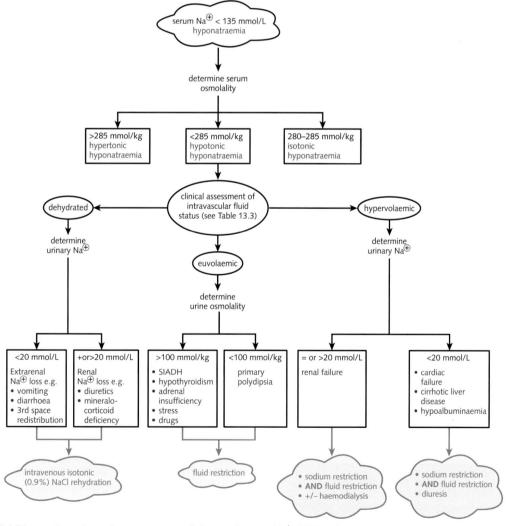

Fig. 13.1 Diagnostic pathway for assessment of abnormal serum Na$^+$. *SIADH*, Syndrome of inappropriate antidiuretic hormone secretion.

Severe, acute hyponatraemia (which may present with seizures) is a medical emergency; initial treatment is with hypertonic saline under senior supervision, followed by isotonic saline. In all other scenarios, correction of abnormal plasma sodium should be performed gradually, due to the risk for central pontine myelinolysis in hyponatraemia or acute cerebral oedema in hypernatraemia.

Potassium

Like sodium, total body deficiency of potassium is very rare, given its abundance in food. However, derangement of plasma K^+ is common, arising from abnormalities of distribution secondary to other pathophysiology (Tables 13.5 and 13.6). Potassium is the predominant intracellular cation, and like sodium is essential for maintaining the resting membrane potential. Because of the influence of plasma K^+ on myocardial excitability – hyperkalaemia and hypokalaemia can both induce life-threatening arrhythmias. For this reason, if symptomatic, urgent action to normalize the serum K^+ is necessary *before* attempting to treat the cause. Serum potassium concentrations less than 3.0 mmol/L or greater than 6.0 mmol/L usually require urgent treatment.

Chloride

As with sodium and potassium, total body deficiency of chloride is very rare due to its abundance in all food. Similarly, a deranged chloride value should prompt identification and treatment of the cause. With chloride, disturbances may be secondary to acid–base disturbance or renal tubular dysfunction – so quantification of serum K^+, renal function as well as blood gas analysis is essential to correctly diagnose the cause.

Table 13.5 Causes of hyperkalaemia according to pathophysiological mechanism

Mechanism	Example causes
Impaired renal excretion of K^+ ions	Renal failure (any cause) Metabolic acidosis Addison's disease Drugs (e.g. spironolactone)
Release of K^+ ions from the intracellular to extracellular compartments	Diabetic ketoacidosis Metabolic acidosis Haemolysis Tumour lysis syndrome Extensive tissue injury (e.g. burns) Digoxin toxicity
Excessive potassium intake	Iatrogenic: excessive oral or intravenous potassium supplementation Excessive consumption of potassium-rich foods
Spurious/misleading elevation of serum K^+	In-needle haemolysis resulting from troublesome venesection Blood drawn from arm with prolonged tourniquet placement In vitro release of intracellular K^+ from overly fragile leukaemic cells

Table 13.6 Causes of hypokalaemia according to mechanism

Mechanism	Example causes
Increased renal K^+ excretion	Thiazide and loop diuretics Diabetic ketoacidosis[a] Acute tubular necrosis Renal tubular acidosis (types I and II) Mineralocorticoid excess Barter, Gitelman and Liddle syndromes
Intracellular movement of extracellular K^+ ions	Hyperthyroidism Metabolic alkalosis Pheochromocytoma Drugs (β-agonists, phosphodiesterase inhibitors, tocolytics) Insulin
Nonrenal K^+ ion loss	Laxatives Diarrhoea Vomiting Nasogastric drainage Enteric fistula Extensive burns
Insufficient dietary potassium intake	Severe malnutrition Generalized malabsorption

[a]Note that diabetic ketoacidosis may present with both hypo-and hyperkalaemia. Total body potassium is usually depleted.

CALCIUM

Calcium is the most abundant mineral in the body. A 70-kg adult contains 1.2 kg of calcium, of which 99% is in bone (as hydroxyapatite). Free ionized calcium is a highly promiscuous signalling ion, and as such its serum concentration is tightly regulated (Table 13.7). RNI is greater during growth, pregnancy, lactation and postmenopause in females.

Active forms and physiological roles

Free ionized calcium ions is the biologically active form of calcium. Calcium ions bound to serum albumin do not exert physiological effects. Calcium is necessary for the following essential physiological processes:

- Neuromuscular transmission
- Neurotransmitter and hormone release
- Muscle contraction (skeletal, smooth and cardiac)
- Neuronal function
- Blood coagulation
- Many intracellular signalling cascades

Absorption and transport

About 1 g of calcium is ingested daily, and approximately 35% of this is absorbed. Gastrointestinal (GI) epithelial absorption of ingested calcium is primarily controlled by vitamin D and parathyroid hormone (PTH). However, GI absorption is also influenced by the presence of other dietary factors. Some (e.g. organic, sugar and citric acids and basic amino acids) promote absorption, whereas others (e.g. fibre, phytates, oxalates, iron, magnesium and an alkaline pH) impair absorption.

Serum calcium ions circulate freely or are bound to albumin at negatively charged binding sites. Albumin therefore acts as a reservoir of calcium ions, attenuating abrupt changes in serum Ca^{++}. The concentration of free ionized calcium does not therefore necessarily reflect the *total* serum calcium. Appreciating the difference is important because it is only *free ionized calcium* that is biologically active. Signs of increased or decreased serum calcium (hypercalcaemia or hypocalcaemia) occur according to the *free ionized* (rather than the total) calcium concentration, *not* the total serum calcium.

Table 13.7 Normal ranges for plasma calcium concentration

Serum parameter	Normal range (mmol/L)
Free ionized calcium	1.0–1.25
Total calcium	2.10–2.60

CALCIUM PARAMETERS

The most common calcium parameter used clinically is the 'corrected' calcium. This refers to the result of a calculation made by the laboratory to 'correct' for the albumin. This limits the confounding influence of a low albumin, which would otherwise imply a low total calcium (i.e. calcium deficiency despite normal levels of (biologically active) free ionized calcium).

Serum *ionized calcium* concentration is highly influenced by pH. Acidosis increases the proportion of free ionized calcium ions, whereas alkalosis decreases it. Thus a change in the pH results in a rapid change in free Ca^{++}, which may cause clinical effects.

CLINICAL NOTES

pH INFLUENCE ON FREE IONIZED CALCIUM

An example of this is seen in hyperventilation. The increased minute volume causes a respiratory alkalosis (a raised pH). This leads to increases in calcium–albumin binding, and to signs and symptoms of hypocalcaemia, despite the total serum Ca^{++} remaining constant.

Calcium homeostasis

Calcium homeostasis is maintained by the integrated action of the kidney, bone and the GI tract. The kidney excretes calcium into the urine. The GI tract absorbs calcium. Calcium may be resorbed or deposited in bone, depending on the hormonal balance. Three main hormones (which also influence serum PO_4^{2-}) influence serum calcium levels:

- PTH: increases serum Ca^{2+}, decreases serum PO_4^{2-}
- Vitamin D: increases both serum Ca^{2+} and PO_4^{2-}
- Calcitonin: decreases both serum Ca^{2+} and PO_4^{2-}

Their actions are summarized in Fig. 13.2.

Clinical features of chronic calcium deficiency

A total body calcium deficiency may occur due to:

- Insufficient dietary intake
- Vitamin D deficiency (see Chapter 12)
- Malabsorption

Longstanding hypocalcaemia is seen in chronic calcium deficiency, but renal disease and impairment of the normal homeostatic mechanisms (e.g. hypoparathyroidism) can also result in hypocalcaemia. Acute hypocalcaemia is usually symptomatic.

RED FLAG

Acute hypocalcaemia. Low serum concentration of free ionized calcium can cause acute neuromuscular symptoms such as paraesthesia, tetany, laryngospasm and bronchospasm, cardiac insufficiency, syncope and seizures. Treatment is with cautious intravenous calcium.

The primary manifestation of chronic calcium deficiency is insufficient bone mineralization. This results in soft, easily deformed bones which fracture easily. Inadequate bone mineralization is common to calcium-deficient adults and children; but in children linear bone growth is affected, resulting in permanent deformities.

COMMON PITFALLS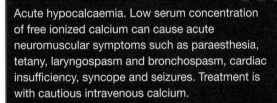

VITAMIN D DEFICIENCY MIRRORING CALCIUM DEFICIENCY

Because calcium deficiency may be secondary to vitamin D deficiency, manifestations such osteomalacia and rickets may be seen with vitamin D deficiency. Thus malabsorption and chronic renal insufficiency, by causing vitamin D deficiency, will also result in calcium deficiency.

Rickets

In children, or adults who were calcium-deficient in childhood, the constellation of permanent skeletal deformities is referred to as 'rickets'. Features of rickets are illustrated in Fig. 13.3.

Osteomalacia

In adults, calcium deficiency results in osteomalacia. This is where bone demineralization increases bone fragility and can manifest with recurrent fractures resulting from minimal or no trauma. There may be widespread bone and joint pain. A dual energy X-ray absorptiometry (DEXA) scan 'Z score' less than -2 indicates bone mineral density reduced for the patient's age.

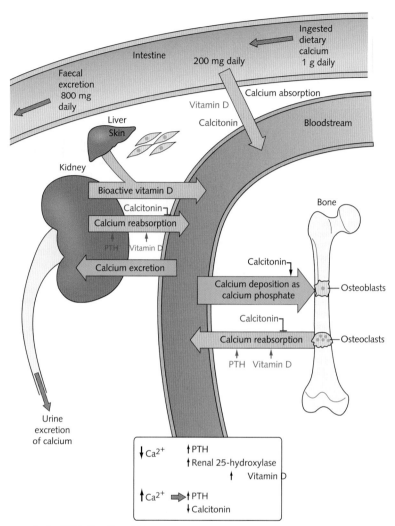

Fig. 13.2 Calcium homeostasis. *PTH,* Parathyroid hormone.

Diagnosis and treatment of calcium deficiency

A dietary history suggesting inadequate calcium or vitamin D, or a fragility fracture(s) (see Chapter 14) should prompt targeted investigations including:

- Serum calcium, vitamin D, phosphate, alkaline phosphatase and PTH
- DEXA scan or long bone radiographs

Treatment is with oral calcium supplementation, in combination with vitamin D if appropriate.

Clinical features of toxicity (hypercalcaemia)

Hypercalcaemia (serum corrected Ca^{++} >2.5 mmol/L) is rarely due to excessive dietary intake. The only

nutritional cause of hypercalcaemia is the 'milk-alkali syndrome'. This is usually due to excessive calcium supplement consumption in the presence of high absorbable alkali such as antacids. The alkalosis impairs renal excretion of calcium and combined with excessive intake leads to hypercalcaemia.

Note that hypercalcaemia is usually secondary to malignancy or disruption of hormonal regulation, for example, hyperparathyroidism. Manifestations of hypercalcaemia include:

- Polyuria, polydipsia, renal calculi and renal impairment
- Fatigue and other neuropsychiatric symptoms
- Abdominal pain, constipation
- Soft tissue calcification ('metastatic' calcification)

Acute hypercalcemia is a medical emergency.

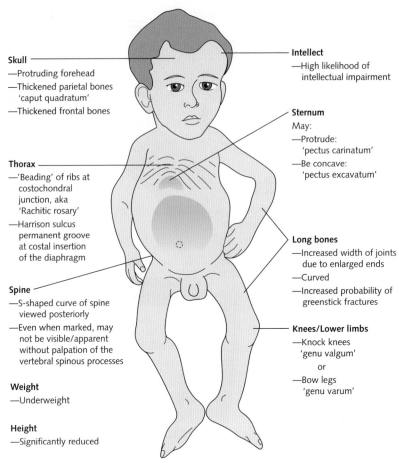

Skull
—Protruding forehead
—Thickened parietal bones 'caput quadratum'
—Thickened frontal bones

Intellect
—High likelihood of intellectual impairment

Sternum
May:
—Protrude: 'pectus carinatum'
—Be concave: 'pectus excavatum'

Thorax
—'Beading' of ribs at costochondral junction, aka 'Rachitic rosary'
—Harrison sulcus permanent groove at costal insertion of the diaphragm

Long bones
—Increased width of joints due to enlarged ends
—Curved
—Increased probability of greenstick fractures

Spine
—S-shaped curve of spine viewed posteriorly
—Even when marked, may not be visible/apparent without palpation of the vertebral spinous processes

Knees/Lower limbs
—Knock knees 'genu valgum' or
—Bow legs 'genu varum'

Weight
—Underweight

Height
—Significantly reduced

Fig. 13.3 Rickets.

RED FLAG

Acute/extreme hypercalcaemia. Ca^{++} up to 3.5 mmol/L may be tolerated chronically, with insidious symptoms development. However, an acute rise to these levels, or even a gradual rise to extremely high levels can cause renal impairment, cardiac arrhythmia and profound muscle weakness. Symptomatic or marked (>3.5 mmol/L) hypercalcaemia is therefore treated with aggressive intravenous (IV) 0.9% saline hydration, IV bisphosphonates and sometimes calcitonin.

PHOSPHORUS

Like calcium, the vast majority of the body's phosphate is incorporated in bone as structural hydroxyapatite. It is also vital for normal cellular function.

Active forms and physiological role

The phosphate ion (PO_4^{2-}) found in biological solutions consists of a phosphorus ion associated with four oxygen atoms. It is termed 'inorganic' to differentiate it from organically bound phosphate such as that in adenosine triphosphate (ATP). It has several fundamental physiological roles:

- Structural – component of bone and teeth
- Genetic – nucleic acid component
- Metabolic – component of ATP and other phosphorylated metabolic intermediates
- Buffering function – phosphate functions as a buffer in urine, bone and serum

Absorption and transport

Phosphate is absorbed from the gut in a vitamin D-dependent manner. Approximately 20% of serum phosphate is protein bound. Phosphate homeostasis is closely linked to calcium homeostasis (see the 'Calcium homeostasis' section). Vitamin D increases serum phosphate by promoting GI absorption, whereas calcitonin and PTH inhibit osteoclast resorption of bone, lowering serum phosphate. PTH also inhibits renal reabsorption of filtered phosphate.

Disorders of serum phosphate

As with other major minerals, derangements of serum phosphate levels are usually a result of abnormal absorption, excretion or distribution of total body phosphate across compartments, rather than an excess/insufficiency of intake in diet. Because of the abundance in all food, dietary phosphate deficiency is extremely rare. Diagnosis of hyperphosphataemia/hypophosphataemia is made based on serum phosphate, which would be measured in patients with risk factors or with suggestive symptoms.

Hypophosphataemia

Moderate hypophosphataemia is often due to chronic ingestion of antacids or phosphate binders, which impair GI phosphate absorption. Hyperparathyroidism and chronic excess alcohol use may also cause hypophosphataemia.

Acute severe hypophosphataemia (<0.3 mmol/L) is an emergency because it causes profound muscle weakness, ultimately leading to respiratory compromise. It is treated with intravenous phosphate. Severe hypophosphataemia, may be present in acute respiratory alkalosis, parenteral insulin administration in diabetic ketoacidosis, and haemofiltration. Severe hypophosphataemia, together with hypokalaemia and hypomagnesaemia, develop in refeeding syndrome (see Chapter 8).

Hyperphosphataemia

Because intact renal excretion ably prevents hyperphosphataemia in the context of normal intake, hyperphosphataemia is most often encountered in renal impairment scenarios. Even with severe hyperphosphataemia, symptoms and signs are usually absent. Paraesthesia and more dangerous neurological symptoms such as convulsions and delirium may develop. Severe hyperphosphataemia can managed with phosphate binders and renal replacement therapy.

MAGNESIUM

A large proportion of the body's magnesium is structurally associated with hydroxyapatite – the mineral component of bone. Dietary magnesium is particularly high in plant matter, as magnesium is a component of chlorophyll.

Active forms and physiological roles

The biologically active form of magnesium is the divalent cation Mg^{++}. As a ubiquitous cofactor, numerous fundamental physiological processes are magnesium ion dependent, including:

- Muscle contraction
- Normal cardiac conduction
- Neurotransmitter release
- Bone formation
- Vascular tone

Absorption and transport

Magnesium is absorbed from the GI tract. In serum, approximately 70% is free ions, the remainder protein bound or complexed. Unabsorbed Mg^{++} is excreted in faeces, whereas any excess absorbed Mg^{++} is excreted in the urine. Bone represents a 'store' of magnesium.

Clinical implications of low serum magnesium

Hypomagnesaemia may be secondary to:

- Excessive renal magnesium loss, as with thiazide and loop diuretics
- Redistribution across body compartments, as in diabetic ketoacidosis
- Chronic alcohol excess
- Inadequate intake (usually as part of generalized nutritional inadequacy secondary to malnutrition or malabsorption)

Manifestations of magnesium deficit (similar to those of acute hypocalcaemia) are cardiac (electrocardiogram changes and arrhythmias, including torsade de pointes) and neuromuscular (weakness, tetany, tremor and convulsions). Hypocalcaemia can arise due to impaired PTH release secondary to low serum Mg^{++}. A refractory hypokalaemia may develop that resolves only with repletion of magnesium levels. Treatment of magnesium deficiency is with oral or intravenous magnesium.

> **RED FLAG**
>
> Magnesium toxicity secondary to intravenous magnesium infusion. Although rare, this is the most commonly encountered scenario of magnesium toxicity. During treatment of severe preeclampsia, an intravenous magnesium infusion may be utilized. Magnesium toxicity can occur rapidly, mandating regular serum Mg^{++} samples and clinical assessment for depression of tendon reflexes.

Magnesium toxicity

This is rarely seen except in profound renal failure, as the kidney is highly competent at excreting excess magnesium. Symptoms and signs of severely raised serum Mg^{++} include muscle weakness, loss of tendon reflexes, respiratory depression and cardiac arrest. Treatment involves resuscitation via an ABC (airway, breathing, circulation) approach, stopping the infusion and immediate intravenous administration of 10 mL of 10% calcium gluconate.

IRON

An essential trace element, iron deficiency is extremely common worldwide, although the causes vary geographically. Total body iron is about 3–5 g. About 60% is found in haemoglobin and the remainder complexed with ferritin and haemosiderin. Iron intake requirements are increased during periods of growth, pregnancy, menstrual or other chronic blood loss (1 mL of blood loss is equal to 0.5 mg of iron). Dietary iron is either:

- 'Haem' iron (iron ions associated with haem-containing proteins such as haemoglobin or myoglobin)
- 'Nonhaem' iron (nonhaem iron-containing proteins)

Active forms and physiological roles

As a transition metal, iron ions can have different oxidation states. This redox property underpins its role in electron transfer reactions. Fe^{2+} (ferrous) ions and Fe^{3+} (ferric) ions are the most common oxidation states in the human body.

The major physiological process requiring iron is haemoglobin synthesis. However, iron ions are also important components of vital redox enzymes and all proteins containing haem moieties.

Absorption and transport

Only 10% of dietary iron is absorbed, thus the RNI is 10 times the actual physiological iron intake requirement. Maximal absorption occurs in the duodenum (Fig. 13.4).

Haem iron is more bioavailable than nonhaem iron, because its GI absorption is less influenced by coingestion of inhibitory dietary factors. Haem iron is absorbed intact within the haem structure via receptor-mediated endocytosis, whereas ferrous (Fe^{2+}) iron ions access the enterocytes via H^+/Fe^{++} symport. Export into the circulation is via an iron exporter.

Once in the serum, ferrous ions (Fe^{2+}) oxidize, becoming ferric (Fe^{3+}) ions. In this form they bind to transferrin, a transport protein. This 'delivers' the iron to:

- Bone marrow, for incorporation into haemoglobin during erythropoiesis
- The liver and reticuloendothelial macrophages, where it is incorporated into ferritin or haemosiderin for storage
- Muscle, where it is incorporated into myoglobin

Importantly, there is no specific mechanism for excretion of excess iron – iron loss occurs only via desquamation of keratinocytes, sloughed mucosal cells and blood loss. Iron levels in the body can only be regulated by modifying the extent of dietary iron absorption from the GI lumen. This is mediated by hepcidin, a protein synthesized by the liver. Hepcidin binds to and internalizes (removes) the iron exporter from the basolateral enterocyte surface, limiting iron's access to the circulation.

Clinical features of chronic iron deficiency

The majority of symptomatic issues pertain to a reduction in haemoglobin, that is, anaemia (see Chapter 14). Anaemia secondary to iron deficiency is microcytic. Iron deficiency as a cause of a confirmed microcytic anaemia is more likely if several additional (nonhaematological) clinical features are also present, including the following:

- Angular stomatitis
- Diffuse hair loss or thinning
- Koilonychia, onycholysis (see Table 14.6)
- Immune dysfunction
- Neurocognitive impairment

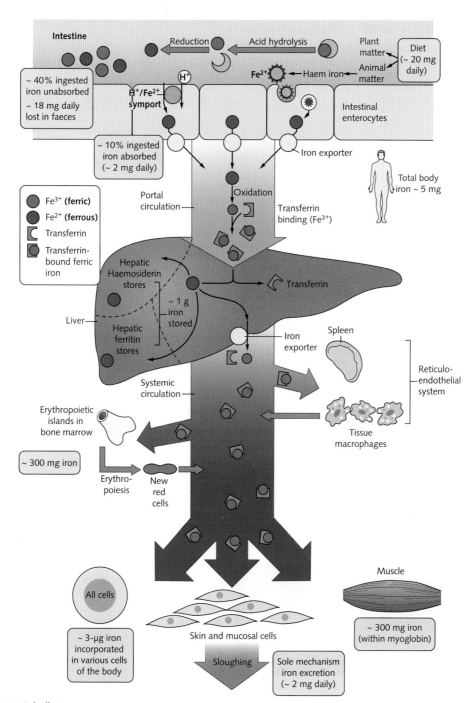

Fig. 13.4 Iron metabolism.

Diagnosis and treatment

Iron deficiency is diagnosed when a microcytic (mean corpuscular volume <80 fL) anaemia (Hb <13 g/dL (M) or <12 g/dL (F)) noted on full blood count is accompanied by characteristic changes seen on a blood film, along with reduced serum iron and ferritin levels, increased serum transferrin and total iron-binding capacity, and an absence of iron stores on bone marrow examination. Treatment is oral iron supplementation. In the UK, dietary deficiency is the commonest cause of iron deficiency, but globally chronic GI blood loss secondary to hookworm infestation is the major cause.

Table 13.8 Other trace elements – background information

Essential trace element (chemical symbol)	RNI (or other intake parameter if RNI not determined)[a]	Known physiological role	Foods rich in element	Deficiency syndrome	Factors carrying risk for deficiency
Selenium (Se)	75 µg (M) 60 µg (F)	Component of glutathione peroxidase Regulation of thyroid hormone synthesis and metabolism	Liver, kidney, Brazil nut, crab, cereals	Keshan disease, Kashin–Beck disease	Long-term renal replacement therapy Living in areas of selenium-poor soil Cisplatin therapy
Fluorine (F)	AI: 4 mg (M) 3 mg (F)	Structurally strengthens teeth enamel and bones	Fluoridated drinking water, tea, grape juice	Increased risk for dental caries	Absence of drinking water fluoridation programmes
Manganese (Mn)	NRV: 5.5 mg (M) 5.0 mg (F)	Enzyme component or cofactor (Mn superoxide dismutase is a principal antioxidant enzyme in mitochondria) Bone development Carbohydrate, amino acid and cholesterol metabolism Wound healing	Pecans, nuts Brown rice, cereals Green vegetables Tea	Not characterized	Long-term total parenteral nutrition (TPN) lacking Mn
Chromium (Cr)	NRV, AI: 35 µg (M) 25 µg (F)	Potentiates insulin action Metabolism of macronutrients	Broccoli, grapes, potatoes, garlic, basil	Not characterized	Long-TPN lacking Cr
Molybdenum (Mo)	RDA 45 µg	Enzyme cofactor (e.g. xanthine oxidase, aldehyde oxide, sulphite oxidase)	Legumes (beans, lentils, peas)	Not characterized	Long-term TPN lacking Mo

[a] RNI values shown here are taken from Department of Health dietary reference values and refer to adults only. Please note that RNI values change often, as nutrition research progresses. Please consult www.BDA.uk.com or other authentic sources for the latest intake recommendations. Where an RNI is not available, alternative parameters are stated and given.

AI, Adequate intake (USA parameter used when insufficient evidence available to set RDA – AI is based on typical average daily intake in a healthy population); NRV, nutrient reference value (Australasian parameter); RDA, recommended daily allowance (USA parameter); RNI, reference nutrient intake.

> **RED FLAG**
>
> Sinister implications of apparently innocent iron deficiency. Always exclude occult blood loss as a cause of a new iron deficiency – gastrointestinal malignancy commonly presents in this way.

Clinical features of toxicity

Because of the absence of an iron excretion mechanism, an excessive iron intake overwhelms the background loss of iron via desquamated cells, leading to toxicity.

Acute iron toxicity

The most common scenario of acute iron intoxication is accidental overdose with iron-containing supplements by young children – this is a leading cause of poisoning fatalities in the <6-year age group. Nausea, vomiting and diarrhoea lead to hypovolaemic shock and metabolic acidosis.

> **RED FLAG**
>
> Emergency treatment of iron toxicity. This is a medical emergency, and treatment is based on oral activated charcoal, gastrointestinal lavage (depending on the time elapsed from ingestion to presentation), intravenous iron chelators and ultimately haemodialysis if needed.

Chronic (transfusional) iron overload

Multiple red cell transfusions (one unit of blood contains 250 mg iron) or excessive parenteral iron therapy may cause iron overload. Certain conditions (e.g. aplastic anaemia) are 'high risk' for iron overload because they impose repeated transfusional requirements. Once the iron 'sinks' (liver, macrophages, bone marrow) are saturated, iron deposits in the heart, liver, pancreas, testes, joints and skin, causing permanent damage. Treatment consists of a combination of:

- Reduction of dietary iron intake
- Increased intake of dietary inhibitors of iron absorption
- Venesection
- Intravenous and oral iron chelators

Haemochromatosis

This autosomal recessive disorder of iron metabolism arises from a failure of hepcidin synthesis due to HFE gene mutations. This results in uncontrolled passage of dietary iron (recall that hepcidin *reduces* iron export from enterocytes to the circulation) into the circulation.

Epidemiology

Around 0.5% of the population are homozygotic for various HFE mutations. However, clinical penetrance shows considerable heterogeneity: only approximately 5% of homozygotes are thought to present symptomatically.

Clinical features

Clinical features arise from inappropriate iron deposition in the relevant organs, and include the following:

- Bronze skin pigmentation
- Hepatomegaly, cirrhosis
- Diabetes mellitus
- Cardiomyopathy, cardiac arrhythmias
- Arthritis (iron deposition in joints)

Treatment is as for transfusional overload.

ZINC

Zinc is an essential trace element. Total body zinc is 2–3 g.

Active forms and physiological roles

Zinc ions (Zn^{++}) are intrinsic components or activating cofactors of numerous enzymes, and important structural components of numerous proteins. Zinc is involved in the immune response to infection, nucleoprotein regulation of DNA, growth, tissue repair and wound healing.

Absorption and transport

Absorption of zinc (in the small bowel) is only approximately 30% effective, thus for a daily intake requirement of approximately 3.3 mg, the RNI is 10 mg/day. Absorption is inhibited by dietary fibre, phytates and iron. Serum Zn^{++} ions circulate bound to albumin and macroglobulin. Zinc

storage zones (where it is bound to metalloproteins) include the liver and kidney. Unabsorbed zinc is excreted in faeces, whereas absorbed zinc is excreted in the urine.

Clinical features of chronic deficiency

Whilst mild or 'marginal' zinc deficiency is not uncommon, severe deficiency is rare. It may, however, be seen in the following situations:

- Conditions of excessive zinc loss, such as severe burns, prolonged diarrhoea and nephrotic syndrome
- Malabsorption
- Alcohol excess
- Zinc-free total parenteral nutrition (TPN)
- Use of metal-chelating drugs (e.g. penicillamine)

The hallmark sign of zinc deficiency is a characteristic skin rash around the mouth, anus and distal extremities. Other symptoms include chronic diarrhoea, immune impairment, prolonged wound healing, night blindness, altered taste and neurocognitive abnormalities. Zinc deficiency in children also causes slowed growth and delayed sexual maturity.

Acrodermatitis enteropathica

This is a rare, autosomal recessive disorder arising from impaired absorption of zinc due to abnormal ZIP4 (a zinc transporter protein fundamental to enterocyte uptake). The symptoms are those of severe zinc deficiency. It is entirely cured with zinc supplementation, but fatal if untreated.

Diagnosis and treatment

Serum Zn^{++} is used as a marker of zinc status. Treatment of deficiency is with oral supplementation, or in the case of TPN-dependent patient with appropriate alteration in the TPN formulation.

Zinc toxicity

Zinc is of low toxicity in overdose, causing mainly GI symptoms. However, long-term consumption of excessive zinc supplements may cause a clinically significant secondary copper deficiency.

COPPER

Copper is an essential trace element.

Active forms and physiological roles

Total body copper is approximately 100 mg. The majority of copper in the human body is in the form of cupric ions

(Cu^{++}). It is a vital component of enzymes underpinning a diverse range of physiological processes including:

- Oxidative phosphorylation
- Connective tissue formation (collagen $\rightarrow$ elastin crosslink formation)
- Neurotransmitter (noradrenaline) synthesis
- Melanin synthesis
- Iron metabolism

Absorption and transport

Absorption occurs in the stomach and duodenum, where approximately 30% of ingested copper is absorbed. Once in the portal vein, copper travels to the liver, bound to albumin, from where it is then incorporated into caeruloplasmin for transport to tissues for utilization in copper-containing enzyme synthesis. Approximately 10% of serum copper consists of free ionized cupric ions (the biologically active form) in equilibrium with the caeruloplasmin-bound remainder. Copper is excreted in bile.

Clinical features of chronic deficiency

Copper deficiency is rare, due to abundance in food and drinking water. It may be acquired or hereditary. Acquired copper deficiency is secondary to generalized malnutrition, malabsorption, nephrotic syndrome, excessive zinc supplement intake or prolonged low-copper TPN administration. Symptoms include the following:

- Microcytic anaemia
- Peripheral neuropathy
- Central nervous system demyelination
- Optic neuritis
- 'Steely' hair depigmentation
- Growth failure

Copper deficiency is diagnosed by low serum copper and treated with oral copper supplementation. The most common (but still extremely rare) hereditary cause of copper deficiency is Menkes kinky hair syndrome.

CLINICAL NOTES

MENKES KINKY HAIR SYNDROME

This is an X-linked disease with incidence of 1 in 50,000 to 100,000. Defective gastrointestinal copper absorption results in symptoms of severe copper deficiency. Copper therapy has no significant effect and sadly the life expectancy is <2 years.

Clinical features of toxicity

Acquired toxicity is extremely rare but can arise rarely in neonates secondary to failure of biliary excretion, or in the context of excessive ingestion of copper supplements. Hereditary copper overload (Wilson disease) is more common than acquired copper toxicity (but is still very rare).

Wilson disease

This is an autosomal recessive disorder of copper metabolism with incidence of 1/100,000. Copper accumulation occurs due to a hepatic failure of biliary copper excretion. It is fatal if untreated. The hallmark is pathological copper deposition, primarily in the liver and brain (especially the basal ganglia). Despite representing the most common abnormality of copper metabolism, it is still rare.

Clinical features

Signs and symptoms of Wilson disease are attributable to liver dysfunction/failure and neuropsychiatric features. Copper deposition in the Descemet membrane results in Kayser–Fleischer rings, which can be seen on slit-lamp examination of the eye (see Chapter 14). The diagnosis is suggested by low serum caeruloplasmin, raised 24-hour urinary copper and raised liver copper on liver biopsy. Treatment is with chelating agents such as penicillamine; however, brain/liver damage is irreversible once sustained.

IODINE

Iodine is an essential trace element. Approximately 80% of the body's approximately 20 mg of iodine is located in the thyroid gland. Iodine is vital for synthesis of thyroid hormones.

Active forms and physiological roles

Iodine is present in the diet as molecular iodine (I_2) or monatomic iodide ions (I^-).

Iodine's key physiological role is as component of thyroid hormones: triiodothyronine (T3) and thyroxine (T4). T3 and T4 synthesis by the thyroid gland utilizes approximately 80 μg of iodine daily.

Absorption and transport

Dietary iodine is ionized in the GI tract and then absorbed. It is 100% bioavailable – all ingested iodine is absorbed as iodide ions, which circulate in plasma. Iodide ions are sequestered by the thyroid gland, excreted renally into urine or, in lactating females, excreted in breast milk.

Clinical features of chronic deficiency

Consequences of iodine deficiency arise secondary to impaired thyroid hormone synthesis. Clinical consequences vary depending on the developmental stage at the time of deficiency.

Goitre

From birth onwards, dietary iodine deficiency usually results in enlargement (hyperplasia) of the thyroid gland. Reduced negative feedback (from low serum (T3) and (T4)) leads to increased hypothalamic thyrotropin-releasing hormone and anterior pituitary thyroid-stimulating hormone release, which drives the hyperplasia. The increase in parenchymal volume increases the gland's capacity to capture available circulating iodide ions, and this may initially compensate for the deficiency, preventing thyroid insufficiency. The enlarged thyroid gland is known as a 'goitre'.

Hypothyroidism

From birth onwards, dietary iodine deficiency that is too extreme to be compensated for by gland enlargement (goitre) alone results in symptoms of hypothyroidism (see Chapter 11) attributable to insufficient thyroid hormone.

COMMON PITFALLS

IODINE DEFICIENCY AS A CAUSE OF HYPOTHYROIDISM

Hypothyroidism is the most common endocrine pathology, but please appreciate that the majority of cases in the UK are secondary to autoimmune disease or to disruption of the hypothalamic–pituitary–thyroid axis rather than iodine deficiency. Presence of a goitre does not necessarily indicate iodine deficiency as this may occur in other types of hypothyroidism.

Cretinism

Fetal iodine deficiency, particularly after the second trimester (prior to this the fetus enjoys maternal thyroid hormones, thus does not need iodine to synthesize its own), leads to a devastating spectrum of irreversible consequences for the fetus. These include neurological and growth deficits. Maternal iodine deficiency is the most common preventable cause of mental retardation, because one-third of the global population live in iodine-deficient zones. Maternal iodine supplementation reliably prevents cretinism.

Diagnosis and treatment

Iodine deficiency is confirmed by low urinary iodide. Treatment is with oral supplementation, which leads to symptoms resolution and normalization of urinary iodide.

Clinical features of toxicity

Iodine toxicity may develop if intake continuously exceeds 1100 µg/day. This may cause hyperthyroidism (see Chapter 11), but often patients remain euthyroid. Confusingly, a paradoxical effect may also occur, when the excess iodine uptake may *inhibit* thyroid hormone synthesis. Iodine toxicity can therefore cause hyperthyroidism, hypothyroidism or no change to thyroid status.

OTHER TRACE ELEMENTS

Recall that 'trace' elements have a daily intake requirement of less than 100 mg and their total body content is <5 g. 'Essential' trace elements are those for which a sustained insufficient intake impairs physiological processes. Iron, zinc, copper and iodine have already been discussed. Others are summarized in Table 13.8.

In the absence of genetic abnormalities of trace element metabolism, toxicity from excessive intake of trace elements in dietary supplements is far more likely than their deficiency (with the exception, of course, of iron and iodine).

● **Chapter Summary**

- Minerals are micronutrients and can be classified as 'major' (also known as 'nontrace') or 'minor' (also known as 'trace') elements according to daily intake requirements. Insufficient or excessive intake is detrimental to health.
- Most clinical issue associated with minerals are related to either total body or serum excesses or deficiencies. Both these scenarios can arise due to insufficient intake or excessive excretion.

- Dietary deficiency of sodium, potassium and chloride is virtually impossible, due to their ubiquitous presence in all foodstuffs. Clinical problems associated with these minerals are usually related to abnormal distribution across body compartments, rather than total body deficiency or excess.
- The concentration of sodium in the bloodstream is a major determinant of fluid distribution between the intracellular, intravascular and extracellular interstitial compartments. As such derangements of plasma sodium concentration have enormous clinical significance in terms of consequences and also diagnostically.
- Potassium is extremely important clinically; even relatively minor abnormalities of plasma potassium concentration can cause dangerous cardiac arrhythmias. Qualified doctors should be confident in the common causes and acute management of hyperkalaemia and hypokalaemia due to these being relatively commonplace within hospitalized patients.
- Calcium homeostasis is closely linked to vitamin D status; many of the calcium deficiency syndromes can arise secondary to vitamin D deficiency. This is because vitamin D is vital for normal absorption of dietary calcium.
- Chronic dietary calcium deficiency causes a characteristic array of clinical abnormalities depending on whether it occurs in childhood (rickets) or adulthood (osteomalacia).
- Serum calcium concentration is affected by multiple factors, primarily due to its association with plasma proteins. Hypocalcaemia and hypercalcaemia have different sets of causes, clinical features and consequences.
- The main clinical relevance of phosphate arises in the context of serum phosphate concentration abnormalities: hyperphosphataemia and hypophosphataemia. Each has distinct causes, signs and symptoms. Phosphate homeostasis, like calcium, is closely associated with vitamin D status.
- Magnesium ions are vital for a diverse and extensive list of physiological functions. Hypomagnesaemia is far more common than hypermagnesaemia, which is only seen in end-stage renal failure.
- Iron is extremely important due to the requirement for haemoglobin synthesis. Deficiency is common and leads to symptoms attributable to low haemoglobin (i.e. anaemia). Pathophysiological excessive absorption of dietary iron is known as haemochromatosis.
- Zinc is required as a component of numerous enzymes. Deficiency manifests with a characteristic rash. The congenital abnormality leading to zinc deficiency due to impaired absorption is known as acrodermatitis enteropathica.
- Copper, like zinc, is an important component of many enzymes, most importantly proteins required for oxidative phosphorylation. Deficiency is very rare. Wilson disease is a genetic disorder leading to copper toxicity as a result of impaired copper excretion.
- Iodine deficiency and excess manifest most commonly with disorders of thyroid function.

USEFUL REFERENCES

https://ods.od.nih.gov/factsheets.
https://www.nrv.gov.au/nutrients.
www.nutrition.org.uk.
www.bda.uk.com.

Clinical assessment of metabolism and nutritional disorders

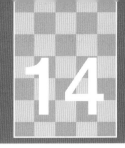

INTRODUCTION

This chapter describes history-taking techniques, relevant examination and appropriate investigations that pertain *specifically* to disorders of metabolism or nutrition. Only information needed to effectively clinically assess these conditions is discussed here. Generic history and examination skills are covered in extensive detail in dedicated textbooks and are not reiterated here: see [1–3] for examples.

HINTS AND TIPS

Throughout this chapter, symptoms, signs and investigations will be discussed in the context of metabolism and nutrition disorders. However, there are nearly always more common causes responsible, and these must always be excluded first. For example, a complaint of abdominal pain is far more likely to be a surgical or medical condition than a presentation of porphyria, which is exceedingly rare.

HISTORY-TAKING

To extract the relevant information needed for a targeted examination and to direct investigations appropriately, certain important components must be covered. These are discussed in the following sections.

COMMON PRESENTING COMPLAINTS

To identify nutritional deficiencies or metabolic disease reliably, be sure to confirm or exclude presence of the following features during a focussed history. As with all positive findings in a history, if a positive feature is identified, establish onset date, duration, exacerbating or relieving factors, symptom severity and impact on the patient.

Weight loss

Unintentional weight loss is deemed clinically significant if it exceeds 5% of usual bodyweight over a 6-month timescale or is relentless and ongoing. It usually indicates serious illness and so a cause must be identified. Before considering pathological causes, rule out calorie reduction (e.g. dieting) or increased energy expenditure (e.g. exercise increase). Directly enquiring if belts, rings and waistbands have become looser may signpost weight loss that the patient has not been aware of themselves.

CLINICAL NOTES

SYSTEMIC CAUSES OF UNINTENTIONAL WEIGHT LOSS (OTHER THAN REDUCED ENERGY INTAKE)

Malignancy, chronic infection and significant heart, lung, renal or gastrointestinal disease comprise the important systemic causes of weight loss. Occult malignancy may be suggested by constitutional symptoms, defined as unexplained weight loss ≥ 10%/6 months, low-grade fever and drenching night sweats.

COMMON PITFALLS

AUTHENTICITY OF REPORTED WEIGHT LOSS

Surprisingly, only around 50% of patients reporting weight loss have genuine weight loss [4] when investigated. Therefore, always confirm that reported weight loss is real. Comparing current weight with previous recorded weights (if available) and obtaining collateral history from friends/relatives may strengthen the authenticity of the symptom.

Important nutritional causes for weight loss include protein–energy malnutrition (see Chapter 9), and nutritional deficiencies (see Chapters 12 and 13). Hypermetabolic states (e.g. diabetes, hyperthyroidism) resulting in excessive energy expenditure also often result in weight loss, but this is lightly to be dramatic (>20% loss from baseline).

Note that weight gain (not attributable to reduction in exercise or increased calorie intake) may also signal disease. Oedema secondary to heart or renal failure is most common, but rarer causes such as Cushing disease can also be to blame. The most common cause of short-term (i.e. over days) weight fluctuation is gain or loss of fluid.

Appetite change

'Appetite' describes the subjective desire to eat. It may be reduced as a manifestation of nearly any acute or chronic disease. Early satiety (feeling full after eating a smaller amount than usual) may hint at abdominal organomegaly or massive tumours. Appetite is notably lost in many malignant states. Appetite may also increase as a side effect of orexigenic medications such as corticosteroids.

An appetite change is most diagnostically significant when unaccompanied by the expected weight change. For example, hypermetabolic states (e.g. hyperthyroidism) increase appetite, but are more likely to be accompanied by weight loss.

Fatigue/weakness

Fatigue is defined as a subjectively perceived lack of energy. It is a normal response to physical or mental exertion. It is a very common symptom, particularly in elderly individuals, where it may represent changes associated with normal ageing.

COMMON PITFALLS

FATIGUE

It is important to differentiate fatigue from shortness of breath, daytime sleepiness and muscle weakness. However, fatigue will often be accompanied by any or all of these associated factors. If arising as a complaint relating to a genuine disease, it will not be an isolated symptom.

Clinically significant fatigue, however, refers to a persistently reduced tolerance of physical/mental exertion in comparison to patient's usual baseline. A useful way to establish this is using quantifiable distances to identify if exercise tolerance is genuinely decreasing (e.g. 'Have you noticed that you are able to walk less far on the flat, or climb fewer stairs than usual before having to stop due to exhaustion?') Causes of fatigue are presented in Box 14.1. It is sometimes easier conceptually for a patient to identify a change in their energy levels if you ask them to compare with a specific earlier time point (e.g. 6 months ago).

Anaemia

Anaemia is defined as a haemoglobin concentration (Hb) less than 13 g/dL (males) or less than 12 g/dL (females). The lower the Hb, the more symptoms the patient is likely to experience. If the Hb falls below 8 g/dL, symptoms will inevitably be present. Iron deficiency (see Chapter 13) is the most common cause in the UK, but note that within the

BOX 14.1 CLINICAL CAUSES OF FATIGUE

Common	Rare
Anaemia	Protein–energy malnutrition
Hypothyroidism	Glycogen storage disorders
Depression	
Chronic cardiac, renal or hepatic failure	
Diabetes mellitus	
Chronic obstructive pulmonary disease, sleep apnoea, hypoxic lung disease	
Chronic fatigue syndrome/ fibromyalgia	
Chronic infection	
Vitamin deficiencies	

inpatient population anaemia secondary to chronic disease may predominate. B12 or folate deficiency (see Chapter 12) and excessive alcohol intake are also important nutritional/metabolic causes of anaemia.

Symptoms and signs of anaemia arise secondary to reduced oxygen delivery to tissues due to a reduced Hb. They include the following:

- Fatigue
- Breathlessness
- Palpitations
- Presyncope/syncope
- Headache
- Pallor
- Tachycardia

Nausea/vomiting

Nausea is the sensation of abdominal discomfort associated with the urge to vomit. Vomiting describes the involuntary muscle contraction of the stomach and oesophagus leading to expulsion of gastric contents.

These distressing symptoms may arise secondary to many nutritional and metabolic disorders, as well as gastrointestinal infection or disease, bowel obstruction, drug side effects, ingested toxins, pregnancy, surgery, anaesthesia, inner ear pathology, raised intracranial pressure, severe pain or systemic disease, particularly hepatic or renal failure. If persistent, ruling out sinister causes with full examination and relevant investigation is mandatory.

Importantly, as well as representing a symptom of nutritional deficiency, nausea and vomiting can cause both macronutrient and micronutrient deficiencies and electrolyte disturbance, particularly if severe and prolonged. If vomiting is severe and clinical signs of dehydration (see the 'Dehydration' section) are present, rehydration is a priority. This scenario also requires prompt electrolyte assessment as marked derangements and renal impairment are likely.

Diabetic ketoacidosis is an important metabolic cause of nausea/vomiting. Significant electrolyte disturbance may also present in this manner, but derangement severe enough to provoke vomiting will inevitably be accompanied by other symptoms and signs suggestive of the specific disturbance. Similarly, excessive intake or deficiencies of most vitamins and minerals can cause nausea and vomiting. Finally, severe hypoglycaemia will often provoke nausea and vomiting until corrected.

Cognitive symptoms

These may include confusion, short-term memory loss, depression or other neuropsychiatric symptoms. B12 and folate deficiencies, as well as exhibiting symptoms of anaemia, are often accompanied by cognitive symptoms. Specific B1 deficiency is notorious for manifesting with cognitive symptoms (see Chapter 12). Endocrine disease too is a common cause of cognitive symptoms – hypothyroidism in particular – often discovered by investigations intended to exclude an organic cause for depression.

Chronic progressive global impairment of cerebral function may, very rarely, represent rare lysosomal storage disorders (e.g. Niemann–Pick type C, Fabry disease, Tay–Sachs or Gaucher disease). Likewise, disorders or carbohydrate metabolism (e.g. Pompe disease or galactosaemia) may present this way. However, these vanishingly rare diseases will almost never present outside of early childhood; other symptoms would be more evident and spontaneous cases unaccompanied by a known family history are rare.

Recurrent fractures

A history of multiple bone fractures, particularly those occurring during normal activities or minor trauma, such as a fall from standing height may be attributable to structural bone weakness as a manifestation of systemic disease. 'Colles' wrist fractures, neck of femur and vertebral fractures occurring in abnormal bone in the absence of severe trauma are termed 'fragility' fractures. It is important to consider and exclude important systemic causes of bone fragility *other than nutritional deficiency*, which is the most common cause. For example, multiple myeloma, metastatic or primary bone cancer may present with fragility fractures.

One of the most common risk factors for fragility fractures is osteoporosis. Calcium or vitamin D deficiency, isolated or combined, as well as causing osteomalacia

(see Chapter 13), is a major contributory factor in development of osteoporosis, as is protein–energy malnutrition.

CLINICAL NOTES

OSTEOPOROSIS

This is a disease where bone density is reduced. Decreased structural integrity leads to an increased risk for fractures. With appropriate treatment and lifestyle alterations, osteoporosis can be effectively managed. Calcium, vitamin D supplementation and bisphosphonates represent the mainstay of pharmacological treatment.

Abdominal pain

Careful examination and history alone are often sufficient to diagnose most causes of abdominal pain. The vast majority of acute abdomen presentations are not due to metabolic/nutritional disease. The most common metabolic causes of abdominal pain are hypoglycaemia and diabetic ketoacidosis. Other rare, but serious metabolic causes include Addisonian crisis, hypercalcaemia (see Chapter 13), porphyria (see Chapter 10), haemochromatosis (see Chapter 13) and Wilson disease (see Chapter 13). Hepatomegaly secondary to various metabolic diseases may be painful. Finally, pancreatitis secondary to hereditary dyslipidaemias (see Chapter 7) or alcohol intake will cause extreme abdominal pain.

Change in bowel habit

As well as a feature of bowel cancer, a change in stool colour, consistency or frequency may be a symptom of nutritional deficiency or metabolic abnormality. Inadequate fibre intake is the most common nutritional cause of constipation. Iron supplementation, thiamine (B1) deficiency and hypercalcaemia may cause constipation. Constipation is often a prominent feature of hypothyroidism, and may arise secondary to autonomic neuropathy in diabetes. B12 deficiency may present with either constipation or diarrhoea. Niacin (see Chapter 12) or zinc deficiency (see Chapter 13) may cause diarrhoea.

Severe diarrhoea unrelated to vitamin or mineral deficiency often *causes* secondary vitamin or mineral deficiency due to malabsorption, particularly if prolonged. Marked electrolyte derangement often occurs, hypokalaemia and hypochloraemia in particular. However, as with vomiting, dehydration is the most dangerous consequence of severe diarrhoea. Vigilant monitoring for clinical and biochemical signs of dehydration is therefore vital in severe diarrhoea.

PAST MEDICAL HISTORY

As with all medical history-taking, identify any significant past illnesses, particularly if they warranted hospital admission, surgical procedures, outpatient appointments or drug treatment. Many conditions have important associations with metabolic disease and others may represent manifestations of an underlying nutritional deficiency. Establish if any of the aforementioned 'common presenting complaints' have been problematic in the past, even if no longer in evidence.

Diet history

Obtain an estimate of daily calorie intake. Establish if fruit and vegetables feature regularly in the patient's diet in reasonable quantities. Identify any exclusion of specific food groups, for example, veganism or vegetarianism. This is important as certain exclusions signal risk for deficiencies; for example, vegans cannot usually obtain adequate iron, calcium, iodine, vitamin D and B12 from their diet alone. Similarly, when documenting allergies, take note if multiple food intolerance/allergies are reported – some people can render themselves deficient in vitamins and minerals due to dietary exclusion.

Identify if the patient follows a calorie-controlled diet, particularly if extreme (e.g. <500 kcal/day), as this may place them at risk for malnutrition even if they appear overweight or obese. Finally, establish if the patient adheres to any other particular style of diet (e.g. Atkins, Dukan, human chorionic gonadotropin (HCG), Paleo, etc.) and clarify exactly what this involves if unfamiliar.

Taking a dietary history relies strongly on the patient's ability to provide useful coherent responses to direct questioning. Sometimes it is impossible to obtain the relevant information simply from discussing with the patient; in these instances, a detailed food diary lasting at least a week will be required for any real diagnostic utility.

Medications

As in a routine medical history, confirm and document regular and occasionally taken (when necessary (PRN)) medications, including their doses and frequencies. Be sure to directly enquire about over-the-counter medicines, herbal remedies, dietary supplements and the oral contraceptive pill. Confirm if a daily multivitamin supplement is regularly taken; this will reduce but not exclude the probability of a vitamin deficiency. Be aware of certain drugs that are known to interfere with normal metabolism in such a way that deficiencies arise. As well as those listed in Table 14.1, two commonly examined examples are:

- Methotrexate: this competitively inhibits dihydrofolate reductase, preventing the dihydrofolate→tetrahydrofolate step in folate

Table 14.1 Drug-induced nutrient/mineral/electrolyte derangements

Drug	Nutrient/mineral derangement
Oral contraceptive pill	B2 and B6 requirement increased
H2-receptor antagonists (e.g. ranitidine, cimetidine)	B12 and zinc absorption impaired
Angiotensin-converting enzyme inhibitors (e.g. Ramipril)	Hyperkalaemia
All diuretics	B1 deficiency
Loop diuretics (e.g. furosemide)	Sodium, potassium, magnesium, calcium depletion by increased renal loss
Spironolactone	Hyperkalaemia
Isoniazid, azathioprine	B6 antagonists; requirement increased Risk for B3 deficiency secondary to B6 deficiency
Methotrexate, trimethoprim, sulphasalazine, phenytoin	B9 (folate) deficiency
Orlistat	Fat-soluble vitamin (A, D, E and K) absorption impaired
Ethambutol	Copper and zinc absorption impaired
Chloramphenicol	B6 and B12 deficiency
Cisplatin	Magnesium depletion
Fluorouracil	Induces B1 deficiency
Foscarnet	Calcium, magnesium, phosphorus, potassium and B12 deficiency

activation, resulting in deficiency. Folate is coadministered with methotrexate to prevent this.
- Isoniazid: this binds and sequesters pyridoxine (B6), which is then lost via urinary excretion. Coadministration of pyridoxine with isoniazid attempts to attenuate isoniazid-induced B6 deficiency.

Alcohol intake

Excessive alcohol intake predisposes to a range of both mineral and vitamin deficiencies as well as macronutrient deficiencies, which are also an issue in severe alcoholism (due to inadequate diet); protein–energy malnutrition (see Chapter 9) is not uncommon in such individuals. An important screening tool for identifying alcohol dependence is the CAGE questionnaire (Box 14.2). Quantify typical alcohol intake in units and be sure to document this clearly in the notes.

CLINICAL NOTES

QUANTIFICATION OF ALCOHOL INTAKE

The definition of a unit of an alcohol is 10 mL (8 g) of pure ethanol. This correlates to a 25-mL measure of liquor (one 'shot'), one-third of a pint of beer or half a standard (175 mL) glass of wine. Current recommendations advise that to keep health risks related to alcohol consumption low, no more than 14 units should be consumed weekly.

Unlike withdrawal from other recreational drugs, sudden abstinence/curtailment of intake in an individual with habitual alcohol intake can be fatal rather than merely unpleasant. Approximately 40% develop an acute withdrawal

HINTS AND TIPS

MECHANISM OF ALCOHOL WITHDRAWAL

Alcohol withdrawal phenomena arise secondary to neuronal hyperactivity. The tonic central nervous system depression maintained by alcohol exposure is lifted on cessation/reduction of intake, leading to a range of symptoms. These include confusion, agitation, anxiety, tremor, tachycardia, hallucinations, nausea, vomiting, diarrhoea, hypertension and hepatic dysfunction. Symptoms usually arise ~6 hours after the last alcoholic drink.

syndrome. Oddly, the risk for withdrawal syndrome is unrelated to the extent of the usual intake. Approximately 5% of individuals experiencing a withdrawal syndrome will suffer delirium tremens, which carries a mortality of up to 20%. Prophylactic reducing courses of benzodiazepines are prescribed for alcohol-dependent inpatients, as are parenteral vitamins (see Chapter 12), to reduce the probability of alcohol withdrawal syndrome.

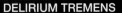

RED FLAG

DELIRIUM TREMENS

This severe manifestation of withdrawal is characterized by disorientation, agitation, diaphoresis, hallucinations, hypertension and hyperthermia. Tonic–clonic seizures may occur. Dehydration and electrolyte derangement must be corrected, and intravenous benzodiazepines are the mainstay of treatment for seizures in delirium tremens. Without treatment death results from cardiovascular and respiratory collapse or arrhythmias.

Family history

Any family history of metabolic disease will usually be well known to the patient. Identifying if any blood relatives have died prematurely should lower your threshold for suspicion of hereditary diseases, which could be metabolic in origin. Premature death: death prior to age 55 years in a male or age 65 years in a female can be considered premature, and will usually be attributable to disease. This can be useful diagnostically if the disease is hereditary. Finally, note that consanguinity significantly increases the probability of rarer inborn errors of metabolism, which are often recessive in inheritance pattern.

Social history

As well as routine enquiry into a person's marital status, accommodation type, employment status and array of dependents or carers, it is always important to qualify and document a patient's functional status. Various indices exist to quantify the activities of daily living that a person can manage independently. This is important for general discharge planning, but also to assess the probability that a person's ability to care for themselves may impact on their capacity to obtain a balanced diet with adequate calories. This is particularly relevant in elderly patients, but also those with a high burden of care responsibilities, such as pregnant women or parents of young children.

Identifying the geographic origin and how recent the immigration is will be significant if the patient originates from a region of the world where particular deficiencies are common due to environment or genetic predisposition. Examples include central African countries, where iodine deficiency is common, and countries where the staple diet consists of polished rice, which have a high prevalence of thiamine deficiency.

Psychiatric history

It is important to identify current or past psychiatric illness. Many metabolic and nutritional disorders may present with neuropsychiatric symptoms (Table 14.2); however, bear in mind that these causes are *much* rarer than primary psychiatric conditions.

It is important to appreciate that psychiatric disease (unrelated to a metabolic or nutritional cause) can itself lead to loss of appetite and weight change. This can be diagnostically confounding as it becomes difficult to differentiate between psychiatric conditions (with secondary insufficient nutritional intake and thus deficiency) and neuropsychiatric symptoms secondary to nutritional deficiency.

General fitness

Objective quantification of an individual's general physical fitness is useful in the context of history-taking in suspected metabolic/nutritional disease. First, the overall impact of the symptoms on the patient's physiology can be assessed and used as a gross marker of impairment. Second, where a complaint of fatigue is reported, the information obtained may help infer the severity of the symptom.

Establish if the patient is capable of climbing two flights of stairs in one go without any untoward effects (such as severe breathlessness, chest pain). If they are able to do this, they are capable of performing four 'metabolic equivalents of task'. This translates to approximately 4 kcal/kg/hour in terms of energy expenditure; less than this is defined as poor exercise tolerance. Alternatively, simply documenting the distance a patient reports they can walk (on a level surface) before they have to stop is often used. It is important to elicit *what* exactly stops them at their distance limit – usually exhaustion but may also be specific symptoms induced by exercise such as chest pain or joint pain.

EXAMINATION

The following section headings will briefly describe features to be identified or excluded from a focussed physical examination. Please note that this is not an exhaustive or comprehensive list of a full general examination, rather a description of examination findings that may be

Table 14.2 Metabolic disorders or nutritional deficiencies presenting with neuropsychiatric features

Deficiency/abnormality	Possible neuropsychiatric manifestations
Hypothyroidism	Depression, memory impairment, coma
Hyperthyroidism	Insomnia, anxiety, agitation
B12 deficiency	Depression, poor concentration, memory impairment, confusion, hallucinations
Folate deficiency	Depression, poor concentration, memory impairment, confusion
B1 deficiency	Wernicke–Korsakoff syndrome, memory impairment, confusion, lack of coordination, paralysis
B3 deficiency	Progressive dementia
B6 deficiency	Depression, convulsions, migraine
Porphyria	Depression, psychosis, anxiety, phobias, agitation, somnolence, catatonia, coma
Magnesium deficiency	Tremor, anxiety, convulsions, tetany, muscle cramps
Zinc deficiency	Irritability, tremors, cerebellar ataxia
Copper deficiency	Seizures, hypotonia, cognitive impairment
Haemochromatosis	Depression, dementia-like illness
Wilson disease	Depression, cognitive impairment, catatonia, psychosis
Cushing disease	Depression, mania, anxiety, cognitive impairment
Urea cycle disorders	Episodic hallucinations, mood disorders
Hyperhomocysteinuria	Learning difficulties, mood disorders, obsessive-compulsive disorder
Niemann–Pick disease (type C)	Learning difficulties, autism-like symptoms, schizophrenia-like symptoms

pertinent to metabolic or nutritional disease. Always remember that with few exceptions (for example, iron deficiency) these diseases are rare, and more common causes must be first excluded before considering metabolic or nutritional disease.

General appearance

This is a summary of your overall impression of the patient from your encounter with them. In the context of nutrition, their body habitus (gross obesity or overt cachexia) and any extremely obvious physical signs that stand out just from looking at them (e.g. extreme pallor or any obvious structural deformities) are significant. Anything striking about their behaviour should be noted, for example, 'the patient has normal physical appearance but during our interaction was noted to be disoriented with rambling speech.'

Always politely introduce yourself, identifying yourself by name and grade. Then confirm the patient's identity, wash your hands and explain what you would like to do and why before obtaining their consent and assisting them with positioning. Ensure you do not provoke or exacerbate any pain they may be in.

In the majority of patients, there is unlikely to be anything hugely dramatic to observe. An example would be: 'Mr X, of normal appearance for a man of 50 years, presents comfortable at rest with no obvious or outstanding abnormalities on general inspection.'

Height/weight

Both height and weight should be accurately measured and documented. The body mass index (BMI) should be calculated (see Chapter 8), allowing objective assessment of weight for a given height, and as such abnormalities such as obesity and cachexia can be identified and monitored. A BMI less than $18.5\,kg/m^2$ suggests inadequate caloric intake, excessive energy expenditure, a combination of both or an underlying disease process resulting in weight loss. A BMI greater than $25\,kg/m^2$ suggests excessive caloric intake, inadequate energy expenditure, a combination of both (most common) or an underlying disease process causing weight gain. A BMI $30\,kg/m^2$ or greater is classed as obesity.

The BMI is a useful tool but can be misleading with patients at extremes of height or with disproportionately muscular individuals such as professional athletes; also important to appreciate is that the lines of division between categories may vary with ethnicity.

Paediatrics

In children, serial measurements of height and weight (and head circumference in infants) are recorded on gender-specific growth charts Fig. 14.1. They are supplied in the 'red book' given to all parents at their child's birth. These exhibit predicted growth curves for different 'centiles' and apply to optimal growth for healthy children born at term. The centile lines on the chart show the expected range of weights and heights and each describes the number of children of that age expected to lie below that line (e.g. 50% of children of that age have weights lying below the 50th centile). About 99% of children growing optimally will be plotted between the 0.4th and 99.6th centile lines, and 50% will lie between the 25th and 75th centile lines.

Cardiovascular system

A routine examination of the cardiovascular system will include inspection of the chest, assessment of heart rate, regularity, auscultation to detect any murmurs and palpation for heaves or thrills and apex beat position. Systolic and diastolic pressure must be recorded, and the pulse pressure calculated. Peripheral pulses should also be assessed. Signs of heart failure (Table 14.3) should be actively sought in all patients:

Nutritional and metabolic causes of cardiac pathophysiology are rare, with some important exceptions:

- Obesity and metabolic syndrome (risk factors for atherosclerotic heart disease)
- Acquired and genetic (see Chapter 7) dyslipidaemias (risk factors for atherosclerotic heart disease)
- Severe anaemia (usually exhibits a resting tachycardia and an ejection-systolic flow murmur, may cause heart failure)
- Alcohol excess and hyperthyroidism, which can each cause atrial fibrillation

Rarer metabolic/nutritional causes of heart failure include the following:

- Genetic dyslipidaemias (see Chapter 7)
- Kwashiorkor (see Chapter 9)
- Beriberi (see Table 12.3)
- Haemochromatosis (see Chapter 13)
- Certain glycogen storage disorders: Pompe disease, Cori disease and Andersen disease (see Chapter 5, Table 5.17)
- Other rare familial storage disorders (e.g. Hurler syndrome and Fabry–Anderson disease)

Respiratory system

All clinical examinations should include assessment of the respiratory system, using standard inspection/palpation/auscultation/percussion techniques described elsewhere [2]. The most important and easiest features to examine are the respiratory rate and pattern. An elevated respiratory rate may occur in response to hypoxia, or as physiological compensation for metabolic acidosis.

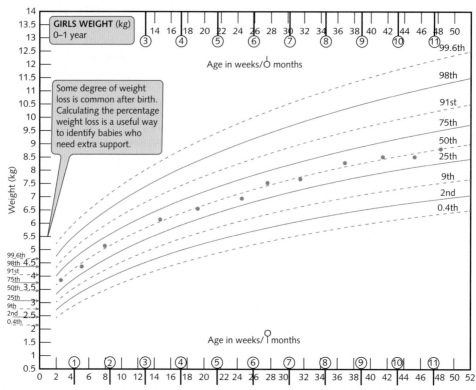

Fig. 14.1 UK paediatric growth chart, females, showing serial measurements plotted. This child is following the 50th centile.

Table 14.3 Cardinal signs of heart failure

Sign	Underlying mechanism
Bibasal crepitations on lung auscultation	Left ventricular failure results in pulmonary oedema
Breathlessness, exacerbated by supine position	Pulmonary oedema impairs oxygenation of the blood by the lungs resulting in hypoxia
Dependent pitting oedema on palpation	Right ventricular failure or congestive cardiac failure results in peripheral subcutaneous oedema
Elevated jugular venous pulse (>4 cm above sternal angle)	Right ventricular failure or congestive cardiac failure results in elevated right atrial pressure. The right atrium communicates with the valveless internal jugular vein
Third heart sound 'S3' – a quiet, very low-frequency sound heard on auscultation in early diastole	Exact cause of sound unclear; however, its presence indicates an increased volume in the left ventricle

RED FLAG

TACHYPNOEA

Apart from extreme anxiety, tachypnoea always has an underlying cause that must be identified. Relative changes in respiratory rate in response to a disease process are proportionally much greater than changes in heart rate or systolic pressure, meaning that an elevated respiratory rate is a more sensitive sign of a patient at risk that often appears earlier than other vital sign changes.

If clinically significant, tachypnoea is usually accompanied by increased work of breathing. This is characterized by use of the accessory muscles of respiration and may be described as 'air hunger'. Increased work of breathing is characterized by use of accessory respiratory muscles. Patients may tolerate the increased metabolic demand initially, but it is a particularly worrisome sign in an unwell patient, as it may indicate that they are tiring and could imminently decompensate further into respiratory failure. Increased work of breathing may also be the first indication of serious illness, especially in children, where head-bobbing, nasal flaring and intercostal, suprasternal and subcostal recession are more apparent than in adults.

Commonly encountered causes in the acute setting include hypoxia, sepsis and systemic shock. Diseases of metabolism/nutrition manifesting with tachypnoea/increased work of breathing are only rarely clinically encountered, with one important exception – diabetic ketoacidosis (see Chapter 6).

HINTS AND TIPS

KUSSMAUL RESPIRATION

This is a deep, laboured, rapid breathing pattern. Whilst the combination of tachypnoea and increased work of breathing is a physiological response to various disease scenarios, the term 'Kussmaul respiration' is used only to describe this pattern when it occurs as a compensatory response to a severe metabolic acidosis (e.g. in diabetic ketoacidosis).

However, pulmonary oedema (which will cause tachypnoea and bibasal crepitations) secondary to cardiac failure may rarely also be due to a metabolic/nutritional cause.

Structural abnormalities of the thoracic cage may be seen in various nutritional or metabolic disease (Table 14.4).

Abdomen

Acute and common surgical or medical causes for an 'acute abdomen' can usually be diagnosed with a combination of history and examination, but investigations, often including imaging, are always used to confirm suspected diagnoses. The abdomen is 'tender' when palpation or percussion elicits pain. Tenderness is therefore elicited by examination rather than abdominal pain, which is reported in the history. Focal tenderness, particularly if accompanied by guarding or worsening when palpating hand is withdrawn (rebound tenderness) is a worrisome sign that may indicate reactive peritonism secondary to a focal surgical condition.

Any palpable organomegaly indicates pathology and a cause must be identified with appropriate imaging and investigations. Ascites similarly is only present in disease; if the underlying diagnosis is not already known, it must be investigated. Metabolic and nutritional diseases that cause hepatomegaly, splenomegaly and ascites are listed in Table 14.5.

Hands and nails

Important information about a myriad of diseases can be gleaned from careful examination of the hands and nails. This holds true for nutritional deficiencies and metabolic disease. Specific nail abnormalities are discussed in Table 14.6. As always, be aware that these abnormalities have many other causes aside from metabolic/nutritional disease, and that these are often more common.

Palmar erythema

This describes a redness of the palmar surface of the hands, particular the thenar and hypothenar eminences. The vasodilation causing this cutaneous erythema arises secondary to a hyperdynamic circulation, most commonly due to pregnancy, hyperthyroidism or liver disease. Alcoholic

Table 14.4 Structural abnormalities of the thorax in nutritional deficiency/metabolic disease

Structural abnormality	Nutritional deficiency/metabolic disease potentially responsible
Pectus carinatum; 'pigeon chest': anterior protrusion of the sternum and medial ribs	Childhood vitamin D deficiency (rickets) Hyperhomocysteinuria Morquio syndrome (mucopolysaccharidosis type IV) Sly syndrome (mucopolysaccharidosis type VII)
Pectus excavatum; 'funnel chest': posterior depression of the central sternum and medial ribs	Osteomalacia Childhood vitamin D deficiency (rickets)
'Rachitic rosary': bilateral row of bony lumps overlying costochondral junction on anterior chest, distributed like beads on a loose-hanging necklace (rosary)	Childhood vitamin D deficiency (rickets)
Harrison sulcus: a horizontal groove delineating the lower border of the ribs, corresponding to the costal insertion of the diaphragm	Childhood vitamin D deficiency (rickets)

Please note that many other, nonmetabolic, nonnutritional causes for the deformities above also exist, but are not included here. Refer to Chapter 13, Rickets and Fig. 13.3 for further discussion of rickets.

Table 14.5 Possible metabolic/nutritional causes for abnormal findings on abdominal examination

Finding	Possible causes
Hepatomegaly; liver margin palpable below costal margin. These metabolic conditions also cause hepatic failure.	*Alcohol-induced hepatitis, steatohepatitis or cirrhosis[a] *Nonalcoholic steatohepatitis[a] Haemochromatosis (see Chapter 13) Wilson disease (see Chapter 13) Glycogen storage disorders (see Chapter 5) Galactosaemia (see Chapter 5) Porphyria (see Chapter 10) Lysosomal storage disorders (e.g. Niemann–Pick diseases, Gaucher disease)
Splenomegaly; palpable spleen (spleen must increase at least threefold to be palpable)	Acute/chronic haemolysis in glucose-6-phosphate dehydrogenase deficiency (see Chapter 5) Pernicious anaemia (see Chapter 12) Galactosaemia (see Chapter 5) Lysosomal storage disorders (e.g. Niemann–Pick diseases, Gaucher disease)
Ascites; generalized distension and shifting dullness to percussion	Metabolic disease leading to congestive cardiac failure (ascites secondary to portal hypertension) Metabolic liver disease (ascites secondary to portal hypertension) Hypoalbuminaemia secondary to protein–energy malnutrition

Please note that only metabolic/nutritional causes of the above findings are listed. With the exception of the starred conditions, all are extremely rare. Always consider more common causes first!

[a] *Cirrhosis may be associated with a liver of normal, enlarged or reduced size depending on the point in the progression of disease when the patient is examined. Any palpable abnormality of size should be further investigated with appropriate imaging, usually ultrasound.*

Table 14.6 Nail abnormalities and associated nutritional/metabolic abnormality

Descriptive term	Description of abnormality	Nutritional/metabolic abnormality
Koilonychia ('spoon-shaped' nails; Fig. 14.2)	Concave nails	Iron deficiency Diabetes mellitus Protein–energy malnutrition (malabsorption, starvation)
Leukonychia (white nails)	Whiteish discolouration of entire nail plate, increased opacity of nail	Hypoalbuminaemia Protein–energy malnutrition (malabsorption, starvation)
Onycholysis (Fig. 14.3)	Painless separation of the nail plate from the underlying nail bed. The separated nail plate appears yellowish or white	Diabetes mellitus Iron deficiency Hyperthyroidism Hypothyroidism Pellagra (B3 deficiency) Erythropoietic porphyria
Terry nails (half-and-half nails; Fig. 14.4)	Proximal part of a nail is white and opacified, distal nail is reddish or dark up to the free edge	Iron deficiency Diabetes mellitus Hyperthyroidism Protein–energy malnutrition (malabsorption, starvation) Zinc deficiency
Hapalonychia (eggshell nails)	Thinning of nails, resulting in easy bending/breaking	Vitamin A deficiency Vitamin B3 deficiency Vitamin B6 deficiency Vitamin C deficiency Vitamin D deficiency Calcium deficiency

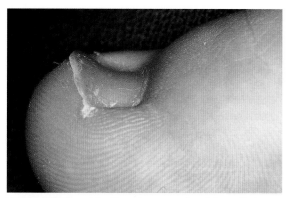

Fig. 14.2 Koilonychia. Note the concavity of the nail plate, with upturned free edge. (Reprinted, with permission, from Schachner LA, Hansen RC: Paediatric dermatology (4th edn), Philadelphia, 2011, Elsevier.)

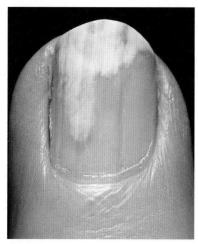

Fig. 14.3 Onycholysis. The free edge (the paler/white part of the nail) occupies proportionally more of the nail, due to separation from the underlying nail bed. (Reprinted, with permission, from Habif TP: Clinical Dermatology (6th edn), Philadelphia, 2016, Elsevier.)

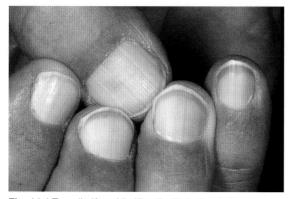

Fig. 14.4 Terry 'half-and-half' nails. Note the darker distal portion of the nail plate, proximal to the free edge (free edge = the white part of the distal nail). (Reprinted, with permission, from Habif TP: Clinical Dermatology (6th edn), Philadelphia, 2016, Elsevier.)

liver disease and nonalcoholic steatohepatitis are the most common of the liver disease causes. Rarer metabolic causes of liver disease include Wilson disease, haemochromatosis, galactosaemia and glycogen or lysosomal storage disorders.

Finger clubbing

Finger clubbing (Fig. 14.5) describes a group of progressive structural changes that develop at the distal joint of the finger. The nail appears bulbous and the nail plate is enlarged in area and excessively curved. There are four aspects to be aware of:

- The nail bed is spongy and fluctuant to pressure.
- The angle between the nail bed and the nail fold (the Lovibond angle, normally ≤160°) increases to ≥180°.
- Nail plate convexity is increased, sometimes dramatically. This is due to subungual nail bed hypertrophy.
- Increased bulk of soft tissue of the terminal phalanx (drumstick clubbing).

Examination of clubbing

To determine if clubbing is present, the index fingers are flexed and placed nail to nail with the cuticles touching each other. Absence of the normal diamond-shaped space (Schamroth window) demonstrates that the nail bed/nail fold angle has been lost; the nails thus demonstrate clubbing.

A common examination question is the causes of digital clubbing: these are therefore listed in Table 14.7. Please note that the most common causes of clubbing are respiratory in nature, and also that the nutritional causes are extremely rare.

Hair

Hair loss is a distressing symptom for both sexes. Normal hair growth requires sufficient levels of iron, folate, vitamin A, vitamin B12 and normal thyroid hormone levels. Deficiencies or abnormalities of these result in reduced new growth of hair whilst the loss rate remains the same. This

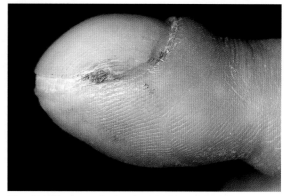

Fig. 14.5 Photograph showing clubbing, lateral view. (Reprinted, with permission, from Habif TP: Clinical Dermatology (6th edn), Philadelphia, 2016, Elsevier.)

Table 14.7 Causes of clubbing by system

System/cause	Disease
Respiratory	Bronchiectasis Chronic infections including tuberculosis Cystic fibrosis Lung tumours Interstitial lung disease Lung abscess Empyema
Cardiovascular	Congenital cyanotic heart disease Right-to-left cardiac shunt Congestive heart disease Infective endocarditis Atrial myxoma
Gastrointestinal	Crohn disease Ulcerative colitis Coeliac disease Cirrhotic liver disease
Malignant	Lung cancer Mesothelioma Thyroid cancer Gastrointestinal cancer Hodgkin disease Disseminated chronic myeloid leukaemia
Endocrine/metabolic	Hyperthyroidism Acromegaly
Nutritional	Hypervitaminosis A Cretinism (childhood iodine deficiency)

RED FLAG

LANUGO HAIR

New growth of lanugo (nonpigmented, soft, fine, downy hair) hair on the abdomen, back and forearms is an important red flag for eating disorders because, bizarrely, it develops in anorexia nervosa, but not in other types of protein–energy malnutrition.

Skin findings

The most important information the skin can provide diagnostically is its colour (Table 14.8). Many metabolic or nutritional diseases will feature specific skin lesions. These are shown in Table 14.9.

Rashes

Certain rashes are characteristic of specific nutrient deficiencies. These are discussed in the relevant sections of Chapters 12 and 13.

gives the appearance of hair 'thinning' or reduced density. This type of acquired, diffuse hair loss is reversible with correction of the underlying abnormality (e.g. with appropriate nutrient supplementation).

Telogen effluvium describes a dramatic increase in the normal overall rate of hair loss. The proportion of hairs growing from follicles in the 'rest' (telogen) phase (usually <10%) is increased. Because telogen phase hairs will fall with mild traction, there is a greater rate of loss overall, and this is noticed by the patient as their hair falling out.

Surprisingly, hair loss can be the sole symptom of early iron deficiency and thyroid disease, thus T3, T4, thyroid-stimulating hormone and ferritin and also a full blood count are important investigations to include when investigating hair loss. Loss of the lateral (outer) third of the eyebrows is a clinical sign of hypothyroidism. Interestingly, an *excessive* intake of vitamin A, B7 (biotin), zinc and selenium can also trigger telogen effluvium.

Eating disorders such as anorexia nervosa or bulimia, dramatic crash diets and starvation result in generalized malnourishment. These scenarios can provoke telogen effluvium of scalp hair, which is compounded by impaired new hair growth.

Table 14.8 Implication of skin colour

Suggest Coloration	Implication	Underlying mechanism
Pale (pallor)	Anaemia or poor perfusion	A low concentration of haemoglobin in the cutaneous vasculature lessens the skin/mucosal membrane's normal pink appearance.
Blue (cyanosis)	Arterial hypoxia	An increase in circulating deoxy-haemoglobin, relative to oxyhaemoglobin
Yellow (jaundice, also known as 'icterus')	Any liver disease, including metabolic liver disease Haemolysis (e.g. in glucose-6-phosphate dehydrogenase-deficient patients undergoing oxidative stress)	Elevated serum bilirubin, either due to reduced clearance from the serum or overproduction
Grey	Haemochromatosis	Cutaneous deposition of iron

Table 14.9 Skin lesions in metabolic or nutritional disease

Lesion	Appearance	Associated conditions
Spider naevi (Fig. 14.7)	Central red area (dilated arteriole) with a halo of wavy fine red lines radiating outward (telangiectasia). Usually located on the abdomen.	Elevated oestrogen levels secondary to liver disease, which may be metabolic in origin Hyperthyroidism
Xanthomata	Yellow-orange (or flesh coloured if located around tendons) nodules or plaques usually situated on dorsal aspects of hands or the Achilles tendons. Please see Fig. 7.24.	Genetic dyslipidaemias
Perifollicular haemorrhages	Pinpoint red areas of subcutaneous bleeding around a hair follicle.	Vitamin C deficiency (scurvy)
Petechiae, ecchymoses	Flat areas, small (<2 mm, petechiae) or large (>2 mm, ecchymoses) of nonblanching subcutaneous or submucosal haemorrhage. Colour evolves with age of lesion.	Vitamin K deficiency
Gouty tophi (Fig. 10.7)	Firm, whiteish-yellow irregular subcutaneous or cartilaginous nodules representing deposition of urate crystals. Ear helix and extensor surfaces of digits are common predilection zones for tophi. In acute gout the skin overlying the tophus will be erythematous.	Gout

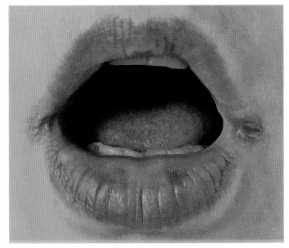

Fig. 14.6 Angular stomatitis. Note the cracked, inflamed corners of the mouth (left of the image in this example has started to heal).

Mouth findings

Signs that can point to nutritional deficiencies in the mouth are shown in Table 14.10.

Breath odour

Acetone-scented breath, often described as smelling like pear drops, arises due to ketone presence (see Chapter 7). An individual in ketosis secondary to starvation, alcohol excess or an extreme low-calorie diet will often have this unusual pear drop-like odour in their breath.

> **RED FLAG**
>
> **KETOACIDOSIS**
>
> Ketoacidosis secondary to new or uncontrolled diabetes (predominantly type 1) will exhibit ketotic breath. This is therefore an important sign not to miss in the dangerous condition of diabetic ketoacidosis.

Thyroid gland

Any assessment of metabolism warrants examination of the neck to assess for presence of thyroid goitre.

Limbs

Limb assessment should include examination of neurological function (power, reflexes, sensation and tone), assessment of peripheral pulses and identification and documentation of any ulcers present as a minimum.

Ulcers

Ulcers are lesions with full-thickness skin loss. They are classified by causative mechanism and are summarized in Table 14.11. When examining an ulcer, it is important (though not always easy) to define whether the ulcer is venous, arterial or neuropathic in nature, because treatment of the ulcer and management implications for the underlying disease will vary accordingly.

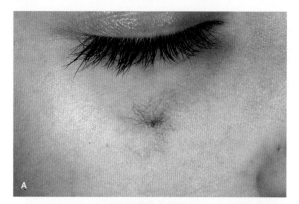

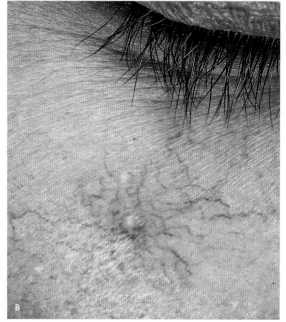

Fig. 14.7 Spider naevus. Note the central feeder arteriole with radiating smaller superficial vessels. (Reprinted, with permission, from Habif TP: Clinical Dermatology (6th edn), Philadelphia, 2016, Elsevier.)

Table 14.10 Oral signs of nutritional deficiencies

Sign	Appearance	Possible nutritional cause
Angular stomatitis (Fig. 14.6)	Inflamed cracks at the junction of the upper and lower lips. Opportunistic candida infection may complicate the focal structural impairment of the skin barrier.	Iron deficiency B12 deficiency Folate deficiency Zinc deficiency Riboflavin (B2) deficiency Niacin (B3) deficiency Pyridoxine (B6) deficiency
Glossitis	Inflamed tongue: appearing red	B12 deficiency Folate deficiency Riboflavin (B2) deficiency Pyridoxine (B6) deficiency
Smooth tongue	Smoother than normal appearance reflecting loss of the usual filiform papillae architecture	Folate deficiency
Gingivitis	Inflamed, possibly bleeding gums	Vitamin C deficiency Niacin (B3) deficiency
Ulcers (aphthae)	Discrete focal painful tender lesions, usually appearing paler than surrounding mucosa	B12 deficiency Folate deficiency
Leukoplakia	A white patch on oral mucosa that cannot be removed by rubbing. Usually asymptomatic	Vitamin A deficiency

In the context of metabolism and nutrition, diabetes is an extremely common cause of all of the aforementioned ulcers, and the most common cause of neuropathic ulcers in the UK (due to diabetic neuropathy). Excessive alcohol intake and protein–energy malnutrition are also important causes of peripheral neuropathy. B12 deficiency is clearly associated with peripheral and central neuropathy, which may manifest with neuropathic ulcers.

Oedema

Distal parts of limbs are useful sites to assess for oedema, because the limited subcutaneous compartments display distension far earlier than, for example, the central abdomen. Progressive dependent oedema in ambulant patients appears first in the feet and gradually progresses upwards, whilst in bedbound patients the sacrum is the first zone affected. Oedema is most commonly associated with organ failure (e.g. heart, renal, hepatic), but is also an important sign in protein–energy malnutrition (kwashiorkor, but not marasmus; see Chapter 9). It may also occur due to hyponatraemia in refeeding syndrome.

Asterixis

Also known as a 'flapping tremor,' asterixis is the abrupt loss of tone during a sustained contraction. It is best observed by asking the patient to hold their arms outstretched with wrists extended. The hands will 'flap', rhythmically flexing at the wrists. Common causes are:

- Carbon dioxide retention in type 2 respiratory failure
- Uraemia in renal impairment
- Hepatic encephalopathy, which is occasionally secondary to a metabolic disease

Table 14.11 Ulcer characteristics

Type	Distinguishing features	Predilection sites	Mechanism
Venous	Often extensive Minimally painful Abundant exudate Poorly defined edges Surrounding skin changes are common, (e.g. haemosiderin pigmentation).	Superior to malleoli (medial > lateral), may involve entire anterior shin.	Arise secondary to pericapillary fibrin deposition-provoked venous hypertension. This fibrin accumulation impairs nutrient and oxygen delivery, leading to cell death.
Arterial	Painful Usually small Well-defined Little exudate Pulses supplying the ulcer zone reduced or absent Distal tissue pale and cold due to arterial insufficiency.	Heel, toe joints, overlying malleoli, anterior shin. Less likely to include proximal shins than venous ulcers.	Develop in areas of arterial insufficiency, resulting in ischaemia and cell death.
Neuropathic	Painless Usually small Well demarcated Granulation tissue covering base Surrounding skin may be callused Distal tissue normally well perfused (unless coexisting ischaemic vascular disease).	Pressure sites, especially soles of feet; particularly the heels and tissue overlying inferior metatarsal surfaces.	Arise from impaired sensation (including to noxious stimuli such as pain from injury, heat and pressure) due to peripheral neuropathy. Because no pain or discomfort is perceived, the patient is unable to take appropriate action to limit the damage.
Pressure	Appearance evolves: initially well-defined nonblanching red area with intact skin, ultimately progressing to full thickness tissue loss with exposure of underlying tissues.	Zones under high external pressure (e.g. bony prominences in contact with an external surface).	Common in immobile and bed-bound patients, prolonged pressure in excess of arteriolar pressure impairs delivery of oxygen and nutrients.

DEHYDRATION

This is an extremely common and potentially life-threatening clinical entity. It occurs when fluid losses exceed fluid intake. This usually arises in the context of disease rather than voluntary insufficient oral intake. The resulting reduction in intravascular volume (intravascular hypovolaemia) compromises tissue perfusion (see Table 13.4), which results initially in reduced urine output due to prerenal impairment. Electrolyte derangement and renal impairment can be severe, and blood should be drawn for these investigations when obtaining intravenous access. Examination findings of dehydration (Table 14.12) are as follows:

- Reduced urine output (<0.5 mL/kg/hour)
- Dry mucous membranes, dry skin (reduced turgor)
- Cool peripheries and reduced capillary refill time
- Tachycardia
- Drowsiness, hypotension (both preterminal signs in dehydration)

In infants, a sunken fontanelle, sunken eyes and absence of tears when crying are useful additional signs signalling dehydration.

Local protocols will be available to guide safe rehydration. As a guide, use the clinical signs to estimate the

Table 14.12 Clinical assessment of dehydration. Estimating the % dehydration clinically is performed using the signs below. If the patient's usual weight is known, the actual % weight loss can be calculated rather than estimated

Extent of dehydration	Accompanying signs
Mild (≤5% usual weight)	Increased thirst, reduced urine output
Moderate (5%–8% usual weight)	Delayed capillary refill time (>2 seconds) Increased respiratory rate
Severe (>8% usual weight)	Tachycardia Reduced consciousness Increased respiratory rate and depth

% dehydration, then using the patient's usual (nondehydrated) weight, calculate the volume of fluid deficit as follows:

- Usual weight × % dehydration × 10
- This gives the total volume in mL that must be replaced. Obtain intravenous access and plan to replace this volume as follows:
- An initial bolus of 10 mL/kg (up to a maximum volume of 1000 mL)

- The remainder of the calculated volume/24 is the hourly rate for the next 24 hours.
- Throughout the 24-hour period continue to give normal maintenance requirements: 1 mL/kg/hour (up to a maximum rate of 125 mL/hour).

> **RED FLAG**
>
> **REHYDRATION FLUIDS**
>
> Isotonic fluid such as 0.9% saline, Plasma-Lyte or Hartmann's should be used for rehydration. Never use hypotonic fluids such as 0.45% saline, as this can lead to fatal hyponatraemia.

A worked example is given here: A 45-kg patient who has had severe vomiting and diarrhoea for 48 hours is drowsy with clinical signs suggesting severe dehydration. The patient is assessed clinically as having greater than 8% dehydration weight loss. The normal weight is known to be 50 kg, so the exact % of weight loss is calculated as 10%: 50 × 10 × 10 = 5000 mL, the total volume to be replaced. An initial bolus is given: 500 mL of 0.9% saline. The remaining 4500 mL of replacement (5000 − 500 = 4500) is given over 24 hours at 187.5 mL/hour. Normal maintenance is given at (1 mL/kg/hour) 50 mL/hour so the total hourly rate is 187.5 + 50 = 237.5 mL/hour.

The example given here would be for appropriate for an otherwise-healthy dehydrated adult patient with normal cardiovascular status. A much slower rate, titrated to clinical response, would be necessary in a patient with cardiac or renal failure. Careful clinical monitoring for signs of intravascular overload is mandatory, as rehydrating too rapidly can cause pulmonary oedema. If the patient is not haemodynamically compromised, rehydration should occur over the same timeframe that the dehydration took to do develop. An exception is the diabetic ketoacidosis. This leads to severe dehydration, with an average fluid deficit of 6000 mL (10% body weight loss!) secondary to both osmotic dehydration from glycosuria and vomiting losses. There are specific, aggressive protocols used for rehydration in the context of diabetic ketoacidosis, available at http://bestpractice.bmj.com/best-practice/monograph/162/treatment/step-by-step.html.

RELEVANT INVESTIGATIONS

Laboratory blood tests

The following investigations are standard as part of an integrated clinical assessment of nutritional and metabolic status. There are more common clinical indications for performing any of these tests, but here we focus on their application of nutritional or metabolic assessment.

Venous blood gas

This assay provides rapid and important information in acute scenarios regarding the following:

- Acid–base status (pH and base excess)
- Global tissue perfusion (suggested by lactate >2 mmol)
- Respiratory function (partial pressure of oxygen (pO_2) and partial pressure of carbon dioxide (pCO_2))
- Electrolytes (Na^+, K^+, Cl^-, HCO_3^- and ionized calcium)
- Glucose level (indicating presence/absence of hypoglycaemia, i.e. <4 mmol) Hypoglycaemia <2.5 mmol requires urgent treatment. Approximately 2 mL/kg of 10% dextrose intravenously is an appropriate bolus dose if oral glucose cannot be tolerated due to reduced consciousness or vomiting.

Of particular note in the context of metabolic disorders are the pH and the base excess, which indicate metabolic acidosis if pH less than 7.35 with a base excess less than −2. In diabetic ketoacidosis, for example, a reduced pH, elevated base deficit, elevated glucose, raised lactate and hypokalaemia would be shown on a blood gas result.

Full blood count

The main parameters that infer useful nutritional information in the full blood count are the Hb concentration and the mean corpuscular volume (MCV). Anaemia is defined as an Hb concentration less than 12 g/dL in females or less than 13 g/dL in males. It is classified by the average red cell volume, which may be reduced (<75 fL (microcytic)), normal (75–100 fL (normochromic)) or raised (>100 fL (macrocytic)).

A macrocytic anaemia is seen in B12 or folate deficiency (chronic haemolytic anaemias may *cause* folate and B12 deficiency as a result of the increased background rate of erythropoiesis). Macrocytosis occurs also in liver disease and alcohol excess. A microcytic anaemia is seen in vitamin C or iron deficiency. The haemolytic anaemia of glucose-6-phosphate dehydrogenase deficiency or pyruvate kinase deficiency may be normocytic, macrocytic or apparently macrocytic due to marrow release of reticulocytes (early nucleated red cell precursors) into peripheral blood.

Caution is required when interpreting normocytic anaemias, because the MCV may be reported as normal range, when in fact the red cell population represents a combination of macrocytic and microcytic red cells (MCV is an averaged value). This scenario may be seen when B12 and folate deficiencies coexist with an iron deficiency. In such cases, the *red cell distribution width* parameter will be raised, indicating coexistence of macrocytic and microcytic red cells.

Blood film

An enormous amount of diagnostic information can be obtained by a haematologist inspecting a blood smear microscopically. Blood films are performed when abnormalities (e.g. low red cell counts) are detected by a full blood count. Specific red cell morphology is associated with certain deficiencies. For example:

- Macrocytic red cells in B12 and folate deficiencies appear oval, and neutrophil nuclei are hypersegmented.
- Macrocytic red cells in alcohol excess and liver disease are round, and there is no hypersegmentation of neutrophil nuclei.
- Lead poisoning is indicated by microcytic red cells with basophilic stippling.

Haematinics

"Haematinics" is a general term for nutrients required for normal synthesis and development of blood cells in bone marrow. Deficiency of haematinics results in anaemia. The serum folate, iron, transferrin and B12 are routine laboratory investigations performed when a full blood count shows anaemia.

Inflammatory markers

These include C-reactive protein (CRP; most commonly used today) and erythrocyte sedimentation rate (ESR). If these are both low, systemic inflammation can be ruled out in nearly all scenarios with the exception of specific unusual immunodeficiency syndromes. In the context of metabolism and nutrition, because these disorders are mostly unusual, excluding inflammation as a component of the underlying pathology is an important initial process.

Liver function tests

These tests are used to diagnose and monitor liver diseases. Components of a standard liver function test panel are discussed in Table 14.13.

Coagulation parameters

Prothrombin time will be prolonged in vitamin K deficiency (see Chapter 12), because clotting factors 2, 7, 9 and 10 are synthesized via a vitamin K-dependent synthetic pathway in hepatocytes. Prolonging of both the prothrombin time and activated partial thromboplastin time is indicative of severely impaired hepatocellular function.

Urea

The urea molecule is the main human mechanism for nitrogen excretion (see Chapter 9, Fig. 9.19). Elevated serum urea most commonly relates to acute or chronic renal impairment. This is often seen in dehydration (a prerenal cause of renal impairment). However, a lowered urea is useful diagnostically in a metabolic/nutritional context, because excessive alcohol, reduced muscle mass and urea cycle disorders (see Chapter 9) result in low urea levels.

Table 14.13 Components of liver function test (LFT) panel

LFT component	Implications of derangement
Alkaline phosphatase (ALP)	ALP is present in the liver and bone, thus elevation may point to a disorder in either of these sites. For example, deficiencies of calcium, phosphate or vitamin D in childhood rickets result in defective bone mineralization with raised ALP levels.
Alanine transaminase Aspartate transaminase	Intracellular liver enzymes whose levels are elevated when there is a higher rate of hepatocyte death than normal, as the enzyme is released by dying cells. They are useful indicators of liver damage.
Bilirubin	Elevated in liver disease, including metabolic diseases such as haemochromatosis and Wilson disease. It is also raised in haemolytic anaemias, including glucose-6-phosphate dehydrogenase or pyruvate kinase deficiencies.
Albumin	Marker of overall hepatic synthetic function. Low (hypoalbuminaemia) in protein–energy malnutrition.
Prothrombin time (PT) and activated partial thromboplastin time (APTT)	PT is a marker of overall hepatic synthetic function (prolonged in liver failure). Surrogate marker of vitamin K status (PT prolonged, APTT normal signifies mild vitamin K deficiency, both PT and APTT prolonged infers severe vitamin K deficiency).

Electrolytes

Serum sodium and potassium are reported routinely, whereas serum magnesium, phosphate, calcium and bicarbonate are usually additional requests. Metabolic acidosis can arise secondary to gastrointestinal bicarbonate losses in acute or chronic diarrhoea; this is therefore important to include in an electrolyte profile investigating gastrointestinal disease. Please see Chapter 13 for discussion and explanation of serum electrolyte derangements.

Glucose and markers of glucose homeostasis

Fasting serum glucose and glycated haemoglobin (HbA1c) are most commonly used to diagnose diabetes. Specific investigations such as an oral glucose tolerance test are also used in this context. When considering hypoglycaemia as a factor in an acutely unwell patient, it is sensible to use a dry test strip, a portable glucose meter or a blood gas to quantify blood glucose, as the results are obtained more rapidly.

Serum lipid profile

A complete lipid profile is usually performed on a fasting sample, and includes total cholesterol (TC), triglycerides, high-density lipoprotein cholesterol (HDL-C), low-density lipoprotein cholesterol and the calculated ratio of TC/HDL-C. Please see Chapter 7 for detail and discussion.

Thyroid hormones

Thyroid-stimulating hormone is usually used as a screening test when hypothyroidism or hyperthyroidism is suspected, and abnormal values are further investigated with T4 and, if necessary, T3. Please see Chapter 11 for clinical inference of abnormalities.

Other biochemical tissue markers

These are shown in Table 14.14.

Urine analysis

A simple multipanelled urine dipstick is a useful and rapid test able to identify abnormalities and direct further investigations or focussed examination. It is semiquantitative; colour intensity corresponds to the magnitude of the detected substance. The following subsections discuss common findings. Sometimes 24-hour urine collections are performed for specific indications, for example, quantification of heavy proteinuria or in investigation of specific micronutrient deficiencies.

Glucose

Glucose in the urine is termed 'glycosuria'. In uncontrolled diabetes mellitus, however, glycosuria is persistent, reflecting the persistently raised blood glucose. When blood glucose is so high that it exceeds the 'renal threshold' for complete reabsorption, glucose is present in the urine. Some individuals have a low renal threshold in the absence of pathology. Moreover, in pregnancy, increased renal blood flow lowers the renal threshold, resulting in glycosuria at normal blood glucose levels.

Alternatively, and usually pathological, when the renal tubules fail to reabsorb a normal quantity of glucose, 'renal glycosuria' occurs. Important (rare) metabolic diseases that feature renal glycosuria include Wilson disease, cystinosis (a lysosomal storage disorder), hereditary tyrosinaemia, glucose/galactose malabsorption and heavy metal poisoning.

Ketones

The most important disease with a positive dipstick for ketones is diabetic ketoacidosis. However, a positive dipstick is also seen in starvation, fasting, high-protein or low-carbohydrate diets, prolonged vomiting and glycogen storage disorders. In addition, an elevated basal metabolic rate (such as seen in pregnancy, hyperthyroidism, fever or lactation) results in ketone presence in the urine. Ketonuria may also accompany renal glycosuria.

> **HINTS AND TIPS**
>
> **KETONURIA**
>
> Ketonuria represents (in the nondiabetic) a relative reduction of carbohydrate catabolism and a relative increase in fat catabolism. In a known diabetic, appearance of ketones in the urine indicated metabolic decompensation.

Protein

Proteinuria is most commonly associated with urinary tract infection (UTI) or renal disease. If persistent, particularly if associated with oedema and low serum albumin, proteinuria should prompt investigation for renal disease. Proteinuria is an important indicator of this dangerous pregnancy-related condition which is easily missed. Assessment of pregnant woman should therefore always include a urine dipstick.

Nitrites/leucocytes

Most gram-negative bacteria (common culprits in UTI) convert nitrates to nitrites. Nitrite-positive urine dipstick

Table 14.14 Other biochemical tissue markers

Marker	Diagnostic utility
Amylase	Pancreatic damage, as in pancreatitis, releases this enzyme from the exocrine pancreas into serum. It is always included in investigations for acute abdominal pain as acute pancreatitis (indicated by raised levels) can be life-threatening if overlooked. Chronic pancreatitis secondary to alcoholism is an important metabolic cause of elevated amylase.
Creatine kinase (CK)	Normal levels are related to muscle mass. Raised CK is indicative of muscle damage, as seen in rhabdomyolysis and myositis. Rhabdomyolysis is seen in prolonged immobility, burns, major trauma, severe infection, following seizures or extreme exercise such as marathons, and following myocardial infarctions. It is also a very rare complication of statin treatment of dyslipidaemia.
Troponin-T	Serum troponin-T is a cardiac-muscle-specific protein that is measured following chest pain to confirm or exclude myocardial infarction in combination with electrocardiogram and examination findings plus history. It is released from damaged cardiac muscle. Aside from ischaemia, myocarditis, acute cardiogenic shock and massive pulmonary embolism may account for a significantly raised troponin.

thus indicates a bacterial UTI. This will usually be associated with a positive dipstick test for leucocytes, where the test assays leucocyte esterase. In the context of metabolism and nutrition, the main diagnostic utility of this dipstick is to rule out infection (the most common cause in a patient with normal renal function) as a cause of proteinuria.

Human chorionic gonadotrophin
HCG is synthesized by the placenta. Pregnancy shares many signs associated with metabolic disease or nutritional deficiency (glycosuria, abdominal swelling, glycosuria, etc.) and symptoms too (fatigue, change in appetite and weight, nausea, vomiting, etc.). It is therefore essential to exclude pregnancy in females of reproductive age with a negative urine HCG dipstick test. It is good practice to inform the patient that you wish to test their pregnancy status and seek consent to do so.

COMMON PITFALLS

PREGNANCY STATUS

In females of reproductive age, despite what the patient may assert regarding their sexually active status, establishing if a pregnancy exists is almost always clinically relevant! The consequences can be devastating if interventions are performed in belief that a patient is not pregnant, as well as causing a delay to appropriate management for either the pregnancy or another disease.

Second-line investigations

The following subsections discuss investigations that would only be performed if specifically indicated by examination, history or first-line investigation results.

Bone marrow iron stores
A bone marrow biopsy is an invasive procedure usually performed by haematologists in the context of suspected bone marrow disorders. It is also the most definitive investigation for differentiating iron-deficiency anaemia from other microcytic causes of anaemia (e.g. sideroblastic anaemia or thalassaemia). In practice, clinical assessment (history and examination) and first-line investigations (serum iron, ferritin, Hb level and MCV) are usually sufficient to confidently diagnose iron deficiency.

Schilling test
This test is performed to confirm/exclude pernicious anaemia (see Chapter 12) as a cause for B12 deficiency. Stages are as follows:
1. Intramuscular injection of nonradioactive B12 (1 mg) is given. This megadose saturates the body's binding

sites, ensuring that any subsequent absorbed oral B12 will be completely excreted via the urine.
2. The patient drinks an oral solution of radiolabelled B12.
3. The urine is collected and quantity of the radiolabelled B12 is assayed.

If no (or reduced) radiolabelled B12 is present in the urine, steps 2 and 3 are repeated after providing oral intrinsic factor. A (normal) patient with endogenous intrinsic factor will have radiolabelled urine after the first test. In pernicious anaemia, a positive test is demonstrated by appearance in the urine of radiolabelled B12 *only after* provision of oral intrinsic factor, because in the absence of exogenous intrinsic factor, the radiolabelled B12 is not absorbed into the bloodstream from the gastrointestinal tract and thus cannot enter the urine.

Serum caeruloplasmin
Serum caeruloplasmin is a copper transport protein that binds 95% of serum copper. Levels are *low* in Wilson disease (see Chapter 13). If not already performed, a slit-lamp examination should be undertaken. This is likely to demonstrate Kayser–Fleischer rings. Contrary to many medical student's belief, these are *not* usually visible simply from looking closely at the eyes. They are usually only visible using a slit lamp, which is able to visualize the layers of the cornea, where the copper deposition occurs. They occur circumferentially at the junction of the cornea with the sclera (the limbus). A liver biopsy is often also performed in suspected Wilson disease.

Serum 25-hydroxy vitamin D
This test would be performed to confirm a suspected diagnosis of vitamin D deficiency (see Chapter 12) inferred by history, examination or first-line investigation results revealing low serum calcium and phosphate and a raised alkaline phosphatase.

Long bone X-rays
Osteoporotic changes seen on long bone radiographs confirm and quantify the extent of the defective bone mineralization seen in identified vitamin D, calcium or phosphate deficiencies. This type of radiological surveying is usually performed following a suspected 'fragility' fracture. Long bone X-rays are also performed in a setting of suspected nonaccidental injury in children, allowing identification of current or previous healed fractures.

Liver biopsy
Histopathological examination of a liver biopsy specimen is conclusively diagnostic in various metabolic conditions (e.g. Wilson disease or haemochromatosis). It is also diagnostic in other more common causes of liver dysfunction or cirrhosis. The procedure carries risk for bleeding and infection, which are significant in patients with delayed clotting from factor deficiencies secondary to impaired hepatic synthetic function.

Ascitic fluid analysis

An ascitic fluid sample, obtained via paracentesis, allows determination of albumin, lactate dehydrogenase, glucose and amylase concentrations. In combination with the serum values, this allows quantification of the serum–ascitic concentration gradients. These gradients (as well as ascitic concentration values) have diagnostic utility for differentiating the pathophysiology of ascites. Portal hypertension, malignancy, hypoalbuminaemia or peritoneal disease account for the majority of cases. This in turn allows exclusion of erroneous differential diagnoses. Cytology and microscopy can also be performed, useful in malignancy or bacterial peritonitis, respectively.

Serum ammonia level

Various inborn errors of metabolism present with elevated ammonia levels, with or without encephalopathy. This test is important to perform in patients presenting with altered consciousness and behaviour, particularly if liver disease is known or suspected, where the cause is likely to be hepatic encephalopathy. Urea cycle disorders exhibit raised ammonia levels. In babies, both haemolytic disease of the newborn and Reye syndrome present with raised ammonia and hypoglycaemia. Large gastrointestinal bleeds are also associated with raised ammonia, even in the absence of primary liver failure.

Enzymatic assays

Direct enzyme assays are used to confirm suspected diagnosis in pyruvate kinase and glucose-6-phosphate dehydrogenase deficiencies (see Chapter 5). Suspicion would arise in confirmed haemolysis with a clinical presentation typical of these conditions (i.e. acute episodes provoked by oxidative stress or other known triggers) for which other causes have been excluded.

CLINICAL NOTES

HAEMOLYSIS

Symptoms and signs are those of anaemia, but jaundice may be present during an acute episode. Investigation findings will reveal low haemoglobin, reduced red cell count, reticulocytosis, elevated serum bilirubin, lactate dehydrogenase and decreased serum haptoglobin.

Urinary porphobilinogen, δ-aminolevulinic acid, total porphyrins

These specific urinary assays would be used as an initial screening investigation where there is clinical suspicion of a porphyria (see Chapter 10) – for example, in patients complaining of blistering, photosensitivity or acute neurovisceral symptoms. If positive, plasma, erythrocyte and stool porphyrins are then quantified to identify the specific porphyria. Urine and stool samples must be immediately placed in a dark environment and refrigerated less than 4°C for porphyrin assays to be accurate.

Urinary galactose, urinary fructose

Galactose is present in the urine (galactosuria) in galactosaemia, so a calorimetric test is used as an initial screen test in infants with suspicious symptoms (see Chapter 5). A positive test (blue copper citrate is reduced by galactose, forming a red-brown precipitate) would prompt red cell galactose-1-phosphate uridyl transferase activity assay, as this will be decreased in galactosaemia.

Fructose is present in the urine in fructose-1-6-bisphosphatase deficiency and fructose-1-aldolase deficiency (see Chapter 5). The urinary assay would prompt a liver biopsy to confirm enzyme absence from hepatocytes and verify the diagnosis. Fructosuria is also present in the benign condition of fructokinase deficiency.

Urine amino acid profile

This may be requested when an inborn error of metabolism is suspected in an infant.

Specific biochemical tests for individual nutrients

The serum level of nearly all vitamins and minerals can be biochemically quantified if required. Some vitamin levels are indirectly quantified, for example:

- Vitamin K status is inferred by the prothrombin time.
- Thiamine; the activity of red cell transketolase is dependent on thiamine levels and the activity therefore corresponds to the patient's thiamine status. This is mentioned as it may be examined; however, nowadays high-performance liquid chromatography is more commonly used to quantify thiamine levels.

Often specific tests are only employed when appropriate supplementation fails to correct the symptoms/signs of a clinical diagnosis. This is because samples may need to be sent to reference laboratories for rarely performed tests, which is costly and time-consuming.

NEWBORN BLOOD SPOT SCREENING

- All newborn babies in the UK are offered a heel prick blood test at 5 days of age. The heel prick test screens for six serious inborn errors of metabolism, as well as sickle cell disease, cystic fibrosis and congenital hypothyroidism. The rationale behind universal screening is that the prognosis for the screened diseases is much more promising if managed appropriately from the neonatal period onwards. If left to develop naturally, babies with these diseases would either suffer severe developmental problems or die. The inborn errors of metabolism screened for in the newborn blood spots are as follows:

- Phenylketonuria
- Maple syrup urine disease
- Isovaleric acidaemia
- Glutaric aciduria type 1
- Homocystinuria (pyridoxine unresponsive)
- Medium-chain acyl-coenzyme A dehydrogenase deficiency (see Chapter 7)

The test is usually performed by a midwife in the baby's home. It is quick and minimally distressing to the baby and his/her parents. The blood is 'spotted' onto a card, which is returned to the screening centre for analysis.

Chapter Summary

- Metabolic diseases and nutritional deficiencies are rare in the UK and usually share many clinical features with more commonly encountered illnesses. Do not consider these as first-line diagnoses!
- History and examination, as always, form the initial part of reaching a diagnosis. The hands, nails, hair and skin examinations are of more significance in the context of nutritional disease.
- If more common causes for an abnormality are excluded, and routine laboratory tests have not yet made a suitable diagnosis, and the signs and symptoms are consistent with a metabolic disease or a nutritional deficiency, specific first- and second-line investigations are then appropriate.

REFERENCES

[1] http://store.elsevier.com/Hutchisons-Clinical-Methods/isbn-9780702067396/.

[2] http://store.elsevier.com/Macleods-Clinical-Examination/Graham-Douglas/isbn-9780702047282/.

[3] http://store.elsevier.com/product.jsp?isbn=9780723438649&pagename=search.

[4] Involuntary weight loss: diagnostic and prognostic significance. Marton KI, Sox HC Jr, Krupp JR, Ann Intern Med. 1981;95(5):568.

SELF-ASSESSMENT

Single best answer (SBA) questions

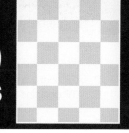

Chapter 1 Cellular biology

1. Regarding components of the cytoskeleton, which of the following options best describes intermediate filaments?
   A. Linear, polymers of actin subunits
   B. Composed primarily of tubulin
   C. The most abundant filament component of the cytoskeleton
   D. A double helical structure
   E. The cytoskeletal feature permitting motility

2. Which of the following best describes the nucleus
   A. Contains genetic material of the cell (chromosomes), delineated by a single phospholipid bilayer
   B. A structure possessing a double membrane containing nucleoli which contain messenger RNAs
   C. A structure possessing a double membrane with an intermembrane space that is consistent with the rough endoplasmic reticulum
   D. The site of ribosome assembly
   E. A structure surrounded by a single membrane containing mitochondria which perform oxidative phosphorylation

3. Which of the following options lists the components of a DNA molecule most accurately?
   A. A phosphate group, a ribose sugar and a nitrogenous base such as cytosine or guanine
   B. A nitrogenous base such as adenine, in combination with three phosphate groups
   C. A nitrogenous base such as guanine, two phosphate groups and a deoxyribose sugar
   D. A deoxyribose sugar, a nitrogenous base (e.g., guanine) and a single phosphate group
   E. A hexose sugar, two phosphate group and a nitrogenous base such as guanine

4. Which option describes the correct sequence of gene expression?
   A. Gene → ribosomal RNA (rRNA) synthesis → ribosomal translation → polypeptide assembly → messenger RNA (mRNA) synthesis → exit from the nucleus
   B. Gene → mRNA synthesis → exit from the nucleus → ribosomal translation → polypeptide assembly
   C. Gene → exit from nucleus → mRNA synthesis → ribosomal translation → polypeptide assembly
   D. Gene → rRNA synthesis → exit from nucleus → mRNA synthesis → ribosomal translation → polypeptide assembly
   E. Gene → mRNA synthesis → exit from nucleus → rough endoplasmic reticulum entry → ribosomal translation → polypeptide assembly

5. Regarding chromosomes, which of the following statements is most true?
   A. They are found in all cells of the human body
   B. A typical human cell (other than a gamete) contains 43 chromosomes
   C. In each cell, all chromosomes are derived from either the mother or the father
   D. Each pair of chromosomes (e.g., chromosome 12) is identical
   E. Chromosomes consist of DNA packaged with associated proteins

6. Concerning the structure of the DNA double helix, which of the options below is most accurate?
   A. A helically coiled single polymer of deoxyribonucleotides
   B. Two intertwined ribonucleotide polymers coiled helically around each other
   C. The phosphate groups of each deoxyribonucleotide protrude inwards
   D. Two closely associated separate nucleic acids forming individual helices
   E. Two deoxyribonucleotide strands coiled around each other to form a helix

7. Regarding mitochondria, which of the following statements is most correct?
   A. Mitochondria possess their own chromosomal DNA
   B. Mitochondria have a single membrane with multiple invaginations
   C. Glycolysis takes part in the matrix of the mitochondria
   D. The outer mitochondria membrane is the site of the electron transfer chain
   E. The tricarboxylic acid (TCA) cycle occurs in the mitochondrial matrix

Chapter 2 Introduction to metabolism

1. Regarding the molecular features of adenosine triphosphate (ATP), which of the following descriptions is accurate?
   A. ATP contains three phosphoanhydride bonds
   B. ATP contains a hexose sugar as a component

C. ATP contains a guanosine base as a component
D. ATP contains four phosphate groups
E. ATP contains a pentose sugar as a component

2. Regarding nicotinamide adenine dinucleotide (NAD$^+$), in which of the following pathways is NAD$^+$ required to act as the oxidant (i.e., NAD$^+$ is reduced to NADH+H$^+$) in a redox reaction?
   A. The tricarboxylic acid (TCA) cycle
   B. Oxidative phosphorylation
   C. Glycerol synthesis
   D. Ketone synthesis
   E. β-oxidation of fatty acids

3. Regarding nicotinamide adenine dinucleotide phosphate (NADP$^+$), which of the following statements most accurately describes molecular features that differentiate it from nicotinamide adenine dinucleotide (NAD$^+$)?
   A. In NADP$^+$ the nucleotides are linked by their phosphate groups
   B. NAD$^+$ is a dinucleotide, whereas NADP$^+$ is a trinucleotide
   C. NADP$^+$ contains an additional phosphate group
   D. In NADP$^+$ there are two ribose groups
   E. In NADP$^+$ the nucleotides are linked by ionic bonds

4. Which of the listed combinations includes only metabolic pathways in which reduced NAD$^+$ (i.e., NADH+H$^+$) is required to act as a reductant?
   A. Ethanol catabolism, glycolysis, the tricarboxylic acid (TCA) cycle
   B. Fatty acid synthesis, cholesterol synthesis, reductive amination
   C. TCA cycle, β-oxidation of fatty acids, mitochondrial component of the carnitine shuttle
   D. Oxidative deamination of glutamate, the pentose phosphate pathway
   E. Glycerol synthesis, ketone synthesis, oxidative phosphorylation

5. Regarding the Michaelis–Menten graph, which of the following statements is accurate?
   A. The graph illustrates both first- and zero-order kinetics
   B. The graph allows easy identification of the Km value
   C. The graph axes are 'velocity' and 'substrate concentration'
   D. The graph curve is described as an exponential
   E. The graph axes are 'enzyme concentration' and 'substrate concentration'

6. Which of the following sentences describes a free radical most accurately?
   A. An indiscriminately reactive redox partner
   B. A molecule containing exclusively paired electrons

C. A molecule which causes damage by reducing intracellular molecules
D. A molecule such as glutathione or vitamin C
E. A powerful redox reductant which reduces other molecules

7. Which of the following mechanisms is not used as a common regulatory mechanism for modulating metabolic pathway activity?
   A. Allosteric inhibition
   B. Phosphorylation
   C. Substrate availability
   D. Hormonal regulation
   E. Free cross-membrane traffic

8. Which of the following pathways are always anabolic?
   A. Ketone oxidation
   B. Glycolysis
   C. Glycogen synthesis
   D. β-Oxidation of fatty acids
   E. Glycogenesis

Chapter 3 The tricarboxylic acid (TCA) cycle

1. Which of the following statements concerning acetyl-coenzyme A (CoA) is most correct?
   A. Acetyl-CoA is an important intracellular donor of methyl units
   B. Catabolism of multiple macronutrients can generate acetyl-CoA
   C. Acetyl-CoA contains a high-energy three-carbon moiety
   D. Intracellularly, acetyl-CoA is found only within mitochondria
   E. The coenzyme component contains vitamin B7 (biotin)

2. Which of the following sequences represents a genuine segment of the tricarboxylic acid cycle?
   A. Citrate ➔ isocitrate ➔ succinyl-coenzyme A (succinyl-CoA)
   B. Oxaloacetate ➔ malate ➔ fumarate
   C. Succinate ➔ fumarate ➔ malate
   D. α-Ketoglutarate ➔ succinate ➔ succinyl-CoA
   E. Isocitrate ➔ α-ketoglutarate ➔ succinate

3. Regarding the generation of high-energy intermediates and reducing equivalents by the tricarboxylic acid (TCA) cycle which of the following statements is most accurate?
   A. Approximately 8 adenosine triphosphate (ATP) equivalents are generated per molecule of acetyl-coenzyme A entering the cycle
   B. ATP in generated by substrate-level phosphorylation, whereas guanosine triphosphate (GTP) is generated indirectly via oxidative phosphorylation

C. One turn of the cycle generates one GTP molecule, one $FADH_2$ molecule and three $NADH + H^+$ molecules

D. The bulk of energy generated by the TCA cycle occurs directly as exemplified by reaction 5

E. The TCA cycle is energetically neutral; the energy consumed is ultimately equivalent to the energy generated

4. Regarding regulation of the tricarboxylic acid (TCA) cycle, which of the following least influences the pathway activity rate?

A. Intracellular sodium ion concentration

B. Isocitrate dehydrogenase

C. Adenosine triphosphate (ATP)

D. $NADH + H^+$

E. Citrate synthase

5. Regarding the anabolic role of the tricarboxylic acid cycle, which of the following is a genuine example of pathway intermediates participating in other synthetic pathways?

A. Oxaloacetate ➔ glycine synthesis

B. Citrate ➔ cholesterol synthesis

C. Succinate ➔ porphyrin synthesis

D. α-ketoglutarate ➔ proline

E. isocitrate ➔ aspartate

Chapter 4 Oxidative phosphorylation

1. Regarding the complexes of the electron transport chain, which of the following options provides an accurate description?

A. Sequential receipt and donation of electron pairs provide chemical potential energy to drive proton accumulation in the intermembranal space.

B. All components reside in fixed locations in the outer mitochondrial membrane except for cytochrome C, which is mobile.

C. The protein complexes number six in total: two are relatively fixed in the inner mitochondrial membrane and four mobile complexes.

D. Each complex spans the inner mitochondrial membrane completely and features an integral hydrogen ion pore.

E. Only complexes I, II and V transduce the redox energy intrinsic to electron receipt/donation into proton transfer.

2. Regarding substrate-level phosphorylation, which of the following statements is most accurate?

A. Adenosine monophosphate (AMP) is a common substrate for this reaction

B. It is limited to mitochondria-containing cells, due to its obligatory spatial location

C. $NADH + H^+$ or $FADH_2$ is required as a redox partner

D. Molecular oxygen is the terminal electron acceptor

E. Creatine phosphate can act as a phosphate donor for this type of phosphorylation

3. Which of the following options describes an *abnormal* 'uncoupling' scenario in the context of adenosine triphosphate (ATP) synthesis?

A. The discharge of the hydrogen ion gradient being intimately associated with ATP synthesis by ATP synthase

B. Compound X imposes a significant increase in the permeability of the inner mitochondrial membrane to hydrogen ions

C. Coupling of the H^+ ion discharge to thermogenesis in the brown fat deposits of a newborn baby

D. Electron receipt and transfer by complex III of the electron transport chain is associated with transfer of protons from the mitochondrial matrix to the intermembranal space

E. Incomplete reduction of molecular oxygen leading to formation of a superoxide radical

4. Which of the following options best describes creatine?

A. Creatine is exclusively obtained from the diet, and is found in particularly high levels in meat products

B. Phosphorylated creatine acts as a phosphoryl donor to adenosine diphosphate (ADP) on initiation of energy-demanding intracellular processes

C. Creatine is first transported to the liver where it enters hepatocytes and is phosphorylated intracellularly

D. Phosphorylated creatine can move freely across cell membranes in both directions

E. Creatine phosphate-mediated substrate-level phosphorylation of ADP occurs if glycolysis upregulation is insufficient to meet intracellular adenosine triphosphate demand

5. Which of the following options refers to the malate–aspartate shuttle?

A. It couples the oxidation of cytoplasmically generated $NADH + H^+$ with generation of $NADH + H^+$ in the mitochondrial matrix

B. The key molecule that traverses the outer mitochondrial membrane to access the intermembranal space is glycerol-3-phosphate

C. The redox potential of cytoplasmic $NADH + H^+$ is associated with generation of $FADH_2$ in the mitochondrial matrix

D. Glycerol-3-phosphate is reconverted to dihydroxyacetone phosphate in the mitochondrial matrix; this reaction's redox partner being flavin adenine dinucleotide

E. Malate exits the mitochondria, whereas aspartate is imported into the mitochondria from the cytoplasm.

Chapter 5 Carbohydrate metabolism

1. Which of the following statements about carbohydrate digestion is accurate?
   A. Salivary disaccharidase action commences carbohydrate digestion in the buccal cavity
   B. Disaccharidase action is terminated by the low pH in the gastric lumen
   C. Polysaccharides are hydrolysed to oligosaccharides by salivary and pancreatic amylases
   D. Sucrase, maltase and lactase are important examples of amylases
   E. Sucrase, maltase and lactase action is prominent in the mouth

2. Regarding adenosine triphosphate (ATP) generation during glycolysis, which of the following options is accurate?
   A. Per molecule of glucose oxidized, four ATP molecules are directly generated by substrate-level phosphorylation
   B. The net yield of ATP generated per molecule of glucose oxidized is 10
   C. One NADH+H$^+$ is generated per molecule of glucose oxidized, representing about 2.5 ATP
   D. Per molecule of glucose oxidized, one ATP molecule is consumed (during reaction 1)
   E. The net yield of ATP generated per molecule of glucose oxidized is 12

3. Which of the following statements best summarizes glycolysis?
   A. An exclusively aerobic anabolic pathway occurring in all cells of the human body
   B. A catabolic pathway for glucose oxidation occurring in cytoplasm in aerobic or anaerobic conditions
   C. A catabolic, predominantly anaerobic pathway occurring in red blood cells
   D. A mitochondrial amphibolic pathway responsible for aerobic glucose oxidation
   E. A cytoplasmic catabolic pathway occurring exclusively in anaerobic conditions

4. Which of the following combinations correctly describes the key regulation points of glycolysis?
   A. Reactions 1, 4 and 10
   B. Reaction 2, 3 and 10
   C. Reactions 1, 3 and 9
   D. Reactions 2, 3 and 9
   E. Reactions 1, 3 and 10

5. Which of the following statements correctly describes pyruvate dehydrogenase (PDH)?
   A. The enzyme catalyses the irreversible oxidative decarboxylation of acetyl-coenzyme A (acetyl-CoA)
   B. Unusually, enzyme activity is not significantly affected by phosphorylation
   C. Multiple coenzymes, including vitamin B2, are needed for normal PDH activity
   D. PDH in fact consists of five physically and spatially associated enzymes
   E. Failure of PDH activity typically results in hyperlactatemia

6. Which of the following statements correctly summarizes the key features of gluconeogenesis?
   A. Occurring exclusively in pancreatic islet cells, gluconeogenesis generates glucose from noncarbohydrate substrates
   B. Gluconeogenesis mostly occurs in hepatocytes and is particularly active immediately after eating
   C. Gluconeogenesis converts fatty acids (derived from lipolysis) into glucose during starvation
   D. The gluconeogenesis pathway contains reactions which occur both cytoplasmically and within mitochondria
   E. Gluconeogenesis activity would be expected to be high in a context of a high insulin:glucagon ratio

7. Which of the following enzymes participates exclusively in gluconeogenesis?
   A. Enolase
   B. Phosphoenolpyruvate carboxykinase
   C. Phosphoglycerate mutase
   D. Phosphoglucoisomerase
   E. Glyceraldehyde-3-phosphate dehydrogenase

8. Which of the following options contains only correct descriptions of the structure of glycogen?
   A. The polymer consists mainly of glucose residues, but also features other hexose residues including fructose and galactose
   B. Branch points occur between C6 of the main-strand glucose residue and C1 of the glucose residue in the branch chain
   C. Branch points occur along the main strand, approximately every 20 residues or so
   D. Main strand glucose residues are linked by glycosidic bonds between C1 and C6 of neighbouring glucose residues
   E. A polymer consisting of multiple glucose and galactose residues, featuring multiple branch points

9. Which of the listed options correctly describes the order of stages in glycogen synthesis?
   A. Elongation, glucose-6-phosphate (Glc-6-P) formation, uridine diphosphate (UDP)-mediated activation, branch formation
   B. Glc-6-P formation, activation, elongation, branch formation

C. Elongation, branch formation, Glc-6-P formation, activation

D. Activation, elongation, branch formation, Glc-6-P formation

E. Glc-6-P formation, elongation, branch formation, activation

10. Which of the following enzymes participates in glycogen synthesis?
A. Glycogen phosphorylase
B. Amylo-α-1,6-glucosidase
C. (1,4)→(1,4) Glucan transferase
D. Uridine diphosphate–glucose pyrophosphorylase
E. Debranching enzyme

11. Which statement correctly refers to/describes the pentose phosphate pathway?
A. The initial reaction uses glucose-1-phosphate as a substrate
B. The pathway is primarily catabolic in nature
C. The principal source of NADPH+H$^+$ and pentose sugars
D. Failure of the pathway is incompatible with life
E. Pathway activity permits glutamate regeneration

12. Which of the following factors would be least likely to trigger an episode of acute haemolysis in a glucose-6-phosphate dehydrogenase-deficient patient?
A. Broad (fava) bean consumption
B. Oral nitrofurantoin
C. Oral sulphamethoxazole (a sulphonamide drug)
D. Intravenous paracetamol
E. Intravenous septrin (cotrimoxazole)

13. Regarding fructose, which of the following statements is most correct?
A. The most common dietary source is the disaccharide lactose
B. It enters enterocytes via the GLUT-2-facilitated diffusion transporter
C. Fructose is phosphorylated by fructokinase, forming fructose-6-phosphate
D. Fructose 1-phosphate is converted to glyceraldehyde-3-phosphate by aldolase A
E. Glyceraldehyde-3-phosphate may enter either the glycolysis pathway or gluconeogenesis

14. Which of the following statements about galactosaemia is accurate?
A. Galactosaemic infants must be exclusively breastfed
B. Toxic galactose accumulation causes irreversible organ damage
C. The inheritance pattern is usually X-linked recessive

D. Galactosaemia is almost unheard of in the Irish Traveller population

E. Onset of irreversible damage occurs in utero

15. Which of the following pathways/reactions is promoted by significant alcohol intake?
A. Glycolysis
B. The pyruvate → acetyl-coenzyme A (acetyl-CoA) reaction
C. Gluconeogenesis
D. Fatty acid synthesis
E. The tricarboxylic acid (TCA) cycle

Chapter 6 Glucose homeostasis and diabetes mellitus

1. Which of the following options best describes type 1 diabetes mellitus?
A. A progressive condition which is usually asymptomatic in the early stages
B. Characterized by a period of impaired glucose tolerance of variable duration prior to frank diabetes
C. Initially, treatment is lifestyle modification, which may escalate to medications drug treatment if unsuccessful
D. Pathologically, it is hallmarked by pancreatic β-cell destruction, which is usually autoimmune
E. Risk factors include obesity, lack of exercise, poor-quality diet and individual genetics

2. Which of the following metabolic/physiological features is *unique* to type 1 diabetes?
A. Impaired glucose entry into cells resulting in hyperglycaemia
B. Impaired suppression of lipid catabolism, gluconeogenesis and ketogenesis
C. Dehydration that results from osmotic diuresis secondary to glycosuria
D. Acute hypoglycaemia is a risk associated with drug treatments
E. Diabetic eye disease and foot ulcers represent major clinical complications

3. Regarding oral hypoglycaemic drugs, which of the following drug classes is *not* listed with its correct mechanism of action?
A. Biguanides: increase in peripheral insulin sensitization sensitivity (attenuation of insulin resistance)
B. Glucosidase inhibitors: retardation of carbohydrate polymer hydrolysis in the gastrointestinal lumen
C. Thiazolidinediones: inhibition of DPP-IV promotes insulin release and inhibits glucagon release
D. Incretin mimetics: functional analogy to glucagon-like peptide 1 (GLP-1)
E. Sulphonylureas: increase in endogenous insulin secretion by K$_{ATP}$ channel activation

219

4. Which of the following options lists investigation results that would be consistent with hyperglycaemic hyperosmolar nonketotic syndrome (HHNS)?
   A. pH 7.20, [H$^+$] 63 nmol/L, [HCO$_3^-$] 12 mmol/L, [glucose] 17 mmol/L, [ketones] 4.5 mmol/L, pCO$_2$ 3.0 kPa, serum osmolality 305 mmol/L
   B. pH 7.40, [H$^+$] 40 nmol/L, [HCO$_3^-$] 26 mmol/L, [glucose] 7 mmol/L, [ketones] 0.5 mmol/L, pCO$_2$ 5.5 kPa, serum osmolality 290 mmol/L
   C. pH 7.40, [H$^+$] 40 nmol/L, [HCO$_3^-$] 12 mmol/L, [glucose] 45 mmol/L, [ketones] 0.9 mmol/L, pCO$_2$ 7.5 kPa, serum osmolality 325 mmol/L
   D. pH 7.30, [H$^+$] 50 nmol/L, [HCO$_3^-$] 18 mmol/L, [glucose] 13 mmol/L, [ketones] 3.5 mmol/L, pCO$_2$ 2.9 kPa, serum osmolality 300 mmol/L
   E. pH 7.40, [H$^+$] 40 nmol/L, [HCO$_3^-$] 23 mmol/L, [glucose] 5 mmol/L, [ketones] 0.2 mmol/L, pCO$_2$ 5.5 kPa, serum osmolality 285 mmol/L

5. A 52-year-old presents to the general practitioner (GP) with a foot ulcer, which has failed to heal after nearly 2 months. He originally stood on a pin but did not realize until he went to put on his socks and had to pull it out. The ulcer developed at the site. He says it has not been bothering him as it does not really hurt, although it is deep and covers about 4 cm^2 of the foot sole. The GP learns that his exercise tolerance has reduced since a day 3 months ago, which he remembers well because he became suddenly short of breath and very sweaty even though it was a really cold day. He passes urine every 20–30 min and has recently found it difficult to read road signs but assumed he was just 'getting old'. A random finger prick reveals blood glucose of 15.1 mmol/L, although he has not eaten anything since breakfast (it is now 14:30 p.m.). He is dizzy and faint standing up to walk to the blood pressure cuff. A full set of investigations reveal moderate renal impairment, early proliferative retinopathy, several poorly healing ulcers and evidence of an old inferior myocardial infarct. What is the most likely underlying diagnosis?
   A. Secondary diabetes
   B. Type 1 diabetes
   C. Impaired glucose tolerance
   D. Type 2 diabetes
   E. Gestational diabetes mellitus

Chapter 7 Lipid metabolism and lipid transport

1. Regarding fatty acid nomenclature, which of the following statements accurately describes the fatty acid 18:4cΔ3,5,9,15?
   A. A polyunsaturated fatty acid with 15 double bonds, including one at carbon-12

   B. A monounsaturated fatty acid with 15 carbons and just one double bond, located at carbon-3
   C. A polyunsaturated fatty acid with 18 carbons and four 'cis' double bonds including one at carbon-3
   D. A polyunsaturated fatty acid with 18 carbons, four 'trans' double bonds including one at carbon-9
   E. A monounsaturated fatty acid with 18 carbons and just one double bond, located at carbon-3

2. Regarding fatty acid synthesis, which of the following statements is entirely correct?
   A. A mitochondrial catabolic process requiring acetyl-coenzyme A (acetyl-CoA) as substrate and NADPH + H$^+$ as a redox participant
   B. A cytoplasmic catabolic process requiring acetoacetate as a substrate and NADH + H$^+$ as a redox participant
   C. A mitochondrial anabolic process requiring acetoacetate as a substrate and NADH + H$^+$ as a redox partner
   D. A cytoplasmic anabolic process requiring acetyl-CoA as a substrate and NADPH + H$^+$ as a redox participant
   E. A cytoplasmic anabolic process requiring acetyl-CoA as a substrate and NADH + H$^+$ as a redox participant

3. Regarding fatty acid oxidation, which of the following sequences defines a segment of the pathway?
   A. Oxidation, hydration, oxidation, thiolysis
   B. Condensation, reduction, dehydration, intentional
   C. Oxidation, reduction, dehydration, reduction
   D. Condensation, hydration, oxidation, thiolysis
   E. Oxidation, hydration, reduction, thiolysis

4. Regarding digestion and absorption of dietary fat, which of the following statements describes the sequence of events?
   A. Bile acid solubilization, amylase-mediated hydrolysis of triacylglycerol, simple diffusion of fatty acids into enterocytes
   B. Pancreatic lipase-mediated hydrolysis of dietary triacylglycerol, receptor-mediated endocytosis of glycerol into enterocytes
   C. Bile acid solubilization, pepsin-mediated triacylglycerol hydrolysis, sodium-coupled import of fatty acids into enterocytes
   D. Bile acid solubilization, lipase-mediated hydrolysis of triacylglycerols, sodium-coupled import of fatty acids into enterocytes
   E. Bile acid solubilization, lipase-mediated hydrolysis of triacylglycerols, diffusion of fatty acids into enterocytes

5. An 18-year-old lady complains of exertional chest pain, sweatiness and breathlessness. On examination she is noted to have corneal arcus, xanthelasma and several tendon xanthomata. She reports that her mother was aged in her 20s when she died of a myocardial infarction, and exhibits the following lipid profile:

Total cholesterol	13 mmol/L
Low-density lipoprotein (LDL)	9.0 mmol/L
Triglycerides (TGs)	1.6 mmol/L
High-density lipoprotein (HDL)	0.9 mmol/L

What would be the best tool or investigation to identify the cause of her lipid profile abnormality?
- A. Serum HbA1C
- B. Glucose tolerance test
- C. Careful dietary history
- D. 24-Hour electrocardiogram (ECG)
- E. Genetic studies

6. A 35-year-old bank clerk who is fit and well has become concerned about his risk of heart attack and stroke after reading a tabloid scare piece. He smokes a pack a day and drinks 8 U of alcohol in a typical week. His parents are alive and aged well in their 80s. His lipid profile is as follows:

Total cholesterol	6.7 mmol/L
Low-density lipoprotein (LDL)	3.9 mmol/L
High-density lipoprotein	1.4 mmol/L
Triglyceride (TG)	3.0 mmol/L

Which of the following options describes the most appropriate management?
- A. Advise him to reduce saturated fat intake, quit smoking and exercise regularly, and repeat lipid profile in 3 months
- B. Commence simvastatin and advise it will be needed for life to reduce his cardiovascular risk to safe levels
- C. Advise him to reduce saturated fat intake, quit smoking and start regular exercise, and start trial of simvastatin
- D. Referral to a geneticist to exclude a genetic dyslipidaemia as the underlying cause of the abnormal results
- E. Reassurance only, including advice about disregarding spurious health-related media articles

7. Regarding ketones, which of the following statements is correct?
- A. Cardiac myocytes preferentially catabolize ketones as their primary metabolic substrate in health

- B. High serum concentrations of ketones in starvation arises from elevated gluconeogenesis and fatty acid oxidation activity
- C. Excessive accumulation of serum ketones, for example in decompensated diabetes, can lead to metabolic alkalosis
- D. The central nervous system (CNS) can completely switch its reliance on glucose to ketones in prolonged starvation
- E. Ketone synthesis generates $NADH + H^+$, which can undergo oxidative phosphorylation

Chapter 8 Bioenergetics and obesity

1. Regarding body composition, which of the following options gives the correct percentages of each component?
- A. Water 61%, Protein 17%, Fat 15%, Bone 7%
- B. Water 55%, Protein 25%, Fat 5%, Bone 15%
- C. Water 75%, Protein 10%, Fat 10%, Bone 5%
- D. Water 45%, Protein 20%, Fat 15%, Bone 20%
- E. Water 58%, Protein 24%, Fat 10%, Bone 8%

2. Regarding lean body mass, what is the most accurate description of the components?
- A. Water, protein, fat
- B. Protein, carbohydrates, bone
- C. Water, carbohydrate, protein
- D. Water, protein, bone
- E. Carbohydrate, bone, protein

3. Which of the following options correctly describes the diet-induced thermogenesis (DIT) component of energy expenditure?
- A. Metabolic energy expended by the body for involuntary organ and cellular processes
- B. It represents approximately 40% of total energy expenditure
- C. Unavoidable heat loss occurring during digestion and absorption of ingested food
- D. It represents approximately 50% of total energy expenditure
- E. It varies with an individual's lean body mass as a proportion of their weight

4. Which of the following is an orexigenic hormone?
- A. Ghrelin
- B. Cocaine/amphetamine-regulated transcript (CART)
- C. Melanocyte-stimulating hormone (MSH)
- D. Cholecystokinin (CCK)
- E. GLP-1

5. Which of the following statements best describes the mechanism of action of cholecystokinin (CCK) in terms of appetite regulation?
   A. Promotes hypothalamic release of agouti-related peptide (AGRP)
   B. Stimulates vagal afferents to the nucleus tractus solitarius (NTS)
   C. Stimulates release of neuropeptide Y (NPY)
   D. Inhibition of ghrelin release
   E. Inhibition of cocaine/amphetamine-regulated transcript (CART) release

6. Which of the following statements about agouti-related protein (AGRP) is correct?
   A. AGRP is anorexigenic and released from the neurons in the arcuate nucleus
   B. Vagal afferent activity stimulates the tractus solitarius to release AGRP
   C. Cocaine/amphetamine-regulated transcript (CART) and AGRP share a common mechanism of action
   D. AGRP is orexigenic and is released by arcuate neurons in the hypothalamus
   E. AGRP is released from P/D1 cells and stimulates neuropeptide Y (NPY) release

7. Regarding obesity treatment strategies, which of the following statements is most correct?
   A. Surgery is the best first-line treatment strategy for the vast majority of patients
   B. Drug treatment should only be considered when lifestyle interventions have been abandoned
   C. The decision to proceed with bariatric surgery is determined by body mass index (BMI) alone
   D. Once surgery is performed, there is no need to adhere to diet or lifestyle interventions
   E. Most obese patients should be educated and motivated to follow a healthy calorie-restricted diet

8. Regarding the causes of obesity, which of the following options represents the most correct answer?
   A. Genetic syndromes
   B. Drug-induced obesity
   C. Social deprivation
   D. Energy expenditure < intake
   E. Endocrine disease

9. A lady is 170 cm and weighs 100 kg. Which class does her body mass index (BMI) fall into?
   A. Normal
   B. Overweight
   C. Class 1 obesity
   D. Class 2 obesity
   E. Class 3 obesity

Chapter 9 Protein metabolism and malnutrition

1. Regarding protein structure, which of the following statements describes both tertiary and quaternary structural characteristics?
   A. β-Sheets are common examples of this stage of structure
   B. Determined by various interactions between R-groups
   C. Arises spontaneously due to hydrogen bond interactions
   D. α-Helices are common examples of this stage of structure
   E. The responsible bonds link amine hydrogen with carbonyl oxygen

2. Regarding protein structure, which of the following options is responsible for a protein's primary structure?
   A. The linear sequence of amino acids defined by the DNA base sequence
   B. Hydrogen bonds between amine hydrogens and carbonyl oxygens
   C. Interactions of various nature between side chain groups
   D. Hydrophobic nonpolar interactions between aliphatic R-groups
   E. Uniting interactions between two separate polypeptides

3. A 5-year-old boy is seen at the Médecins Sans Frontières (MSF) base in Darfur, Sudan. Predicted weight is 20 kg. He weighs only 11 kg and appears skeletal. In terms of protein–energy malnutrition, what best describes this clinical presentation?
   A. Underweight
   B. Kwashiorkor
   C. Marasmus–kwashiorkor
   D. Marasmus
   E. Cretinism

4. Regarding parenteral and enteral nutrition, in which of the following cases would total parenteral nutrition (TPN) be the preferred form of nutritional support?
   A. A 35-year-old intensive care unit patient on mechanical ventilation for acute respiratory failure in the context of lower respiratory tract infection
   B. A sectioned 19-year-old patient on psychiatric ward with a body mass index (BMI) of 13 kg/m^2 due to severe anorexia nervosa
   C. A 94-year-old on medical ward awaiting residential placement: BMI 18 kg/m^2 (due to inability to self-care) but otherwise well

D. A 75-year-old patient with right-sided cerebrovascular accident and dysphasia, dysphagia and dense left hemiplegia

E. A 36-year-old with acute flare-up of Crohn syndrome postsignificant bowel resection

5. Regarding phenylalanine, which of the following descriptions is accurate?

A. Nonessential, endogenous synthesis possible, purely glucogenic, negatively charged R-group, shares a transporter with glutamate and aspartate

B. Essential, endogenous synthesis impossible, positively charged R-group, shares a transporter with histidine and lysine

C. Essential, endogenous synthesis possible, ketogenic and glucogenic, aromatic R-group, shares transporter with valine and tyrosine

D. Nonessential, endogenous synthesis impossible, 'imino' R-group, purely ketogenic, shares transporter with proline and glycine

E. Essential, endogenous synthesis possible, purely glucogenic, shares transporter with alanine and serine

6. Regarding individuals with phenylketonuria (PKU), which of the following statements is correct?

A. Inheritance is usually autosomal dominant

B. It is almost always fatal to sufferers

C. Tyrosine takes on 'essential' status

D. The affected enzyme is tyrosinase

E. It cannot be detected by newborn blood spot screening

7. Regarding catecholamine synthesis, which of the following sequences describes the correct order of the synthetic pathway?

A. Tyrosine, phenylalanine, noradrenaline, dopamine, dihydroxyphenylalanine (DOPA), adrenaline

B. Phenylalanine, tyrosine, dopamine, DOPA, noradrenaline, adrenaline

C. Phenylalanine, tyrosine, DOPA, dopamine, adrenaline, noradrenaline

D. Tyrosine, phenylalanine, dopamine, DOPA, adrenaline, noradrenaline

E. Tyrosine, phenylalanine, DOPA, dopamine, noradrenaline, adrenaline

8. Which of the following clinical situations are scenarios of positive nitrogen balance?

A. Multiple, large third-degree burns in a house fire victim

B. An intensive therapy unit patient with septicaemia secondary to extensive chronic leg ulcers

C. An elderly patient admitted with fractured neck of the femur with a long lie before rescue

D. A healthy, well 12-year-old child

E. A severely malnourished 18-year-old with a chronic eating disorder

9. Which of the following amino acids is both glucogenic and ketogenic?

A. Serine

B. Alanine

C. Proline

D. Isoleucine

E. Glutamate

Chapter 10 Purines, pyrimidines, haem and one-carbon transfer

1. A 75-year-old plumber presents to his general practitioner (GP) with his wife who has forced him to consult, citing his gradual-onset lethargy, fatigue, insomnia and forgetfulness as the main issues making him difficult to live with. He was recently started on mirtazapine for depression, but this has not helped. He admits to recent breathlessness on exertion, intermittent abdominal pain and numbness and tingling of his hands and feet. He is very pale, with symmetrical decreased light touch sensation and sluggish ankle reflexes. The GP notes a blue line where his teeth meet the gums. A recent routine full blood count included a peripheral blood film which referred to 'basophilic stippling' of red cells. What is the most likely diagnosis?

A. Vitamin B12 deficiency

B. Folate deficiency

C. Iron deficiency

D. Lead poisoning

E. Copper toxicity

2. A 22-year-old girl presents with severe abdominal pain. She has epilepsy, which is poorly controlled; her neurologist has recently started valproate to try and reduce her fitting. Otherwise she is well, and takes only the oral contraceptive pill, which is a recent addition as she has entered a committed relationship. She has no abnormalities on examination, and is discharged with diclofenac for analgesia. Eight hours later she is brought in by the police under a section 136 of the mental health act, raving and incoherent, having stripped in public and wandering down the main road at risk from traffic. Urinary [porphobilinogen] is 40 times the normal reference range. Which of the following diagnoses is most likely?

A. Porphyria cutanea tarda

B. Lead poisoning

C. Erythropoietic protoporphyria

D. Acute intermittent porphyria

E. Congenital erythropoietic porphyria

3. A 55-year-old publican presents with an acutely painful, inflamed erythematous big toe. Serum urate is significantly elevated. His symptoms resolve with colchicine and allopurinol is commenced. Which of the following features from his background is most likely to be a risk factor for his hyperuricaemia?
   A. Type 1 diabetes (insulin deficiency)
   B. Low dietary purine intake
   C. Low body mass index (BMI; i.e., <18 kg/m^2)
   D. Five beers and two whiskeys a day
   E. Lesch–Nyan syndrome

4. Regarding urate, which of the following statements is accurate?
   A. Urate is synthesized from hypoxanthine via two sequential reduction reactions
   B. Xanthine oxidase contains molybdenum and copper ions
   C. Urate is predominantly excreted in the bile and is lost in faeces
   D. Urate exists as urate (rather than uric acid) at physiological pH because its $pK_a = 5.4$
   E. Urate represents the main metabolic by-product of pyrimidine catabolism

5. Which of the following statements regarding the porphyrias is accurate?
   A. All are characterized by varying degrees of photosensitivity
   B. All porphyria patients must avoid hormonal contraceptives
   C. All porphyria patients with skin rashes must avoid fasting
   D. All porphyrias confer absolute contraindication to barbiturates
   E. A blistering skin rash can occur in most of the porphyrias

6. Which of the following nucleotides is a purine derivative?
   A. Thymine
   B. Cytosine
   C. Adenine
   D. Uracil
   E. Uridine diphosphate

7. Regarding haem synthesis, which of the following represents the rate-limiting enzyme of the pathway?
   A. δ-Aminolevulinic acid (δ-ALA) dehydratase
   B. Ferrochelatase
   C. δ-ALA synthase
   D. Uroporphyrinogen III cosynthase
   E. Protoporphyrinogen IX oxidase

8. Regarding haem catabolism, which of the following statements is correct?
   A. The glucuronidation of haem increases its lipid solubility
   B. Catabolism of haem generates ferric iron, biliverdin and carbon dioxide
   C. Biliverdin is generated in the cytoplasm from reduction of bilirubin
   D. Cleavage of the porphyrin ring forms bilirubin
   E. Haem catabolism mainly occurs in reticuloendothelial macrophages

Chapter 11 The thyroid gland

1. Which of the following most accurately describes the location and anatomical relations of the thyroid gland?
   A. Anterior to the oesophagus, posterior to the trachea and medial to the carotid sheaths
   B. Posterior to the inferior belly of the omohyoid strap muscles
   C. Anterior to the trachea, posterior to the sternohyoid and sternothyroid muscles
   D. A midline structure lying inferior to the superior thyroid arteries
   E. Anterior to the thyroid cartilage and superior to the cricoid cartilage

2. Which of the following statements is most correct regarding the different thyroid hormones T4, T3 and reverse triiodothyronine (rT3)?
   A. T4 is more potent than T3 and rT3 and is presents at the highest total concentration in plasma
   B. rT3 is more metabolically active than either T4 or T3, and is a structural isomer of T4
   C. T3 and rT3 are structural isomers, but T3 is more potent than both T4 and rT3
   D. T3 is secreted in greater quantities than T4 as it is far more metabolically active
   E. T4 is secreted at a ratio of 10:1 compared with T3, reflecting the plasma ratio of T4:T3

3. Regarding the molecular synthesis of the thyroid hormones, which of the following is most accurate?
   A. Reverse triiodothyronine (rT3) is synthesized by inner ring deiodination of T4 and contains three iodine atoms
   B. T3 is synthesized by outer ring deiodination of rT3 and contains three iodine atoms
   C. T4 is synthesized from either T3 or rT3 and contains four iodine atoms
   D. T4 contains two tyrosine residues and three iodine atoms
   E. T3 contains two tyrosine residues and four iodine atoms

4. Regarding thyroid hormone homeostasis, which of the following statements is most correct?
   A. Thyroid-stimulating hormone (TSH) acts on thyroid parafollicular cells, promoting synthesis and secretion of T4 and T3
   B. Thyrotropin-releasing hormone (TRH) acts on the anterior pituitary cells, promoting TSH synthesis and secretion
   C. The predominant negative influence on TRH secretion is exerted by TSH
   D. TSH acts on hypothalamic TRH-releasing cells, stimulating TRH release
   E. T3 and T4 exert negative feedback on TSH release, but not on TRH release

5. Regarding the metabolic effects of T3 hormone, which of the following statements is correct concerning macronutrient metabolism?
   A. Anabolic pathways such as gluconeogenesis are suppressed, whereas catabolic pathways such as lipid synthesis are activated
   B. Lipolysis, protein synthesis, glycogenolysis and gluconeogenesis are all upregulated
   C. Lipolysis and triglyceride hydrolysis are promoted, with liberated glycerol largely diverted towards gluconeogenesis
   D. Proteolysis of skeletal muscle is inhibited, whereas protein synthesis is promoted
   E. Lipid synthesis, lipolysis, proteolysis, glycogenolysis and gluconeogenesis are all suppressed

6. Which of the following descriptions is most consistent with sick euthyroid syndrome?
   A. Fatigue, weight gain, raised serum [TSH] and low [T3]
   B. Diarrhoea, weight loss, significantly raised [T4] and [T3], low [TSH]
   C. Thyroid symptoms absent, low [T3], and [TSH] and [T4] mildly raised
   D. Cold intolerance, depression, raised [TSH] and low [T4]
   E. Nervousness, irritability, sweating, high [TSH] and raised [T4] and [T3]

Chapter 12 Vitamins and their deficiencies

1. Which of the following statements correctly describes a feature of fat-soluble vitamins?
   A. They are minimally toxic in excess, causing few symptoms
   B. Reliant on normal gastrointestinal lipid absorption for their absorption
   C. Regular intake is necessary as no significant stores are laid down by the body

   D. They are easily degraded by various cooking techniques
   E. Absorption is typically either sodium coupled, active or via simple diffusion

2. A strict vegan presents with fatigue, breathlessness on exertion and palpitations. A vitamin deficiency is suspected to be the underlying cause. Which of the following investigations would typically accompany these results on a full blood count and film: Mean corpuscular volume, 110 fL; haemoglobin (Hb), 95 g/L, megaloblastic changes seen on film?
   A. Elevated serum [homocysteine]
   B. Low leucocyte [ascorbic acid]
   C. Decreased 24-hour Urinary niacin metabolite excretion
   D. Low serum [pyridoxal-5'-phosphate]
   E. Low serum [retinol-binding protein]

3. A 24-year-old female has her 12-week ultrasound for her first pregnancy. Devastatingly, the fetus is noted to be anencephalic, and she chooses to terminate the pregnancy. A deficiency of which of the following vitamins could potentially represent the primary cause of this fetal manifestation?
   A. Vitamin A
   B. Vitamin B6
   C. Vitamin C
   D. Vitamin E
   E. Vitamin B9

4. Which of the following feature in the history in a 26-year-old immigrant female would increase your suspicion of vitamin D deficiency in a patient with osteomalacia, generalized muscle weakness and pain?
   A. Use of tanning beds at least once a week
   B. Regular consumption of 10 cups of tea and coffee a day
   C. Strict observance of the Wahabi interpretation of Islam
   D. Staple diet consisting of primarily maize products
   E. Having very pale skin, light eyes and red/blonde hair

5. A 25-year-old patient presents with forgetfulness and diarrhoea. A symmetrical erythematous scaling rash is noted, which appears to be worse on his forearms and face. He did not mention it because he is so forgetful, and apart from looking awful does not itch or hurt. He has recently commenced treatment for pulmonary tuberculosis with quadruple therapy (rifampicin, ethambutol, isoniazid and pyrazinamide). He is also on long-term dialysis whilst awaiting renal transplant and takes azathioprine for his rheumatoid

arthritis. Which vitamin deficiency is most likely to be responsible for his skin, gastrointestinal and cognitive symptoms?

A. Vitamin B9 (folate)
B. Vitamin B12
C. Vitamin B3
D. Vitamin C
E. Vitamin E

Chapter 13 Minerals and their deficiencies

1. A well patient presenting for an elective cystoscopy is noted at preassessment to have a [Na$^+$] of 118 mmol/L. Which of the following statements is most appropriate regarding clinical management of this patient?

A. Serum sodium should be normalized as rapidly as possible with hypertonic saline
B. As the patient is well, and hyponatraemia mild, it can be safely ignored
C. The first priority is clinical assessment of intravascular fluid status
D. Gradual normalization of the value should be attempted with cautious administration of 5% dextrose solution
E. If euvolaemic, intravenous 0.9% NaCl is an appropriate treatment strategy

2. You are asked to review a ward patient, as her [Na$^+$] is 125 mmol/L. On examination, the patient has well hydrated mucous membranes, peripheral oedema to midthigh, bibasal crepitations on auscultation and her jugular venous pressure is at 8 cm above the sternal angle. Urine output has persistently exceeded 100 mL/hour. Which of the following options combines the correct diagnosis and treatment strategy?

A. Hypovolaemic hypernatraemia: intravenous dextrose saline
B. Hypovolaemic hyponatraemia: fluid restriction
C. Hypervolaemic hyponatraemia: fluid restriction ± diuresis
D. Euvolaemic hyponatraemia: fluid restriction
E. Hypovolaemic hyponatraemia: intravenous isotonic saline

3. You are urgently called to review an intensive care unit patient, as the patient's recent arterial blood gas has revealed [K$^+$] to be 7.5 mmol/L. You note widening of the QRS complex on the cardiac monitor. What is the most appropriate immediate action?

A. Oral calcium resonium
B. Intravenous (IV) insulin/dextrose infusion
C. IV 10% calcium gluconate
D. Nebulized salbutamol
E. Oral sando-K

4. Which of the following patients would you expect to exhibit hypokalaemia?

A. A hypertensive patient taking angiotensin-converting enzyme inhibitors
B. A patient with norovirus
C. A patient with severe acute kidney injury
D. A patient presenting with Addison disease
E. A patient with significant metabolic acidosis

5. Which of the following results are most consistent with iron deficiency?

A. Mean corpuscular volume (MCV) 105 fL, Haemoglobin (Hb) 9 g/L
B. MCV 85 fL, Hb 13.5 g/L
C. MCV 70 fL, Hb 8.5 g/L
D. MCV 80 fL, Hb 7 g/L
E. MCV 90 fL, Hb 12.5 g/L

6. You are called to assist at a cardiac arrest on labour ward. The midwife informs you that the arrested lady was being treated for severe preeclampsia but was otherwise well, then 'went to sleep' just before handover, and was later found unresponsive. The anaesthetist has given 10 mL of 10% calcium gluconate intravenously, and the patient now has a pulse and is beginning to recover. What electrolyte disturbance is most likely to have led to the cardiac arrest?

A. Hypocalcaemia
B. Hypermagnesemia
C. Hypophosphatemia
D. Hyperkalaemia
E. Hyponatremia

7. Which of the following mineral deficiencies are those adhering strictly to a vegan diet least likely to develop?

A. Iron
B. Calcium
C. Magnesium
D. Zinc
E. Iodine

8. Regarding dietary iron absorption, which of the following statements is most correct?

A. Nonhaem iron is generally better absorbed than haem iron
B. Ferric iron is better absorbed by enterocytes than ferrous iron
C. Coingestion of phytates, zinc and calcium improves haem iron absorption
D. Coingestion of copper and vitamin C improves nonhaem iron absorption
E. Haem iron is absorbed by a symport

9. Regarding the hormonal regulation of calcium metabolism, which of the following statements is most correct?
   A. Vitamin D deficiency leads to excessive calcium absorption by gut enterocytes
   B. Parathyroid hormone and calcitonin both decrease serum $[Ca^{++}]$
   C. Parathyroid hormone and vitamin D both increase serum $[Ca^{++}]$
   D. Calcitonin and parathyroid hormone both increase serum $[Ca^{++}]$
   E. Calcitonin and vitamin D both lower serum $[Ca^{++}]$

Chapter 14 Clinical assessment of
metabolism and nutritional disorders

1. A 16-year-old female presents to the emergency department in severe abdominal pain. She is agitated, sweating and unable to provide a coherent history. Her worried mother tells you she has always been well and the only notable change has been that she recently entered a relationship and started to take the oral contraceptive pill. Her boyfriend informs you in confidence that they had drunk quite a lot of alcohol together earlier that day. Her abdominal examination is normal, and vital signs are normal aside from mild tachycardia (95 beats/minute). Her urine appears dark red, but the standard dipstick panel does not reveal any positive findings. Alanine transaminase (ALT) is slightly raised, but other liver function tests (LFTs) are normal. What would be the most appropriate next investigation?
   A. Red cell porphobilinogen deaminase levels
   B. Toxicology screen for substances of abuse
   C. Chest radiograph
   D. Urinary porphobilinogen
   E. Liver ultrasound

2. A 35-year-old male presents with fatigue, poor appetite, tingling extremities and weight loss of 5 kg over 6 months. He has hypothyroidism and vitiligo, but no other medical history. On questioning he admits to recent reduced exercise tolerance, becoming breathless whilst walking his usual route to work. On examination he is pale, with prematurely grey hair and very subtle scleral icterus. Investigation results are shown below:
   Haemoglobin: 9 g/L
   Mean corpuscular volume: 108 fL
   Platelets: 125×10^9
   White cell count: 3.0×10^9
   Thyroid-stimulating hormone: 2.5 mU/L
   Which of the following investigation would conclusively diagnose the disease responsible for the symptoms, signs and investigation results?

   A. Peripheral blood film
   B. Serum B12
   C. Schilling test
   D. Bone marrow examination
   E. Intrinsic factor antibodies

3. A 35-year-old patient presents with gastroenteritis. He reports he has not passed urine in the last 12 hours and is complaining of severe thirst. His partner explains that he has been vomiting every time he tries to drink, and also that he has had diarrhoea for 48 hours. During the history-taking he becomes progressively more confused and drowsy. On clinical examination:

Lips and tongue:	Dry and cracked
Heart rate	120 beats/minute
Respiratory rate	22 breaths/minute
Blood pressure	85/30 mmHg
Peripheries	Cool to touch, capillary refill time >4 seconds

   Which of the following options represents an appropriate clinical assessment of his condition?
   A. Hydration status normal
   B. Mildly dehydrated
   C. Moderately dehydrated
   D. Severely dehydrated
   E. Preterminally dehydrated

4. A 25-year-old female presents with nausea and vomiting, fatigue, swollen ankles and polyuria. She also affirms recent weight gain of around 10 kg over 3 months despite having little appetite. She is very worried as her mother died of polycystic kidney disease when she was aged in her 30s, and she thinks her symptoms resemble those her mother experienced, although she has been tested and was told she does not have the disease. On examination she has a palpable mass in the suprapubic/umbilical region, oedema up to her lower calves and pigmented vertical line on her abdominal midline. Urine dip shows +ve glycosuria but no other abnormalities. She adamantly denies the possibility she could be pregnant because she states that she and her partner are sexually abstinent for religious reasons.
   What is the most appropriate investigation?
   A. 24-hour Urinary collection for protein
   B. Serum urea and electrolytes
   C. Renal ultrasound
   D. Urinary human chorionic gonadotropin (HCG)
   E. Abdominal computed tomography (CT)

5. A pleasant 75-year-old lady is admitted with community-acquired pneumonia and commenced on oral antibiotics. She has well-controlled hypertension and no other medical conditions. Approximately 6 hours after admission, she begins to behave strangely, shouting at the nurses that a large bear is menacing her, and rushing about the ward trying to get into other patients' beds. You are asked to attend urgently. She refuses to interact with you and no bear can be located so it is assumed she is hallucinating. She is tremulous, sweating profusely and obviously agitated. She vomits whilst you are present. She then falls to the floor and has a tonic–clonic seizure lasting 4 minutes. Her drug chart has only antibiotics and her usual antihypertensive. Her most recent observations were:

Blood pressure	180/110 mmHg
Heart rate	160 beats/minute
Respiratory rate	26 breaths/minute
Temperature	38.5°C
Glucose	6.5 mmol/L

As part of an ABC approach, what is the most urgent drug to administer?

A. Intramuscular Pabrinex
B. Oral chlordiazepoxide
C. Intravenous (IV) diazepam
D. IV dextrose
E. IV haloperidol

Extended-matching questions (EMQs)

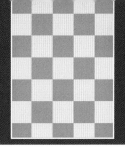

Each answer can be used once, more than once or not at all.

Chapter 1

Role of intracellular organelles

A. Lysosome
B. Peroxisome
C. Golgi apparatus
D. Smooth endoplasmic reticulum
E. Rough endoplasmic reticulum
F. Nucleus
G. Mitochondria

For each scenario below, choose the most likely corresponding option from the list given above.

1. A double-membraned organelle, with internal circular DNA specific to this organelle, that is responsible for oxidative phosphorylation, and furthermore the interior is the site of the tricarboxylic acid cycle.
2. A double-membrane-bound structure, with transiently associated ribosomes and an intermembrane space continuous with the nuclear intermembrane space.
3. A vesicular structure containing enzymes of the pentose phosphate pathway that is also the main intracellular site of very long-chain fatty acid oxidation.
4. A double-membrane-enclosed organelle that contains ribosome assembly zones and the genetic material of the cell.
5. A vesicular organelle containing a large array of hydrolases.

Chapter 2

Enzyme nomenclature

A. Kinase
B. Phosphatase
C. Dehydrogenase
D. Mutase
E. Decarboxylase
F. Carboxylase
G. Transferase
H. Isomerase
I. Hydroxylase

For each scenario below, choose the most likely corresponding option from the list given above.

1. An enzyme which catalyses the incorporation of a phosphate group to a substrate.
2. An enzyme which removes a methyl group from one molecule to a different molecule.
3. An enzyme which incorporates an oxygen covalently bonded to a hydrogen into a molecule.
4. An enzyme which rearranges the molecular structure of a molecule without adding in or removing any new atoms.
5. An enzyme which transfers a functional group from one location to another, within the same molecule.

Chapter 5

Carbohydrate metabolism

A. Glycolysis
B. Ethanol metabolism
C. Gluconeogenesis
D. Glycogen synthesis (glycogenesis)
E. Glycogenolysis
F. The pentose phosphate pathway
G. Fructose catabolism
H. Galactose catabolism
I. Sorbitol catabolism

For each scenario below, choose the most likely corresponding option from the list given above.

1. This pathway ensures that the blood [glucose] is maintained once glycogen reserves are exhausted if fasting continues.
2. This pathway is the main mechanism responsible for ensuring a continuous supply of the reducing equivalent necessary for glutathione regeneration.
3. An autosomal recessive defect in a gene responsible for this pathway requires lifelong dietary exclusion of lactose.
4. This pathway is the only mechanism for adenosine triphosphate (ATP) generation in erythrocytes and cells lacking mitochondria.
5. Aldolase B deficiency leads to toxic intracellular phosphate sequestration due to failure of this pathway. The hallmark clinical feature is fasting hypoglycaemia, which arises due to a functional impairment of aldolase A and glycogen phosphorylase.

Chapter 6

Different causes of diabetes

A. Type 1 diabetes mellitus (T1DM)
B. Impaired glucose tolerance
C. Type 2 diabetes mellitus (T2DM)
D. Diabetes mellitus in pregnancy

E. Gestational diabetes
F. Acromegaly
G. Cystic fibrosis
H. Haemochromatosis
I. Alcoholic pancreatitis
J. Gallstone pancreatitis

For each scenario below, choose the most likely corresponding option from the list given above.

1. A 3-year-old with chronic respiratory failure, recurrent chest infections and multiple vitamin deficiencies secondary to malabsorption and growth retardation presents extremely unwell. She is acidotic, dehydrated, hyperglycaemic and has raised ketones.
2. A 45-year-old female with pyruvate kinase deficiency, a disease characterized by haemolytic anaemia, has been suffering with recurrent episodes of right upper quadrant pain and pale, offensive stools. She now complains of worse than usual fatigue and constant thirst.
3. A 55-year-old with slate-grey skin discolouration, cardiomyopathy, mild hepatosplenomegaly and arthralgia of numerous joints complains of a recent onset of weight loss, fatigue, polyuria and thirst.
4. A 26 weeks' pregnant 18-year-old female is currently well but was found to have a fasting blood glucose of 6.0 mmol/L.
5. A 62-year-old who is generally well despite having had body mass index of 42 kg/m^2 for at least 30 years presents for an elective knee replacement. Her body mass on the ward preoperatively after 6 hours of fasting is found to be 6.8 mmol/L.

Chapter 7

Lipid transport particles

A. Nascent chylomicrons
B. Mature chylomicrons
C. High-density lipoprotein (HDL)
D. Low-density lipoprotein (LDL)
E. Intermediate-density lipoprotein (IDL)
F. Very-low-density lipoprotein (VLDL)
G. Mixed micelles
H. Chylomicron remnants
I. VLDL remnants

For each of the following descriptions, please select the lipid transport particle it refers to from the list above.

1. This particle is assembled in the liver and delivers endogenously synthesized cholesterol and lipids to peripheral tissues.
2. This particle is the lower-density particle of the two types that evolve from VLDL as it progressively offloads its lipid cargo in the periphery.
3. This particle is assembled in enterocytes and subsequently extruded into the lymphatic circulation via the lacteals.
4. This particle has acquired apoproteins from HDL particles it encountered in the vascular circulation.
5. This particle represents the only vehicle for cholesterol transport from the periphery to the liver for excretion.

Chapter 8

Obesity treatment strategies

A. Dietary advice
B. Exercise programme
C. Orlistat
D. No intervention
E. Gastric band
F. Roux-en-Y procedure

For each scenario below, choose the most likely corresponding option from the list given above. It will help if you calculate the body mass index (BMI) before choosing an option.

1. A 32-year-old female weighing 104 kg who is 1.66 m tall with haemophilia, Crohn disease, severe anxiety and type 2 diabetes mellitus (T2DM) presents to her general practitioner (GP) expressing a wish to lose weight. She is unwilling to change her current diet and refuses to consider an exercise programme as she has significant bilateral knee osteoarthritis.
2. A 25-year-old male shift worker is concerned about his weight and attends the GP. He weighs 113 kg and is 1.89 m tall. He relies on takeaways and fast food for nourishment as he is often too tired to prepare meals from scratch. He cycles 5 miles to work and back at least five times a week.
3. A 52-year-old lady weighs 132 kg and is 1.6 m tall. She has been following a 700 kcal/day diet religiously for several months and is attending a gym daily since being signed off work 2 months previously with severe anxiety, for which she takes 100 mg OD of sertraline (a selective serotonin reuptake inhibitor). She has a terrible fear of surgery and absolutely will not consider any kind of operation, but is desperate to lose weight.
4. A 36-year-old female receptionist weighing 122 kg and 1.78 m tall approaches her GP, keen for weight reduction surgery. She is in good health and on no regular medications. She adheres closely to a low-calorie diet and has done for the last year. She is sedentary both at work and at home, and her main activities outside work include watching TV and surfing the Internet.
5. A 28-year-old man weighing 162 kg and 1.67 m tall attends his GP to discuss his parents' concern about his weight. He has previously been prescribed Orlistat, but found the side effects intolerable. Despite

his obesity he recently safely underwent a recent emergency open cholecystectomy. He rarely exercises as he dislikes getting hot and sweaty and says he enjoys his food too much to comply with the hospital nutritionist's recommendations.

Chapter 9

Biochemical features of amino acids

A. Leucine
B. Tryptophan
C. Tyrosine
D. Phenylalanine
E. Arginine
F. Glutamate
G. Glycine
H. Proline
I. Cysteine
J. Valine
K. Alanine
L. Methionine
M. Lysine
N. Glutamine

For each scenario below, choose the most likely corresponding option from the list given above.

1. This large, neutral, both ketogenic and glucogenic, essential amino acid is a precursor for the neurotransmitter serotonin. It can also act as a precursor for an important B vitamin.
2. This nonessential amino acid has the smallest molecular weight of the amino acids. In muscle tissue, this amino acid is important in nitrogen excretion, incorporating excess amino groups and entering the circulation destined for the liver, where it may enter the urea cycle or alternatively gluconeogenesis.
3. This glutamate-derived amino acid is the only amino acid where component atoms of the R-group are bonded with the α-carbon of the amino acid 'skeleton'. This cyclic nature confers a high conformational rigidity to the molecule. When hydroxylated, this amino acid is an important component of stability of collagen.
4. This nonessential amino acid is a component of glutathione, and possesses a sulphur-containing R-group responsible for many of its structural roles in proteins. Two key enzymes in its biosynthesis (which requires methionine and serine) are pyridoxal phosphate (vitamin B6) dependent.
5. This nonessential ketogenic and glucogenic amino acid shares a transporter with phenylalanine, as well as a phenyl component within the R-group. It is a precursor for thyroid hormone, catecholamines and melanin.

Chapter 10

Causes of hyperuricaemia

A. Tumour lysis syndrome
B. Polycythaemia rubra vera
C. Lesch–Nyhan syndrome
D. Rhabdomyolysis
E. Haemolysis
F. Renal insufficiency
G. Ketogenic diet
H. High dietary purine intake
I. Metabolic syndrome
J. Loop diuretics

For each scenario below, choose the most likely corresponding option from the list given above.

1. An 8-week-old baby boy with an orange-coloured sand-like precipitate in his nappy.
2. A forklift driver is involved in an accident where he was trapped for several hours whilst the fire brigade struggled to clear a route to release him following a collapse of warehouse crates onto him. He has extensive crush injuries.
3. A bodybuilder has been following a strict dietary plan which only allows minimal carbohydrate intake. His urate is significantly elevated.
4. A haematology inpatient who has recently commenced induction chemotherapy for acute myeloid leukaemia develops acute kidney injury with associated hyperphosphataemia and hyperuricaemia.
5. An obese 65-year-old male with type 2 diabetes and hypertension (for which he is taking atenolol) is found to have hyperuricaemia.

Chapter 12

Symptoms, signs and treatment of abnormal vitamin status

A. Vitamin A deficiency
B. Hypervitaminosis A
C. Thiamine deficiency
D. Vitamin D deficiency
E. Vitamin C deficiency
F. B12 deficiency
G. Folate deficiency
H. Niacin deficiency
I. Vitamin E deficiency
J. Vitamin K deficiency
K. Vitamin B6 deficiency

For each scenario below, choose the most likely corresponding option from the list given above.

1. A baby born at 30 weeks' gestation is noted to be extremely pale and icteric, and also in significant

respiratory distress, despite receiving the standard intramuscular parenteral vitamin given to all newborns postdelivery. Haemoglobin (Hb) is found to be 95 g/L with evidence of haemolysis on the blood film and hyperbilirubinaemia. Serum [α-tocopherol] is extremely low. Parenteral vitamin supplementation successfully treats the cause.

2. A strict vegan with a medical history notable for hypothyroidism, diabetes, rheumatoid arthritis and Crohn disease presents complaining of a sore mouth, general fatigue and tingling in her hands and feet. She takes regular folate supplements as folate deficiency was suspected as a cause of her tiredness. On neurological examination, joint position and vibration are impaired, ankle reflexes are absent but knee reflexes are abnormally brisk. She has lemon-yellow skin and marked glossitis and angular stomatitis. Although she is 24 years of age, she has silver hair. Hb is 85 g/L, mean corpuscular volume is 105 fL with a megaloblastic red cell appearance on blood film. Serum and red cell [folate] are within the normal range. Serum [lactate], [homocysteine] and [methylmalonic acid] are elevated. A Schilling test is +ve.

3. A 32-year-old homeless man attends the outreach clinic complaining of widespread joint pain and recurrent nosebleeds. He drinks 30–40 U of cider daily and smokes 40–50 rollies a day. He relies on discarded unsold burgers from a fast-food venue to survive. On examination he has widespread bruising, perifollicular haemorrhages, several large joint-effusions and severe gingivitis with several teeth missing. He is admitted to hospital and intravenous Pabrinex is commenced. He becomes better over the following weeks, and is given oral supplements, dietary advice and found hostel accommodation.

4. A 52-year-old female horse rustler with chronic pancreatitis and Crohn disease presents with difficulty seeing while driving at night. She attributes this to having had sore eyes for a while. On examination Bitot spots, angular stomatitis and very dry skin are noted. The gastroenterologist suspects a vitamin deficiency.

5. A 23-year-old legal secretary is referred to hospital by her psychiatrist with a right-sided *Haemophilus influenzae* pneumonia. The referrer believes that there may be an organic cause for her bizarre behaviour and would like this to be investigated. She had complained of severe tingling and numbness of hands and feet before becoming acutely confused. On examination, her body mass index is 14 kg/m^2, and she has auscultatory signs supporting the known diagnosis of lower respiratory tract infection. She is staggering about, and her right eye is laterally deviated. She is rambling and confabulatory and complies poorly with the examination, but her reflexes are sluggish and she has decreased light touch

sensation and reduced motor power 3/5 in her lower limbs. Her psychiatrist's letter states that she suffers from severe anorexia and has been a long-term abuser of diuretics for weight control. In an effort to limit her food intake, she drinks over 10 cups of tea and coffee a day. When she does eat, she will only eat uncooked fresh prawns and oysters, believing them to be calorie free. Her symptoms improve rapidly with intravenous Pabrinex.

Chapter 13

Symptoms and signs of abnormal mineral status

A. Haemochromatosis
B. Calcium deficiency
C. Magnesium toxicity
D. Hypophosphataemia
E. Hypocalcaemia
F. Hypercalcaemia
G. Wilson disease
H. Iron deficiency
I. Iodine deficiency
J. Acrodermatitis enteropathica
K. Hypernatraemia

For each scenario below, choose the most likely corresponding option from the list given above.

1. A 45-year-old lady presents unwell following 48 hours of severe diarrhoea and vomiting. She says that she has lost 5 kg (her usual weight is 50 kg). Her heart rate is 140 bpm and capillary refill time is 4 seconds. On examination she has sunken eyes and very dry mucous membranes with reduced skin turgor. Once catheterized her average urine output is <10 mL/hour. She has a postural drop in systolic blood pressure of 20 mmHg.

2. A 6-year-old girl, recently immigrated from Saudi Arabia, is seen by the general practitioner (GP) as her mother is concerned about some symmetrical lumps on her anterior ribs. The GP notes bilateral bowing of her legs, protruding abdomen and a rachitic rosary on examination. History is notable for lactose intolerance and strict observance of the family's religious custom to be fully covered head to toe at all times when outside the house.

3. A 24-year-old vegan presents to her general practitioner with menometrorrhagia. Her mean corpuscular volume is 70 fL, Hb is 96 g/L and ferritin is 5 μg/L. On examination koilonychia, angular stomatitis, pallor and diffuse hair thinning were noted. She admits to chronic breathlessness on exertion, fatigue and occasional palpitations.

4. A 17-year-old male is referred to gastrointestinal outpatients with deranged liver function tests. He has severe depression and his general practitioner wanted to exclude any underlying

organic pathology, particularly as he complained of tremor and was noted to have a mildly ataxic gait. Slit-lamp examination reveals circumferential brownish discolouration at the limbus, and his serum caeruloplasmin was low. Once the correct diagnosis was confirmed with a liver biopsy, penicillamine treatment was commenced.

5. A 60-year-old man with a new diagnosis of multiple myeloma presents to emergency department with severe flank pain. Computed tomography reveals a large obstructing ureteral calculus. He is listed for urgent ureteral stenting, but first treatment commences for a marked electrolyte disturbance noted on his admission blood tests. Treatment (vigorous intravenous isotonic saline, bisphosphonates and calcitonin) is started immediately.

Chapter 14

Investigations in metabolic/nutritional disease

A. Genetic testing
B. Liver biopsy
C. Glycated haemoglobin
D. Venous blood gas
E. Newborn blood spot
F. Serum caeruloplasmin
G. High-performance liquid chromatography serum thiamine
H. Serum and faecal porphyrins
I. Serum ammonia
J. Serum B12
K. Serum magnesium

For each scenario below, choose the most likely corresponding option from the list given above.

1. A 39-week pregnant lady with confirmed preeclampsia is being managed with fluid restriction and the continuous intravenous infusion that is standard management in severe preeclampsia. She becomes drowsy, tachycardic and her blood pressure becomes unrecordable. On examination, no tendon reflexes can be elicited. The infusion is stopped, the patient is treated with calcium gluconate and resuscitated with an ABC approach. Blood drawn during the acute resuscitation is sent for investigations to confirm the suspected diagnosis.

2. An asymptomatic newborn baby undergoes a routine screening test at 5 days of age.

3. An 18-year-old male is brought to the emergency department by his worried girlfriend. They have both had a chest infection recently, but he has suddenly become first strangely agitated and then drowsy. She also tells you that he seemed to be up and down repeatedly overnight to pass urine. He is now unconscious. He has no known medical history. On examination:

Glasgow Coma Score	13 (E3V5M5)
Respiratory rate	35 breaths/minute
Heart rate	130 beats/minute
Blood pressure	90/50 mmHg
Peripheries	Cool; capillary refill time >5 seconds
Peripheral capillary oxygen saturation (SpO_2)	92%
Urinary glucose	+++
Urinary ketones	+++

4. A recent immigrant from rural Philippines presents with bilateral lower limb paraesthesias and burning pain, anorexia and constipation. His wife comments on his recent poor memory and irritability, and comments that over the last few months he becomes breathless at the slightest exertion and on lying flat. Dietary history indicates they had recently been on a staple diet of white rice. On neurological examination, joint position and vibration sensation are impaired and lower limb reflexes are absent. He is tachycardic, with clinical evidence of heart failure including pulmonary oedema, oedema to mid shin, raised jugular venous pressure and displaced apex beat.

5. A 25-year-old male presents with recurrent severe poorly localized abdominal pain. Examination is notable only for extensive chronic blistering lesions on the dorsal hand and forearms and mild tachycardia. Hyponatraemia is the sole finding from routine serum investigations. However, a urinary porphobilinogen test is strongly positive.

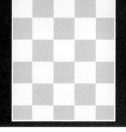

Chapter 1 Cellular biology

1. C. Intermediate filaments are the most abundant. (A) describes F-actin. (B) refers to microtubules. (D) describes the structure of DNA and (E) describes microfilaments, the main component of which is F-actin.

2. C. The nuclear intermembrane space is indeed continuous with the interior of the rough endoplasmic reticulum. The nucleus does contain chromosomes, but has a double membrane not a single membrane. Nucleoli are present, but represent ribosome assembly zones, not messenger RNA (mRNA) synthesis. Ribosomes are assembled in the nucleus, and mRNA synthesis takes place, but translation occurs in the cytoplasm. Mitochondria are located in the cytoplasm, not the nucleus.

3. D. The DNA consists of a deoxyribose sugar, a single phosphate group and a nitrogenous base (guanine, adenine, cytosine or thymine).

4. B. Only option B gives the correct (much simplified!) sequence of events of gene expression. All the other options are incorrect.

5. E. It describes chromatin, which makes up chromosomes. This is the most accurate from the listed options. Chromosomes are absent from nonnucleate anucleate cells (e.g., mature red blood cells and platelets). In each somatic cell, there are 46 chromosomes, or 23 pairs of chromosomes. Each member of a pair is derived from the person's mother, and the other from the person's father.

6. E. The structure of the double helix involves two separate nucleic acid chains (deoxyribonucleotide polymers). These coil around each other, forming the double helix. Phosphate groups of each deoxyribonucleotide protrude outwards from the helix, not inwards.

7. E. Option E is correct because this is the only intracellular site containing all necessary enzymes to allow the TCA cycle to occur. Mitochondria do possess their own DNA, but it is in circular form rather than the chromosomal form seen in the nucleus. They have a double membrane, where the inner membrane has multiple protrusions and invaginations. The inner (not outer) mitochondrial membrane is the site of the electron transport and is where oxidative phosphorylation occurs. Glycolysis occurs in the cytoplasm, not within mitochondria.

Chapter 2 Introduction to metabolism

1. E. ATP contains three (not four) phosphate groups. These are attached to the C5 of the ribose (a pentose, not a hexose) sugar component. There are two phosphoanhydride bonds, not three. The base component is an adenine ring, not a guanosine.

2. A. Although NAD^+ required to act as the oxidant, be aware that the TCA cycle additionally requires flavin adenine dinucleotide (FAD) as well. Both act as oxidants (i.e., redox partners for an oxidation reaction). When NAD^+ functions as an oxidant, NAD^+ itself is reduced to $NADH + H^+$. Options B, C and D require the $NADH + H^+$ to act as reductants. Option E requires FAD as an oxidant.

3. C. Look back to Figs 2.16 and 2.14. Only option C describes the true difference between the two electron acceptor molecules. Options A and D are features that apply to **both** molecules. Option B is false; both are dinucleotides. Option E is false; the two nucleotides (adenine and nicotinamide) are linked by their phosphate groups.

4. E. Only Option E lists only pathways/processes requiring $NADH + H^+$. Option A lists pathways requiring nicotinamide adenine dinucleotide (NAD^+), option B lists pathways requiring $NADPH + H^+$, option C lists pathways/processes requiring flavin adenine dinucleotide (FAD) whilst option D requires nicotinamide adenine dinucleotide phosphate ($NADP^+$).

5. A. The initial portion of the graph follows first-order kinetics, that is, as one parameter increases, the dependent parameter increases by a constant proportion. However, the plateau of the graph exhibits zero-order kinetics – as one parameter increases, the dependent parameter remains constant regardless of the change in the first. This phenomenon arises once the reaction velocity becomes limited by enzyme concentration. The shape of the curve is a rectangular hyperbola (not an exponential). K_m is not easy to precisely determine

from the Michaelis–Menten graph, hence the need for manipulation to form the Lineweaver–Burk plot. The axes are the reciprocals of the parameters listed in option C.

6. A. The best description is option A (i.e., the opposite of B). A free radical contains an unpaired electron, and causes damage by causing oxidation of intracellular molecules. Option D gives examples of antioxidants, which oppose free radical damage by scavenging free radicals. Options C and E both describe reductants, whereas free radicals are oxidants.

7. E. Options A–D are all major regulatory mechanisms. Free cross-membrane traffic (option E) would make regulation of intracellular pathways **more** challenging, because traffic in both directions across the membrane would be determined solely by concentration gradients rather than specific mechanisms determined in part by the cell.

8. C. The other options list catabolic pathways. Remember that anabolic pathways consume energy and are usually synthetic pathways.

Chapter 3 The tricarboxylic acid (TCA) cycle

1. B. Acetyl-CoA is synthesized by different macronutrient catabolic pathways, for example, β-oxidation of fatty acids and glycolysis. Because pathways that produce acetyl-CoA occur in both cytoplasm and mitochondria, its occurrence is not restricted to either location. The acetyl-CoA molecule 'delivers' the high-energy acetyl group to the tricarboxylic acid cycle for oxidation and liberation of chemical potential energy: being 'acetyl' – it contains two carbons, not three and so can only act as a donor of acetyl, not methyl units. The coenzyme component of acetyl-CoA includes pantothenic acid (vitamin B5; Fig. 2.18) not vitamin B7 (biotin).

2. C. Please refer to Fig. 3.1. for revision.

3. C. The ATP is generated indirectly, after the $FADH_2$ and three $NADH + H^+$ molecules go on to participate in oxidative phosphorylation. This is where the bulk of energy 'generation' of the TCA cycle is realized. GTP (not ATP) is generated directly by substrate-level phosphorylation in reaction 5 of the cycle; this 'direct' generation only represents the minority of the energy-generating potential of the cycle. In total, the equivalent of 10 ATP (not 8) molecules is the net output of the cycle.

4. A. It is the intracellular Ca^{++} (not sodium) concentration that exerts a powerful regulatory stimulus on the main rate-limiting enzymes, reflecting the need for upregulation of TCA cycle activity in a context of highly active energy-demanding processes such as muscle contraction. All of the other options contribute to TCA cycle regulation. The three rate-limiting enzymes (options B, E and α-ketoglutarate dehydrogenase) are strongly influenced by [ATP] intracellular concentration and $NADH + H^+$ in an example of negative feedback [these molecules are products generated either directly ($NADH + H^+$) or indirectly (ATP) by pathway activity].

5. D. Please refer to Fig. 3.3 for a list of genuine examples.

Chapter 4 Oxidative phosphorylation

1. A. This option summarizes the functions of the complexes of the electron transport chain. All are embedded within the inner (not outer) mitochondrial membrane. Complexes I, II, III, IV and V are relatively fixed, whereas ubiquinone (coenzyme Q) and cytochrome C are both mobile. Complexes I, III and IV pump protons from the mitochondrial membrane into the intermembranal space, accumulating a gradient which then 'discharges' through complex V (adenosine triphosphatase synthase).

2. E. Creatine phosphate or phosphocreatine acts as a phosphate donor to adenosine diphosphate (ADP) in the immediate aftermath of high-intensity metabolic demand onset once adenosine triphosphate is exhausted, but before upregulation of glycolysis and other catabolic pathways can meet the new increased demand. Option A is false because ADP (not AMP) is the most common substrate. Options B, C and D refer to oxidative phosphorylation, rather than substrate-level phosphorylation.

3. B. Only option B describes an abnormal uncoupling scenario (see discussion in Uncoupling). Option C describes 'physiological' (not abnormal) uncoupling, A and D describe components of normal oxidative phosphorylation, and E, although detrimental to intracellular molecules, is a consequence of oxidative phosphorylation rather than being related to coupling.

4. B. Creatine is obtained from the diet but is also endogenously synthesized in the liver. It then travels to skeletal muscle tissue, where it enters myocytes. Once phosphorylated, creatine is 'trapped' intracellularly. Creatine phosphate-mediated ADP phosphorylation occurs immediately after the onset of an increased demand, before (not after) glycolysis activity upregulation has had time to occur.

5. A. Options B, C and D refer to the glycerol-3-phosphate shuttle. Option E describes the opposite directions of travel to the genuine movements within the malate–aspartate shuttle.

Chapter 5 Carbohydrate metabolism

1. C. Options A and B refer to salivary amylase (not disaccharidase). Option D lists key examples of disaccharidases (not amylases) whose actions are prominent in conversion of disaccharides to monosaccharides in the small intestine (not the mouth, as stated in option E).

2. A. Option A occurs during reactions 7 and 10 of glycolysis. However, 2 ATPs are consumed by reactions 1 and 3 of glycolysis (not one, as in option D). Two (not one, as stated in option C) $NADH + H^+$ molecules are generated per molecule of glucose oxidized, representing approximately 5 ATP (2.5 ATP per $NADH + H^+$). The net ATP generation is therefore approximately 7 ATP per molecule of glucose oxidized.

3. B. Glycolysis is a catabolic pathway, sequentially oxidizing glucose molecules. It occurs in both aerobic and anaerobic conditions; indeed, it is the only adenosine triphosphate generation mechanism in anaerobic conditions. It is particularly relevant therefore in cells lacking mitochondria such as red blood cells, however it takes place in all cells of the body.

4. E. Phosphorylation of glucose (reaction 1), phosphorylation of fructose-6-phosphate (reaction 3) and conversion of phosphoenolpyruvate to pyruvate (reaction 10) are the key regulatory points of glycolysis.

5. E. Reduction of PDH activity results in accumulated pyruvate, which is then converted to lactate. PDH is a complex of three associated enzymes. Mandatory coenzymes and cofactors include vitamin B1 (not vitamin B2), CoA, lipoic acid, nicotinamide adenine dinucleotide and flavin adenine dinucleotide. Phosphorylation status significantly affects PDH activity and represents the primary regulatory influence. The reaction mediated by PDH is an irreversible oxidative decarboxylation, but it is pyruvate → acetyl-CoA, rather than the reverse reaction quoted in option A.

6. D. Most reactions of gluconeogenesis occur within the cytoplasm, but two occur in the mitochondrial matrix, thus only option D is correct. Gluconeogenesis occurs mainly in hepatocytes.

Gluconeogenesis is active during fasting (not the fed state), particularly prolonged fasting, and generates glucose from many ubiquitous noncarbohydrate substrates. Fatty acids are a notable exception – they are not gluconeogenic substrates. Because insulin inhibits gluconeogenesis, but glucagon promotes gluconeogenesis, a high insulin:glucagon ratio would be expected to lower gluconeogenesis pathway activity.

7. B. Option B is a gluconeogenesis enzyme. Phosphoenolpyruvate carboxykinase converts oxaloacetate to phosphoenolpyruvate. All the other listed enzymes participate in both glycolysis and gluconeogenesis. The other enzymes that participate in gluconeogenesis but not in glycolysis are glucose-6-phosphatase, fructose-1,6-bisphosphatase and pyruvate carboxylase. These enzymes mediate the reactions of gluconeogenesis: recall that this pathway is not simply a reversal of steps of the glycolysis pathway (see the 'Gluconeogenesis' section).

8. B. Branch points integrate via glycosidic bonds between C6 of the main strand residue and C1 of the terminal residue of the branch. Glycogen is a polymer consisting of glucose residue monomers (not galactose). Branch points occur every 8–12 (not 20) residues. Neighbouring residues are linked by glycosidic bonds between C1 and C4 (not C1 and C6).

9. B. Phosphoglucomutase-mediated Glc-6-P formation is followed by activation (attachment of UDP) of Glc-6-P, allowing the incoming residue to integrate into a growing chain (elongation). Branch formation requires branching enzyme to excise a segment (soon to become a branch) from an existing elongated chain and integrate it to a main-strand residue (via a 1–6 glycosidic bond) as a new branch.

10. D. Option D participates in stage 2, 'activation', of glycogen synthesis. The other listed enzymes participate in glycogen degradation (glycogenolysis). Note that options C and E are in fact craftily synonymous.

11. C. The initial substrate for reaction 1 is glucose-6-phosphate (not glucose-1-phosphate). The pathway is primarily anabolic (not catabolic) in nature. Pathway failure is not incompatible with life as evidenced by the existence of patients with glucose-6-phosphate dehydrogenase deficiency. In these individuals, the citrate shuttle bears sole responsibility for generating $NADPH + H^+$; however, this is a mitochondria-associated shuttle and thus consequences of glucose-6-phosphate dehydrogenase deficiency are prominent in cells lacking mitochondria such

as erythrocytes, hence haemolysis is the clinical hallmark of the condition. An intact pathway enables glutathione (not glutamate) regeneration by providing a supply of $NADPH + H^+$.

12. D. Paracetamol is safely used in these patients. It is exposure (rather than the route of administration) that is relevant. Nitrofurantoin and sulphonamide drugs have a high probability of precipitating haemolysis in these patients and should be avoided. Septrin (cotrimoxazole) contains sulphamethoxazole and should be avoided. Fava beans are a classic 'exam' precipitant, although sensitivity to their vicine compounds varies among glucose-6-phosphate dehydrogenase-deficient individuals.

13. E. The most common dietary source of fructose is sucrose, not lactose. Fructose is absorbed into enterocytes via GLUT-5 (not GLUT-2), and *leaves* enterocytes into the blood of the portal vein via GLUT-2. In hepatocytes, fructose is phosphorylated by fructokinase, but to fructose-1-phosphate (not fructose-6-phosphate). This is then converted to glyceraldehyde-3-phosphate by aldolase B (not A).

14. B. Galactose accumulation starts postnatally (not in utero), as soon as the infant is fed galactose-containing formula or breastmilk, which contains lactose and therefore galactose. Breastfeeding offers no benefits in the context of galactosaemia. Inheritance is typically autosomal recessive. This condition occurs at a particularly high incidence in the Irish Traveller community (1 in approximately 450 versus 1 in approximately 36,000).

15. D. Fatty acid synthesis activity is upregulated due to increased acetyl-CoA availability. This increased availability occurs because of reduced activity of the TCA cycle, glycolysis and gluconeogenesis pathways and impairment of the pyruvate → acetyl-CoA reaction. These pathways/reactions are all suppressed due to nicotinamide adenine dinucleotide (NAD^+) depletion, which occurs due to NAD^+ participation in ethanol detoxification (catabolism). The other options all list pathways/reactions with significantly reduced activity in the context of NAD^+ scarcity.

Chapter 6 Glucose homeostasis and diabetes mellitus

1. D. All other options refer to type 2 diabetes.

2. C. All other features are common to *all* types of diabetes, whether type 1, type 2, gestational or secondary.

3. C. All options list correct associations, except option C – the mechanism of action listed here describes the action of gliptins (such as vildagliptin and sitagliptin), whereas thiazolidinediones such as pioglitazone activate the peroxisome proliferator-activated receptor-γ.

4. C. Option C exhibits extreme hyperglycaemia and raised osmolality in the *absence* of ketonaemia or metabolic acidosis. The raised partial pressure of carbon dioxide (pCO_2) suggests an element of hypoventilation, consistent with the drowsy or stuporous state seen in severe HHNS, which is an acute complication of type 2 diabetes mellitus. Options A and D show the characteristic derangements associated with a diabetic ketoacidosis [an acute complication of (almost always) type 1 diabetes mellitus]. Osmolality is mildly elevated due to dehydration. pCO_2 is low due to Kussmaul respiration: a physiological response to metabolic acidosis. Option B and E are normal results.

5. D. This gentleman gives a history of a silent myocardial infarction (MI) 3 months ago – in advanced autonomic neuropathy (evidenced by his postural hypotension) pain and other usual MI symptoms may be absent. Only shortness of breath and usually sweating signal an MI in patients with autonomic neuropathy, emphasizing the importance of electrocardiography in diagnosis of MI in the diabetic population. The infarct impaired his cardiac function and thus reduced his exercise tolerance. The polyuria is evidence of osmotic diuresis from the glycosuria seen in chronic hyperglycaemia, rather than the age-related changes in bladder control that he self-diagnosed. The vision impairment is also a complication of untreated chronic hyperglycaemia with microvascular diabetic eye disease. His fasting finger prick blood glucose places him unambiguously in the 'diabetes' category rather than the impaired glucose tolerance category (please see the 'Impaired glucose tolerance' section). The slow insidious onset suggests type 2 diabetes mellitus (T2DM) rather than type 1 diabetes mellitus. There is no history of a primary disease impairing the pancreas, and secondary diabetes is also much rarer than T2DM. Multiple end-organ impairments secondary to untreated diabetes have accumulated, but fortunately the peripheral neuropathy and nonhealing ulcer have brought him to medical attention. This late presentation, only after disease has progressed sufficiently as to cause various end-organ complications, is unfortunately not unusual in T2DM.

Chapter 7 Lipid metabolism and lipid transport

1. C. This notation describes an 18-carbon fatty acid. The number after the colon indicates the number of double bonds (any more than one makes it a polyunsaturated) – four in this case. The numbers following the 'Δ' sign indicate the carbon positions of the double bonds. The 'c' indicates the geometric configuration of the double bond as the 'cis' rather than the 'trans' isomer.

2. D. Biosynthetic pathways are typically anabolic. Fatty acid (FA) synthesis occurs in the cytoplasm, hence the need to export acetyl-coenzyme A (the main substrate) from the mitochondrial matrix where it is generated by the tricarboxylic acid cycle as a first step in FA synthesis (via the citrate shuttle). The redox partner is $NADPH + H^+$, which is oxidized in parallel with the two reduction steps in the pathway.

3. A. Option B describes fatty acid synthesis. The remainder are not typical of any major catabolic pathway.

4. E. Without bile acid solubilization, lipases can only hydrolyse a minute proportion of triacylglycerols (i.e., those located at the very surface of fat globules). Being hydrophobic, fatty acids diffuse freely into enterocytes down their concentration gradient without the need for specific carrier import. This is followed by chylomicron assembly and extrusion into the lymphatic system, ultimately entering the venous circulation via the thoracic duct.

5. E. A premature death in a first-degree relative warrants further investigation, particularly as the patient gives a typical history of angina and exhibits a dyslipidaemic phenotype despite her very young age. Her cholesterol and LDL are significantly elevated, despite relatively normal [TG] and [HDL] – suggesting familial hypercholesterolaemia. Only genetic studies (option E) will conclusively identify this. A 24-hour ECG may identify changes typical of myocardial ischaemia and HbA1C or glucose tolerance test would confirm/refute a diagnosis of diabetes or insulin resistance, respectively, but neither can diagnose the cause. Dietary history would be helpful, but less conclusive, particularly as a genetic dyslipidaemia is likely (young age, symptomatic of vaso-occlusive disease, positive family history, extremely deranged lipid profile).

6. A. This is the best course of action, with appropriate follow-up allowing recourse to adding in a drug if behavioural change was unsustainable or ineffective.

Option B is premature as statins are not without their complications and side effects, and this gentleman's lipid profile may normalize with appropriate advice. His cholesterol is not grossly elevated and he has no family history of premature atherosclerosis-related events, and there are no other results that would point to a genetic dyslipidaemia, so tertiary referral (option D) would be inappropriate. Option E dismisses a potentially modifiable risk factor for cardiovascular disease (raised cholesterol, LDL and TG) and could embarrass the patient.

7. B. Option B gives the most prominent cause of ketone elevation in starvation. Cardiac myocytes preferentially catabolize fatty acids in health. Excessive serum ketone concentrations result in metabolic acidosis, not alkalosis. The CNS can switch to utilizing ketones in starvation, but never completely – glucose is always required as well. Ketone catabolism generates $NADH + H^+$; ketone synthesis generates nicotinamide adenine dinucleotide (NAD^+).

Chapter 8 Bioenergetics and obesity

1. A. See the 'Body composition' section.

2. D. Bone, protein and water comprise lean body mass. This represents approximately 85% of body mass in a normal adult male.

3. C. Regarding metabolic energy expenditure: 50% is lost as heat, 10% by DIT and the remaining 40% of energy expenditure is represented by the sum of the basal metabolic rate (BMR) and physical activity. Options A and E described the BMR. Option D refers to involuntary heat loss.

4. A. The only listed orexigenic hormone above is ghrelin, which has both central and gastrointestinal effects. Ghrelin also inhibits release of the anorexic CART and MSH and enhances release of the orexigenic neuropeptide Y (NPY) and agouti-related peptide (AGRP). CCK and GLP-1 also reduce appetite, but via different mechanisms.

5. B. CCK is a gastrointestinal hormone, released postprandially, which supresses appetite. Option B is correct, as it accounts for the communication to the NTS, which is the underlying mechanism for appetite suppression: the NTS then stimulates melanocyte-stimulating hormone and CART release, not AGRP or NPY release (which would be highly orexigenic). Inhibiting ghrelin would supress appetite, but this is not the mechanism of CCK.

6. D. AGRP is a potent orexigenic neurohormone and is a peptide. AGRP shares a mechanism of action with NPY, not CART or melanocyte-stimulating hormone. Option E refers to ghrelin, not AGRP. Cholecystokinin stimulates the nucleus tractus solitarius (NTS) via vagal afferents, but the NTS then increases AGRP release from the hypothalamic neurons, specifically those located in the arcuate nucleus, thus B is incorrect.

7. E. Surgery is only a first-line therapeutic strategy in patients with BMI exceeding 50 kg/m^2, that is, not the majority of obese patients. In other obese patients, BMI is an important factor in considering surgery, but presence of severe and reversible obesity-related complications is also important. Drug treatment is an adjunctive treatment which should be implemented in conjunction with diet and exercise. A healthy diet and regular exercise should be recommended even after bariatric surgery.

8. D. Option D is the cause of the bulk of clinically encountered obesity. Option C is an association not a causation. The other options are rarer causes of obesity.

9. C. 100 divided by 1.7 squared (2.89) = 34.6. A BMI of 34.6 places her in the class 1 obesity category.

Chapter 9 Protein metabolism and
malnutrition

1. B. All other options describe secondary structural features, where β-sheets and α-helices are the common structural motifs, formed due to hydrogen bonds between the amine group hydrogen and carbonyl group oxygen of component amino acids.

2. A. B gives rise to secondary structure, C and D determine tertiary and quaternary structure and E is a feature of quaternary structure.

3. D. This patient weighs <60% of predicted weight. Oedema is absent. The diagnosis is thus marasmus (D). If he were 80%–100% of predicted weight, this would be classed as underweight (A). If oedema were present, the diagnosis would be marasmus–kwashiorkor (C). He could not be diagnosed with kwashiorkor or marasmus–kwashiorkor, because oedema is absent and his weight should be between 60% and 80% of predicted (12–16 kg) to fit their criteria. Cretinism (E) does cause growth retardation, but not with such emaciation and skeletal appearance.

4. E. Patient E has a dysfunctional shortened bowel. TPN would be needed in this patient to maintain nutrition until gastrointestinal (GI) absorption had recovered sufficiently. The patients described in options A, B and D are ideal candidates for enteral nutrition. If the respiratory sepsis was overwhelming in patient A and enteral nutrition failed due to impaired GI absorption, TPN would be appropriate, but TPN is only an option when the enteral route is not appropriate. Patient C should do well with fortification supplements and encouragement as a first-line approach.

5. C. Phenylalanine is considered essential despite endogenous biosynthesis being possible (eliminating B) as the physiological requirement exceeds maximum synthetic output. It is both ketogenic and glucogenic (eliminating options A, D and E) and is an important precursor for tyrosine. The R-group is large and contains a phenyl group, thus it shares the large and neutral/aromatic amino acid transporter (again excluding B, A, D and E).

6. C. Endogenous tyrosine synthesis is impaired, making dietary intake of tyrosine essential. Tyrosine is synthesized from phenylalanine by phenylalanine hydroxylase (not tyrosinase), which is the enzyme affected in PKU. Phenylketonuria is an autosomal recessive (excluding A) inborn error of metabolism. It is included in the newborn blood spot screening (excluding E), because if diagnosed this early, with strict dietary rules a sufferer can have a normal healthy lifespan (excluding option B).

7. D. The enzymes responsible are phenylalanine hydroxylase, tyrosine hydroxylase, DOPA decarboxylase (vitamin B6 cofactor), dopamine-β-hydroxylase, phenylethanolamine-N-methyltransferase (vitamin B12 cofactor).

8. D. Growth (option D) and pregnancy are the most representative scenarios of positive nitrogen balance (i.e., where nitrogen assimilation exceeds excretion). The other options are all good examples of negative nitrogen balance; in options A, B and C from excess nitrogen loss due to significant tissue damage and in option E due to insufficient nitrogen intake.

9. D. Amino acids are either ketogenic (their catabolized skeletons ultimately enter ketogenesis) or glucogenic (catabolized skeletons can participate in gluconeogenesis, i.e., glucose synthesis). Isoleucine is catabolized to succinyl-coenzyme A (succinyl-CoA), which may enter gluconeogenesis via the tricarboxylic acid (TCA) cycle, giving it glucogenic status, or acetyl-CoA, which may participate in ketogenesis. Serine (A) is dehydrated to pyruvate. Alanine (B) is transaminated to pyruvate.

Pyruvate is a gluconeogenic substrate. Proline (C) is dehydrogenated, then oxidized to glutamate (E), which is then oxidatively deaminated to form α-ketoglutarate, which enters the TCA cycle, ultimately forming oxaloacetate, another gluconeogenic substrate.

Chapter 10 Purines, pyrimidines, haem and one-carbon transfer

1. D. All of the above conditions could have caused this gentleman's anaemia. This in itself could cause many of his symptoms. However, the combination of the 'Burton line' and the blood film comment on red cell basophilic stippling make lead poisoning the most likely diagnosis. The symptoms of peripheral neuropathy and subtle neuropsychiatric symptoms (refractory depression, sleep disturbance, cognitive impairment and personality change) support this diagnosis.

2. D. This lady initially presented with abdominal pain due to an acute porphyria attack provoked by commencing both hormonal contraceptive and valproate, two drugs that are absolutely contraindicated in the acute porphyrias. Not unusually, porphyria was not considered, and unfortunately, she was discharged with diclofenac for analgesia (another contraindicated drug in acute porphyria), which exacerbated the acute attack resulting in acute psychosis. The dramatic elevation of urinary porphobilinogen (PBG) confirms an acute episode of one of the acute porphyrias. Of those listed, only acute intermittent porphyria (the most common porphyria; option D) is an 'acute' porphyria, that is, features acute attacks that may be precipitated by drugs. Lead poisoning could also elevate urinary [PBG], but tends to present insidiously and is not precipitated by particular drugs in this manner.

3. D. Option D represents a high purine intake – a risk factor for increased urate production and the clinical manifestation of gout. Insulin resistance (not insulin deficiency as in option A) and obesity (not a low BMI as in option C) are risk factors for impaired urate excretion, and high (not low as in option B) purine diets cause increased urate production. Lesch–Nyhan syndrome (option E) sufferers do not survive into late adulthood – this gentleman is aged 55 years (although they do exhibit marked hyperuricaemia).

4. D. Option D is correct – above its pK_a (i.e., a pH 7.4 in plasma) the weak acid is deprotonated, forming the urate anion. A product of purine (not pyrimidine) catabolism, urate is synthesized from hypoxanthine via two sequential oxidation (not reduction) reactions. Xanthine oxidase contains molybdenum and iron (not copper) ions. Urate is primarily excreted by the kidneys in urine (not faeces).

5. E. Options B and D refer to only the acute (i.e., not cutaneous) porphyrias. Option A is incorrect because acute intermittent porphyria lacks this feature. Option C is inaccurate, because porphyria cutanea tarda, erythropoietic porphyria and congenital erythropoietic porphyria exhibit rashes but are cutaneous (not acute) porphyrias and therefore certain drug avoidance and fasting avoidance are not mandatory.

6. C. Adenine is a purine derivative. All the others are pyrimidine derivatives.

7. C. It is inhibited by haem and requires pyridoxal phosphate as a cofactor. The other options are indeed enzymes of the haem synthesis pathway but are not rate limiting.

8. E. The majority of haem catabolism occurs in macrophages of the reticuloendothelial system; only ~15% occurs in hepatic Kupffer cells. Haem glucuronidation renders it water soluble, not lipid soluble. Catabolism generates carbon monoxide (not dioxide). Bilirubin is reduced in the cytoplasm from biliverdin, not the other way round. Biliverdin (not bilirubin) is formed by cleavage of the porphyrin ring of haem.

Chapter 11 The thyroid gland

1. C. The median isthmus of the bilobed thyroid gland structure is a midline structure. The thyroid is superficial to and anterior to the trachea. Each lobe lies anteromedial to the ipsilateral carotid sheaths. Muscles overlying and anterior to the thyroid (i.e., the thyroid is posterior to these structures) are the sternothyroid and sternohyoid strap muscles. The thyroid and cricoid cartilages also lie superficial to (i.e., anterior) to trachea.

2. C. T3 is three to four times more potent than T4. rT3 is metabolically inactive. It is a structural isomer of T3. The ratio of total T4 to total T3 in plasma is 50:1, however the physiologically relevant fractions are the unbound or 'free' hormones. Free T4 is present at a ratio around 3:1 relative to free T3. The thyroid gland secretes 10 times the amount of T4 as it does T3.

3. A. T4 functions as a precursor to rT3 and T3. Outer ring deiodination of T4 generates T3, whereas inner ring deiodination generates rT3. T4 contains four

iodine atoms, whereas T3 and rT3 contain three iodine atoms. T4, T3 and rT3 all contain two tyrosine residues; these are derived from thyroglobulin and paired together following iodination.

4. B. Hypothalamic TRH promotes synthesis and release of TSH from thyrotrophic cells of the anterior pituitary. TSH stimulates synthesis and secretion of T3 and T4 by thyroid follicular cells (not parafollicular cells of the thyroid; these secrete calcitonin). T4 and T3 also exert the primary negative feedback on both TSH and TRH synthesis and secretion (not TSH).

5. C. Anabolic pathways are mostly stimulated by T3, whereas catabolic pathways are activated (A incorrect). Option B would be correct but for the inclusion of protein synthesis, which is suppressed by T3. Option D describes the opposite scenario: in fact, T3 suppresses protein synthesis but promotes skeletal muscle proteolysis. Option E gives a list of pathways that are promoted (not suppressed) by T3.

6. C. The key to a diagnosis of sick euthyroid syndrome is that despite mildly deranged T3, T4 and thyroid-stimulating hormone (TSH) parameters, clinical symptoms that would be expected in this context are absent, thus eliminating all other options. However, because sick euthyroid is typically precipitated by other illness, symptoms specific to the precipitating disease would be expected. Options A and D refer to hypothyroidism, whereas option 2 might be seen in Graves disease, and option E might be seen in hyperthyroidism secondary to an adenoma of thyrotrophic cells of the anterior pituitary (typically elevation of T4 would suppress TSH release).

Chapter 12 Vitamins and their deficiencies

1. B. The other options all describe different features specific to water-soluble vitamins.

2. A. The symptoms are typical for anaemia. Vegans are at high risk of vitamin B12 deficiency. The full blood count/film results are consistent with megaloblastic anaemia, which is a feature of B12 deficiency. The only investigation finding consistent with this is option A. Option B would be seen in vitamin C deficiency, option C in B3 deficiency, option D in B6 deficiency and option E in vitamin A deficiency.

3. E. Neural tube closure defects such as anencephaly are strongly associated with folate deficiency. Folate is also known as 'vitamin B9', thus option E is the correct answer. Note that vitamin A deficiency is also significant in embryogenesis and excess vitamin

A results in teratogenicity, but fetal abnormalities arising from these conditions tend to be craniofacial and cardiac rather than neural tube defects.

4. C. This cultural belief advocates limited skin exposure for modesty reasons, thus preventing sun exposure, impairing endogenous ultraviolet-dependent synthesis of vitamin D. This shifts the vitamin D requirement to diet alone; however, few foods are sufficiently high enough in vitamin D to compensate for negligible endogenous synthesis. There should therefore be a low threshold for suspicion of vitamin D deficiency and supplement prescription in this population. Option A would ensure vitamin D deficiency was highly unlikely, though risk of skin cancer would be high. Likewise, option E would not confer risk of deficiency – it is darker pigmentation that carries the increased risk. Option B would possibly place the enthusiastic tea/coffee drinker at risk of B1 deficiency (high thiaminases intake in the form of tannin and caffeic acid polyphenols). Option D carries risk of B3 deficiency (the 'classical' cause).

5. C. This gentleman is likely to be at risk of vitamin D and calcium deficiency (renal failure), but this is not given as an option and would not cause these symptoms. The triad of skin symptoms combined with diarrhoea and neuropsychiatric impairment is due to pellagra, from niacin (vitamin B3) deficiency (option C). The rash is photosensitive, hence worse on sun-exposed areas. The specific risk factors in this case are renal replacement therapy, azathioprine and isoniazid use. These latter drugs should always be co-prescribed with vitamin B6 to prevent a secondary B3 deficiency.

Chapter 13 Minerals and their deficiencies

1. C. Clinical assessment of fluid status is the first step in directing further investigations and/ or interventions. Option A is incorrect – when attempting to normalize [Na$^+$] it must be undertaken gradually; over-rapid correction is associated with central pontine myelinolysis. This correction strategy would only be appropriate if the patient presented with seizures. Option B is not appropriate – this is significant hyponatraemia and a cause must be identified with clinical assessment and further investigations. Option D is incorrect – this is the treatment strategy in hypernatraemia. Option E is incorrect – fluid restriction would be the appropriate treatment strategy in euvolaemic hyponatraemia and would exacerbate the hyponatremia.

2. C. Her clinical signs suggest hypervolaemia and the hyponatraemia is likely secondary to intravascular volume expansion. This is a typical example of

a patient with congestive cardiac failure. Note that options A, D and E describe an appropriate strategy for the stated abnormality except option B – hypovolaemic patients should never be fluid restricted and would exacerbate their dehydration.

3. C. The priority in a severe hyperkalaemia (particularly with worrisome electrocardiogram changes) is the stabilization of the myocardium with immediate intravenous calcium. Potassium-lowering treatment should then be implemented. Option E is incorrect, as this would worsen the hyperkalaemia. Options A, B and D will lower the serum potassium – option A by eliminating potassium faecally, and options B and D by driving serum potassium intracellularly, but too slowly for this scenario.

4. B. Norovirus infections causes severe vomiting, which leads to acute hypokalaemia. All other options would cause hyperkalaemia, not hypokalaemia.

5. C. Option C is a microcytic anaemia, of which the most common cause is iron deficiency. Option A is a macrocytic anaemia, which would be see in vitamin B12 or folate deficiency; options B and E are normal values and option D would imply acute blood loss or anaemia of chronic disease (i.e., a normocytic anaemia).

6. B. Severe preeclampsia is treated with a magnesium infusion. The 'antidote' is calcium gluconate, which has contributed to her recovery. Magnesium toxicity is a rare complication of magnesium infusions – parturients are vigilantly monitored to try to prevent it occurring, as severe toxicity can manifest with cardiac arrest as with this patient.

7. C. Only the intake of magnesium, option C, is not limited by a vegan diet. Iron deficiency often arises due to lack of the more easily absorbed haem iron. Zinc absorption is impaired by phytate intake (typically high in vegan diet) and zinc-rich shellfish/meat/offal (other rich sources of zinc) are shunned by vegans. Calcium intake is often inadequate in vegans, who also avoid dairy products. Dairy exclusion also limits access to dietary iodine, as does seafood omission.

8. D. Haem is absorbed intact by receptor-mediated endocytosis (E incorrect) and is thus less sensitive to other ingested foods. Phytates, zinc and calcium impair absorption of nonhaem iron (C incorrect). Ferrous (Fe^{2+}), not ferric (Fe^{3+}), ions are taken into enterocytes via a symport (B incorrect). Ferric ions cannot access enterocytes and thus cannot be absorbed. Haem iron is better absorbed that nonhaem iron (A incorrect).

9. C. Vitamin D and parathyroid hormone both increase serum $[Ca^{++}]$ and calcitonin lowers serum $[Ca^{++}]$ (A, B, D and E incorrect).

Chapter 14 Clinical assessment of metabolism and nutritional disorders

1. D. This lady presents with neurovisceral symptoms and acute behavioural disturbance due to acute intermittent porphyria (AIP). In this instance the exposure to alcohol and the oral contraceptive pill have provoked the episode. The urine is dark red from accumulation of porphyrins/porphyrin precursors. It is not haematuria because the standard dipstick is negative. Typically for AIP, most examination findings and investigations are normal, although note the slightly raised ALT from hepatic involvement and the tachycardia, which may be secondary to catecholamine release or autonomic hyperactivity. The correct option is therefore D – an appropriate initial second-line investigation. A liver ultrasound (E) would be inappropriate in absence of hepatomegaly or marked derangement across the LFT panel. Option B could be reasonable, but for the suspicious urine. Option C would be appropriate to exclude free air under the diaphragm in suspected acute surgical condition, but the normal abdominal examination makes this extremely unlikely. Option (A) would not be appropriate without having first screened for porphyrias with the urinary assay (although even in absence of an acute episode red cell porphobilinogen deaminase levels are decreased in 90% of patients with AIP).

2. C. This gentleman presents with symptoms secondary to B12 deficiency and anaemia. The coexisting hypothyroidism and vitiligo should raise suspicion of an autoimmune predilection. Pallor combined with mild jaundice in a prematurely grey-haired individual should raise suspicion of pernicious anaemia. The thyroid-stimulating hormone is normal, suggesting adequate control of hypothyroidism, thus this is less likely to be the cause of the symptoms. The investigations show macrocytic anaemia with mild thrombocytopenia and leucopenia, typical of pernicious anaemia. Option C will differentiate between pernicious anaemia and other causes of B12 deficiency. Option A, the blood film, would show megaloblastic changes in white cells and macrocytic anaemia, but would not be able to differentiate between folate and B12 deficiency. Option B would show low B12, but would not identify whether this was dietary, due to malabsorption or pernicious anaemia. Option D, bone marrow examination, would confirm megaloblastic change, but would not be able to differentiate between the causes of B12

deficiency. Option E would be positive in only 50% of individuals with pernicious anaemia so this is a less accurate response.

3. E. Your clinical priority should be acute resuscitation via an ABC approach, obtaining intravenous access, commencing rehydration, performing a blood gas, catheterizing to monitor urine output and requesting urgent urea and electrolytes as the 12-hour anuria indicates severe acute kidney injury (prerenal, secondary to dehydration). Rehydration should commence with a rapid bolus. If his blood pressure does not respond to the initial bolus, repeat boluses may be required. From the clinical signs, this patient presents with severe dehydration (>8%) secondary to substantial gastrointestinal losses and needs urgent rehydration. Because he is drowsy, vomiting and critically ill, oral rehydration would be inappropriate. Recall that hypotension and drowsiness are dangerous signs of decompensation in extreme dehydration – critical care input should be requested. Once initially stabilized, his maintenance rates should be calculated to fully correct the deficit over the 48-hour period it has taken to develop. Only isotonic fluids such as 0.9% saline are appropriate. Intravenous potassium supplementation should be guided by regular electrolytes, but as this patient is likely to have marked acute kidney injury, his potassium may well be dangerously elevated, so potassium should not be added until his serum [K$^+$] is known.

4. D. This lady presents with symptoms and signs consistent with pregnancy. This must be excluded in a female of reproductive age with suggestive symptoms and signs, even if the patient states they are sexually abstinent, hence option D is the right answer. Option B would be appropriate after confirming she is nonpregnant with the urinary HCG. Option A would be appropriate only if heavy proteinuria was seen on dipstick and pregnancy excluded. Option C would be appropriate if there was evidence of urinary obstruction or the patient had not been confirmed negative for polycystic kidney disease, but not until B had been performed. Option E would be appropriate to investigate a palpable abdominal mass once pregnancy had been excluded; CT is contraindicated in pregnancy.

5. C. This elderly lady is experiencing delirium tremens (DT). When taking a history, respectable elderly ladies are not often pressed about their alcohol intake as it can seem somehow disrespectful – however, they absolutely should be offered the same right to correct inpatient management as anyone else; this includes taking a comprehensive history to identify risk factors such as regular alcohol intake. In this instance, prophylactic chlordiazepoxide and Pabrinex were not prescribed and thus are absent from the drug chart. Hallucinations, nausea, vomiting, agitation, diaphoresis and ultimately seizures are typical features of DT. The picture is clearly that of alcohol withdrawal and therefore option C is correct. Option A will not address the seizures, which will recur without benzodiazepine administration, although it should be prescribed to reduce the probability of Wernicke encephalopathy. Option B will not take effect rapidly enough, plus the patient is postictal and oral medication would not be safe or practical. Option D would be appropriate if hypoglycaemia were the cause for the lady's condition, which would be a reasonable explanation but for the hypertension/tachycardia/fever (hypoglycaemia does not cause these features) and the normal BM. Option E would be acceptable only if the patient were severely agitated and all reversible provocative causes had been excluded.

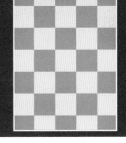

EMQ answers

Chapter 1 Cellular biology

Role of intracellular organelles

1. **G:** This description defines only the mitochondria, which is the only structure responsible for oxidative phosphorylation, the site of the tricarboxylic acid cycle and the only organelle aside from the nucleus to contain DNA. Other double-membraned structures include the nucleus and rough endoplasmic reticulum.

2. **E:** The rough endoplasmic reticulum appears rough due to the presence of associated ribosomes. The intermembrane space communicates with the nuclear intermembrane space at distinct locations.

3. **B:** The main differential for vesicular organelles is between lysosomes and peroxisomes. Lysosomes, unlike peroxisomes, contain hydrolases and do not participate in the pentose phosphate pathway.

4. **F:** This describes the nucleus. As well as chromosomes, it features nucleoli in its interior. These represent areas of ribosome assembly (from ribosomal RNA).

5. **A:** Lysosomes contain hydrolases, which differentiates them from peroxisomes

Chapter 2 Introduction to metabolism

Enzyme nomenclature

1. **A:** Incorporation of a phosphate group (phosphorylation) is mediated by kinases. These are ubiquitous in human physiology.

2. **G:** This question describes the transfer of a methyl group, but any transfer of a functional group between molecules is catalysed by transferase enzymes. In this example, the enzyme would be a methyltransferase.

3. **I:** This process is hydroxylation: the substrate has an '–OH' group attached, often to a carbon atom. Under physiological conditions, the hydrogen dissociates, leaving a charged negative oxygen atom behind. Phenylalanine hydroxylase is an important example of this enzyme, which is deficient in phenylketonuria.

4. **H:** This question describes isomerization, which unsurprisingly is mediated by isomerases. Glucose-6-phosphate isomerase is an example,

a key enzyme which interconverts fructose-6-phosphate and glucose-6-phosphate.

5. **D:** This defines a mutase. If the question had stated between molecules, it would refer to a transferase. An example is phosphoglycerate mutase, which features in glycolysis.

Chapter 5 Carbohydrate metabolism

Carbohydrate metabolism

1. **C:** On commencement of fasting, initially, glycogen reserves in muscle and liver cells are consumed by glycogenolysis. In the absence of gluconeogenesis, once these finite depots are depleted, hypoglycaemia would ensue. However, gluconeogenesis (a primarily anabolic pathway) converts noncarbohydrate substrates such as the products of other macronutrient catabolism (e.g., glycerol from lipolysis) into glucose to ensure blood [glucose] is maintained above the minimum levels.

2. **F:** Glutathione regeneration requires $NADPH + H^+$. The main mechanism of generation of $NADPH + H^+$ is the pentose phosphate pathway. It also converts dietary pentose sugars into hexose and triose intermediates which can participate in glycolysis.

3. **H:** This question describes galactosaemia. Patients lacking any of the three enzymes are unable to catabolize galactose, which results in toxic accumulation and irreversible damage to specific organs, for example, the central nervous system. The condition is managed by complete exclusion of galactose, which occurs primarily in lactose-containing food such as dairy products.

4. **A:** Cells lacking mitochondria cannot undertake oxidative phosphorylation. ATP generation is exclusively via substrate-level phosphorylation. Glycolysis is the only pathway that can operate in the absence of mitochondria. The anaerobic environment of mitochondria-free cell interiors (as for example red blood cells) is therefore deeply reliant on glycolysis for ATP generation for ATP-requiring intracellular processes, in particular maintenance of membrane integrity.

5. **G:** Aldolase B (also called 'fructose-1-phosphate aldolase') deficiency results in an accumulation of fructose-1-phosphate when

individuals consume fructose. This effectively sequesters intracellular phosphate. Glycogen phosphorylase and aldolase A enzymes are reliant on phosphorylation for their activation, thus glycogenolysis and gluconeogenesis, respectively, are impaired in this context. This results in fasting hypoglycaemia.

Chapter 6 Glucose homeostasis and diabetes mellitus

Different causes of diabetes

1. G: This child presents acutely with diabetic ketoacidosis. The history is typical for cystic fibrosis. This disease causes progressive pancreatic damage. Exocrine failure (impaired digestion and thus malabsorption and growth retardation) precedes endocrine failure. The secondary diabetes that develops is clinically identical to the more common autoimmune T1DM and is managed the same way with insulin injections.

2. J: Any disease known to affect the pancreas should lower the threshold of suspicion for T1DM. Gallstone pancreatitis is one of the most common causes of acute pancreatitis. This history of intermittent RUQ pain and steatorrhea in a patient with a predisposing tendency to (chronic haemolytic anaemia) gallstones means that the thirst and fatigue could well represent symptoms of new secondary diabetes.

3. H: This patient is presenting with new symptoms of diabetes. The skin discolouration and evidence of infiltrative disease (represented in this case by iron deposition in the heart, liver, spleen and joints) are suggestive of haemochromatosis. Progressive deposition of highly toxic free iron in organ parenchyma causes organ failure, as has occurred in this gentleman's pancreas and other organs.

4. E: New evidence of impaired glucose intolerance from investigations (fasting hyperglycaemia and hyperglycaemia post oral glucose tolerance test) is often clinically asymptomatic, as in this example of gestational diabetes mellitus. More severe hyperglycaemia (i.e., ≥ 7.0 mmol/L) would place the patient within the World Health Organization diagnostic criteria for diabetes in pregnancy.

5. B: An otherwise well and asymptomatic patient with fasting hyperglycaemia that is not quite severe enough to categorize the patient as diabetic (for diabetes the fasting blood [glucose] must be >7 mmol/L); this lady has a value of 6.8 mmol/L, which fits the criteria of impaired glucose tolerance. This can be thought of as an early developmental stage of T2DM; the risk factors are the same (obesity in this example). Her 2-hour postoral glucose tolerance test blood [glucose] being in the range 7.8–11.1 mmol/L would confirm impaired glucose tolerance.

Chapter 7 Lipid metabolism and lipid transport

Lipid transport particles

1. F: VLDL is the particle from which IDL and LDL evolve from as they offload their lipid cargo. Only chylomicrons are less dense.

2. E: IDL and LDL evolve from VLDL via progressive reduction in the hydrophobic lipid cargo, increasing the relative density of the particle. LDL is actually of higher density, hence IDL being the correct answer.

3. A: This defines a nascent chylomicron. It has not yet entered the vascular system (via the thoracic duct into the subclavian vein) and thus has not yet encountered HDL particles to appropriate apoprotein E and CII from.

4. B: This describes a mature chylomicron because it is within the vascular system where it has borrowed apoprotein E and CII from HDL particles. CII allows it to interact with LDL receptors and switch from transport to delivery mode.

5. C: All the other lipid transport vehicles confer net movement of their cargo lipids in the opposite direction, that is, towards the peripheral tissues where they deposit their lipids and cholesterol. Only HDL collects lipids/cholesterol from the tissues and exports it to the liver for excretion.

Chapter 8 Bioenergetics and obesity

Obesity treatment strategies

1. E: As her BMI exceeds 35 kg/m^2 (BMI 37 kg/m^2) and she has a reversible complication due to her obesity (T2DM) she is a candidate for bariatric surgery. The knee osteoarthritis at such a young age is likely to be weight related as well, though not reversible. A Roux-en-Y procedure requires a laparotomy with a large abdominal incision and would be hazardous for a patient with increased risk of bleeding, thus favouring the less invasive (laparoscopic) gastric band procedure. Nonetheless, a healthy diet and exercise should be strenuously recommended prior to surgery. Orlistat would be contraindicated in Crohn disease, so this option is not a viable alternative to surgery in her case.

2. A: This man is already exercising well, and his obesity (BMI 32 kg/m^2) is likely related to a significant energy intake excess rather than a lack of energy expenditure. The practice dietician or hospital nutritionist will be able to provide him with guidance and appropriate ideas for quick but healthy nutritious low-calorie meals to reduce his energy intake so that it no longer exceeds his energy expenditure. This will lead to weight loss if he complies.

3. C: This lady's BMI is 51 kg/m^2. Accordingly, her first-line treatment would ideally be bariatric surgery, however if she has capacity and refuses, this is not a viable option. Drug treatment would be appropriate, so Orlistat is therefore the best option for this lady who is already dieting and exercising.

4. B: This lady is in the BMI bracket 35–40 kg/m^2 (her BMI is 39 kg/m^2) where she would only be eligible for bariatric surgery if she had a reversible complication such as (as with the patient in question 1) T2DM. In her situation, an exercise programme would most likely confer maximum benefit to risk ratio, particularly when compared with surgery or drugs. As she is sedentary at work and at home even with a reduced energy intake, it still exceeds her energy expenditure. Exercise will remedy this.

5. C: Even if this young man had not already effectively exhausted all other treatment avenues, with his BMI at 58 >40 bariatric surgery would be offered as a first line treatment strategy. As he has recently survived a significant operative procedure and anaesthetic without complication despite, a Roux-en-Y procedure would represent the most effective approach in this gentleman.

Chapter 9 Protein metabolism and malnutrition

Biochemical features of amino acids

1. B: Tryptophan is also a melatonin precursor. Where dietary B3 is absent/severely restricted, endogenous B3 synthesis must occur, and this requires available tryptophan as a biosynthetic pathway substrate or 'raw material'.

2. B: With a single 'H' atom comprising the R-group, this small, aliphatic amino acid takes a prominent position in nitrogen excretion in muscle tissues via the glucose–alanine cycle. It is also the most abundant amino acid produced from muscle catabolism in starvation, when it is diverted to gluconeogenesis in the liver.

3. H: Proline, a nonessential amino acid derived by reduction of glutamate, shares a transporter with glycine. Multiple sequential proline residues in the primary structure form 'polyproline' helices, which are the predominant secondary structures seen in collagen, a vital structural protein. The hydroxylation of these prolines is vitamin C dependent, accounting for manifestations of defective collagen in vitamin C deficiency (scurvy).

4. I: This question describes cysteine. Oxidation of the thiol group of this sulphur-containing amino acid allows formation of disulphide bridges, a key component of tertiary and quaternary structure in proteins. Glutathione is a vital antioxidant and is of clinical significance in paracetamol overdose. Around 5% of ingested paracetamol is converted to a highly toxic metabolite [N-acetyl-p-benzoquinone imine (NAPQI)]. This is usually detoxified by glutathione conjugation. In overdose, the usual glucuronidation/sulphation pathways are saturated and greater amounts of paracetamol are metabolized to NAPQI, overwhelming the available pool of glutathione and resulting in hepatotoxicity. Intravenous acetylated cysteine is given as an antidote to replenish glutathione.

5. C: Tyrosine is usually derived from phenylalanine (by phenylalanine hydroxylase, deficient in phenylketonuria), hence its common molecular features. It is usually nonessential, but in phenylketonuria it cannot be synthesized endogenously and thus it becomes essential in the diet.

Chapter 10 Purines, pyrimidines, haem and one-carbon transfer

Causes of hyperuricaemia

1. C: Although enzyme deficiencies as a cause of (nearly absent hypoxanthine guanine phosphoribosyl transferase activity) of excessive urate production are an extremely rare cause of hyperuricaemia, this example describes a classic presentation.

2. D: This poor man has suffered crush injuries. Muscle death (rhabdomyolysis) results in large-scale release of intracellular contents, including nucleic acids into the circulation. Purine catabolism activity is extremely high, resulting in high urate production.

3. G: He has been consuming a high protein, low carbohydrate diet, which is ketogenic. Ketosis impairs urate excretion. High protein diets are usually also high in purines, increasing his risk for hyperuricaemia.

4. A: This patient is a victim of tumour lysis syndrome. Large numbers of neoplastic cells are killed by the induction chemotherapy, resulting in release of their intracellular contents causing acute kidney injury and the described electrolyte derangements. Renal insufficiency in this example is secondary to the tumour lysis syndrome: the urate is elevated due to the lysed tumour cell content liberation (intracellular contents including nucleic acids have their component purines catabolized, forming urate) rather than the failure to excrete the urate, although this will exacerbate the hyperuricaemia.

5. I: This gentleman has all the features of metabolic syndrome, which is strongly associated with hyperuricaemia. Loop and thiazide diuretics are a known cause of hyperuricaemia: but the question states he is using a β-blocker for control of his hypertension.

Chapter 12 Vitamins and their deficiencies

Symptoms, signs and treatment of abnormal vitamin status

1. I: Preterm babies are at particular risk of deficiency of fat-soluble vitamins. Haemorrhagic disease of the newborn (vitamin K deficiency) is not the cause in this instance; the baby received intramuscular vitamin K and furthermore this scenario typically manifests with gastrointestinal bleeding. This case is typical for severe vitamin E deficiency, and is effectively treated with parenteral vitamin E.

2. F: Vegans are at risk of B12 deficiency due to exclusion of the vast majority of B12-rich foods. Crohn disease compounds the risk. This lady with multiple autoimmune diseases is at risk of developing further autoimmunity. In this case, she has developed pernicious anaemia (PA; positive Schilling test) that has caused megaloblastic anaemia (macrocytic anaemia), which has led to the fatigue. The premature greying is a 'classical' sign of PA. Her folate status is normal due to supplementation, but she is B12 deficient due to PA, as evidenced by the elevated lactate, methylmalonic acid and homocysteine. The neurological symptoms represent typical signs of early subacute combined degeneration of the cord (see Box 12.13). This example illustrates the danger of blind folate supplementation without first confirming whether B12 deficiency is not also contributing to the symptoms: the neurological symptoms have progressed.

3. E: Scurvy (vitamin C deficiency) is rare in the UK, except in the elderly, homeless vagrants and alcohol dependent. Smoking increases the risk. This man has no access to fresh fruit or vegetables, and has manifested with typical symptoms of severe vitamin C deficiency. Intravenous Pabrinex is the acute treatment for repletion of exhausted vitamin C, but regular intake needs to be maintained (water-soluble vitamin) hence the supplementation and dietary advice.

4. A The symptoms are consistent with vitamin A deficiency; night blindness and evidence of deficient epithelialization of cornea and skin. Terminal ileal disease such as Crohn impairs micellar absorption, presenting risk of fat-soluble vitamin deficiency; in this lady this risk is compounded by exocrine pancreatic insufficiency: impaired lipase secretion leads to fat malabsorption as well.

5. J: This poor lady was generally malnourished from the anorexia, but also had specific risk factors for thiamine deficiency in particular (thiaminase-rich food, extremely high tea/coffee intake and chronic diuretic use). She exhibits neurological symptoms of chronic thiamine deficiency (dry beriberi), superimposed with acute exacerbation (Wernicke encephalopathy), precipitated by the acute infection developed on the psychiatric ward. The triad of ataxia, ophthalmoplegia (in particular a VI nerve palsy) and acute confusional state is the hallmark of Wernicke, and these symptoms rescind rapidly with parenteral B1, which is a component of Pabrinex.

Chapter 13 Minerals and their deficiencies

Symptoms and signs of abnormal mineral status

1. K: This lady is severely dehydrated from gastroenteritis, as suggested by the tachycardia, prolonged capillary refill, postural hypotension and oliguria as well as the 10% weight loss. She needs urgent rehydration and resuscitation. Intravascular hypovolaemia will result in serum hypernatraemia. Hypokalaemia is also likely, but is not listed above.

2. B: Absent sun exposure and exclusion of dairy products plus dark skin and high-latitude migration places this child at high risk for vitamin D deficiency. Because vitamin D drives calcium absorption, deficiency leads to secondary calcium deficiency. In adults, this causes osteomalacia, whereas in children rickets results. This child exhibits some of the characteristic bony deformities.

3. **H:** Vegans are at risk of iron deficiency, as are those suffering chronic blood loss. This lady exhibits typical microcytic anaemia with associated symptoms as well as signs specific to iron deficiency.

4. **G:** Wilson disease should be your first thought in this young patient with neurological symptoms (severe depression and tremor in this example) and hepatic dysfunction (as indicated by deranged liver function tests). Raised serum and urinary copper would also be noted. Treatment is with a metal chelator such as penicillamine.

5. **F:** This gentleman has experienced a renal stone as a complication of insidious hypercalcaemia secondary to malignancy. The electrolyte disturbance, very common in malignancy and particularly myeloma, is treated appropriately.

Chapter 14 Clinical assessment of metabolism and nutritional disorders

Investigations in metabolic/nutritional disease

1. **L:** The lady is being treated with a magnesium infusion. This reduces the hypertension and chance of intraventricular haemorrhage in severe preeclampsia unresponsive to first-line antihypertensives. Magnesium toxicity is a dangerous complication of the treatment; thus regular assessment for signs of toxicity and monitoring of vital signs is mandatory. In this scenario, magnesium toxicity should be the first suspected cause for her collapse, and appropriate treatment (stopping the infusion, airway support, oxygenation, calcium gluconate, etc.) should be immediately undertaken before serum confirmation of elevated magnesium. Retrospective analysis may be needed, however, and as such the only appropriate investigation is L.

2. **E:** The newborn blood spot test is performed on all babies in the UK. It screens for congenital hypothyroidism, cystic fibrosis, sickle cell disease and six serious inborn errors of metabolism.

3. **D:** The patient is critically ill with diabetic ketoacidosis: his first presentation of new type 1 diabetes, provoked by the acute chest infection. The polyuria was secondary to glycosuria from elevated blood sugar. He is acutely unwell, clinically severely dehydrated and exhibiting Kussmaul respiration, suggesting metabolic acidosis. He requires aggressive rehydration, insulin replacement, potassium replacement guided by an appropriate diabetic ketoacidosis emergency protocol. The best and most appropriate investigation above is D; this will rapidly quantify the glucose levels, extent of metabolic acidosis, hypokalaemia, raised anion gap and give all the information needed to guide immediate resuscitation. Option C is a monitoring investigation used to assess adequacy of therapy in diabetics over the long term, and would not add anything to the clinical diagnosis or urgent management.

4. **G:** This gentleman is exhibiting classic neurological, cardiovascular and gastrointestinal signs and symptoms of thiamine (B1) deficiency or 'wet' beriberi. White rice has been 'polished', that is, the thiamine-rich husks removed, which puts people at risk of thiamine deficiency if the remainder of the diet is not suitably diverse to compensate. A serum thiamine level would be more usual as a first-line treatment but is not included above. The only investigation above that would diagnose thiamine deficiency is serum thiamine which is measured by high-performance liquid chromatography; therefore G is the correct option. Historically, red cell transketolase activity (which would be decreased) would have been the investigation of choice. Given the high likelihood of the diagnosis from the history and examination, most practitioners would commence thiamine replacement without waiting for the result, but in the event that this did not begin to correct the reversible symptoms a negative result would be clinically valuable, allowing consideration of alternative diagnoses.

5. **H:** Urinary porphobilinogen test is positive, identifying a porphyria. The symptoms presenting here are manifestations of variegate porphyria, although presentation is often clinically indistinguishable from acute intermittent or hereditary coproporphyria. Episodic abdominal pain is due to enteric nervous system involvement, and the low $[Na^+]$ secondary to syndrome of inappropriate secretion of ADH, which is associated with acute episodes in many of the porphyrias. The chronic blistering lesions represent skin photosensitivity, which features in variegate porphyria, porphyria cutanea tarda, hepatoerythropoietic porphyria and congenital erythropoietic porphyria. Option H is the only option which allows further differentiation between hereditary coproporphyria and variegate porphyria according to the relative patterns of elevation in plasma and faecal porphyrins. This is therefore the correct option.

Glossary

Acyl carrier protein A protein or a domain of a protein that contains thiol groups which provide attachment sites for malonyl-coenzyme A (malonyl-CoA) and growing fatty acid chains.

Adenosine diphosphate (ADP) A ribonucleotide diphosphate in which two phosphoryl groups are successively linked to the 5′ oxygen atom of adenosine.

Adenosine monophosphate (AMP) A ribonucleotide monophosphate in which a phosphoryl group is linked to the 5′ oxygen atom of adenosine.

Adenosine triphosphate (ATP) A nucleotide containing a purine base (adenine), a five-carbon sugar, ribose and three phosphate groups.

Adenosine triphosphatase (ATPase) An enzyme that catalyses hydrolysis of ATP to ADP + inorganic phosphate (P_i).

Adipose tissue Also known as 'fat tissue'. Animal tissue composed of specialized triacylglycerol-storage cells known as adipocytes. There is growing evidence that adipocytes are hormonally active secreting a range of so-called adipokines (e.g. leptin is an adipokine).

Aerobic Occurring in the presence of oxygen.

Amino acid An organic acid consisting of an α-carbon atom to which an amino group, a carboxyl group, a hydrogen atom and a specific side chain (R-group) are attached.

Anabolism The synthesis of complex molecules from simpler ones. Anabolism is associated with energy entrapment and storage.

Anaemia The blood haemoglobin below the normal range for the patient's age and sex. The normal range in males is 13.5–18.0 g/dL and in females is 11.5–16.0 g/dL.

Anaerobic Occurring in the absence of oxygen.

Atherogenic Able to start or speed up the process of atherogenesis, which is the inflammation-driven formation of lipid deposits in the arteries leading to thickening and hardening of the arterial wall.

Autophosphorylation Phosphorylation of a protein kinase catalysed by the same kinase.

Bioenergetics The study of the energy changes accompanying biochemical reactions.

β-oxidation A cyclical sequence of reactions that degrade fatty acids to acetyl-CoA. It consists of four steps: oxidation, hydration, further oxidation and thiolysis.

Carbohydrate A complex molecule in which the molar ratio of C:H:O is 1:2:1.

Carnitine shuttle A pathway that shuttles acetyl-CoA from the cytosol to the mitochondria through the formation of acyl carnitine.

Catabolism The breakdown of energy-rich complex molecules (e.g. carbohydrate) to simpler ones (e.g. CO_2, H_2O). Catabolism is associated with energy release.

Chaperone A protein that forms complexes with newly synthesized polypeptide chains and assists in their correct folding into biologically functional conformations.

Chylomicron A plasma lipoprotein that transports dietary lipids absorbed from the intestine to the tissues.

Citrate shuttle A pathway that shuttles acetyl-CoA from the mitochondria to the cytosol providing a substrate for fatty acid synthesis.

Condensation A reaction involving the joining of two or more molecules accompanied by the elimination of water.

Cori cycle An interorgan metabolic loop that distributes the metabolic burden between the muscle and the liver. Lactate, which builds up in muscle during intense activity, is taken to the liver to be converted back to glucose via gluconeogenesis. This replenishes fuel for the muscle and prevents lactic acidosis. The produced glucose returns to muscle as an energy source, completing the cycle.

C-terminus The amino acid residue bearing a free carboxyl group (–COOH) at one end of a peptide chain.

Cytochrome A haem-containing protein that is an electron carrier in processes such as respiration and photosynthesis.

Deaminase An enzyme that catalyses the removal of an amino group from a substrate, releasing ammonia.

Dehydrogenase An enzyme catalysing oxidation–reduction reactions involving addition or extraction of hydrogen atoms.

De novo pathway A metabolic pathway in which a biomolecule is formed 'from scratch', from simple precursor molecules.

Diabetes mellitus A syndrome caused by the lack, or diminished effectiveness, of insulin, resulting in a raised blood glucose (hyperglycaemia) and the presence of chronic vascular complications.

Dyslipidaemias A group of disorders caused by a defect in lipoprotein formation, transport or degradation.

Electron transport chain A series of mitochondrial enzyme complexes and associated cofactors that are electron carriers, passing electrons from reduced CoAs or substrates to molecular oxygen (O_2), the terminal electron acceptor of aerobic metabolism.

Endergonic reaction A reaction during which there is a net gain of free energy, $\Delta G > 0$. Such reactions do not occur spontaneously.

Endocytosis Process by which matter is engulfed by a plasma membrane and brought into the cell within a lipid vesicle derived from the membrane.

Endothermic reaction A reaction during which there is heat absorption – a positive enthalpy change ($+\Delta H$).

Enthalpy change (ΔH) A measure of the heat released or absorbed during a reaction.

Entropy change (ΔS) A measure of the change in disorder or randomness in a reaction.

Enzyme A biological catalyst that is almost always a protein.

Essential amino acid An amino acid that cannot be synthesized by the body and must be obtained from the diet.

Essential fatty acid A fatty acid that cannot be synthesized by the body and must be obtained from the diet.

Exergonic reaction A reaction during which there is a net loss of free energy, $\Delta G < 0$. Such reactions proceed spontaneously.

Exothermic reaction There is a release of heat during the reaction – a negative enthalpy change ($-\Delta H$).

Fatty acid breakdown The process in which a molecule of fatty acid is degraded by the sequential removal of two carbon units, producing acetyl-CoA, which is then oxidized to CO_2 and H_2O by the tricarboxylic acid (TCA) cycle.

Fatty acid synthesis A cyclical reaction in which a molecule of fatty acid is built up by the sequential addition of two carbons units derived from acetyl-CoA.

Feedback inhibition Inhibition of an enzyme that catalyses an early step in a metabolic pathway by an end product of the same pathway.

Free energy change A thermodynamic state that defines the equilibrium in terms of the changes in enthalpy and entropy of a system at constant pressure, $\Delta G = \Delta H - T \times \Delta S$.

Free radical A highly reactive atomic or molecular species with unpaired electron.

Gluconeogenesis Production of glucose from noncarbohydrate sources (e.g. amino acids, lactate, glycerol).

Glucose–alanine cycle An interorgan metabolic loop that transports nitrogen (as alanine) to the liver and transports metabolic fuel (glucose) from the liver to the peripheral tissues.

Glycation Nonenzymatic reaction resulting in binding of a sugar molecule to a protein.

Glycogen A large, highly branched polymer of glucose molecules joined by α-1,4 linkages with α-1,6 linkages at branch points.

Glycolysis Catabolic pathway consisting of 10 enzyme-catalysed reactions by which one molecule of glucose is broken down into two molecules of pyruvate.

Glycoprotein A complex protein molecule containing carbohydrate residues, produced through the glycosylation of proteins in the endoplasmic reticulum or in the Golgi apparatus.

Glycosaminoglycan Long unbranched polysaccharides consisting of repeating disaccharide units. The disaccharide unit consists of an N-acetyl-hexosamine and a hexose or hexuronic acid, either or both of which may be sulphated.

Glycosides A group of organic compounds, occurring abundantly in plants, that yield a sugar and one or more nonsugar substances on hydrolysis.

Glycosylation The enzymatic addition of glycosyl groups to a protein to form a glycoprotein.

Haemoglobin A tetrameric, haem-containing globular protein in erythrocytes that carries oxygen to cells and tissues.

High-density lipoprotein (HDL) A type of plasma lipoprotein that is rich in protein and transports cholesterol and cholesteryl esters from tissues to the liver (this is known as the 'reverse cholesterol transport').

Hydrolase An enzyme that catalyses the hydrolytic cleavage of its substrate.

Hydrophilic 'Water loving'. A molecule that interacts with polar solvents, in particular with water, or with other polar groups.

Hydrophobic 'Water fearing'. Nonpolar compounds that do not dissolve in water, such as oil.

Intermediate-density lipoprotein (IDL) A type of plasma lipoprotein that is formed during the transformation of very-low-density lipoprotein (VLDL). IDLs are also called 'remnant lipoproteins' and are atherogenic.

Isomerase An enzyme that catalyses a change in geometry or structure within one molecule.

Isozymes Enzymes from a single biological species that catalyse the same reaction.

Ketogenesis A five-step pathway that synthesizes ketone bodies from acetyl-CoA in the mitochondrial matrix.

Ketone bodies Small molecules that are synthesized from acetyl-CoA in the liver (acetoacetic acid, acetone, 3-hydroxybutyric acid).

Kinase An enzyme that catalyses the transfer of a phosphoryl group to an acceptor molecule.

Lipase An enzyme that catalyses the hydrolysis of triacylglycerols.

Lipid A water-insoluble organic compound found in biological systems.

Lipolysis The hydrolysis of triacylglycerols by lipase. (Note that lipolysis is different from fatty acid breakdown.)

Lipoprotein A macromolecular assembly of lipid and protein molecules with a hydrophobic core and a hydrophilic surface, present in plasma. Lipoproteins transport triacylglycerols (triglycerides) and cholesterol between tissues.

Low-density lipoprotein (LDL) A type of plasma lipoprotein that is formed during the breakdown of IDL and is enriched in cholesterol and cholesteryl esters. LDL is atherogenic. The measurement of plasma cholesterol reflects mainly the concentration of LDL.

Lysosome A specialized digestive organelle in eukaryotic cells.

Metabolism An integrated set of chemical reactions occurring in the body. The sum of chemical reactions in the body.

Micelle An aggregation of amphipathic (both water-repellent and water-friendly) molecules in which the hydrophilic portions of the molecules project into the aqueous environment and the hydrophobic portions point into the interior of the structure.

Mitochondrion An organelle that is the main site of oxidative energy metabolism in eukaryotic cells.

Nonessential amino acid An amino acid that can be produced in sufficient quantity to meet metabolic needs.

N terminus The amino acid residue bearing a free α-amino group ($-NH_2$) at one end (conventionally a beginning) of a peptide chain.

Nucleophilic A chemical compound or group that is attracted to nuclei and tends to donate or share electrons.

Nucleoside A compound containing a purine or pyrimidine and a sugar: a purine or pyrimidine N-glycoside of ribose or deoxyribose.

Nucleotide The phosphate ester of a nucleoside, consisting of a nitrogenous base linked to a pentose phosphate.

Oxidase An enzyme that catalyses an oxidation–reduction reaction in which O_2 is the electron acceptor.

Oxidation The loss of electrons by a molecule, atom or ion. Gain of oxygen or loss of hydrogen by a molecule.

Oxidative deamination The removal of an amino group from an amino acid, which leaves behind the oxidised carbon skeleton.

Oxidative phosphorylation A process in which ATP is formed as electrons are transferred from NADH and $FADH_2$ to molecular oxygen, via a series of electron carriers that make up the electron transport chain.

Pentose phosphate pathway A pathway by which glucose-6-phosphate is metabolized to generate nicotinamide adenine dinucleotide phosphate (reduced form of $NADP^+$; 'NADPH') and ribose-5-phosphate.

Peptide Two or more amino acids covalently joined in a linear sequence by peptide bonds.

Peptide bond The covalent secondary amide linkage that joins the carbonyl oxygen atom, the amide hydrogen atom and the two adjacent amino acids in a peptide.

Peroxidase An enzyme that catalyses a reaction in which hydrogen peroxide is the oxidizing agent.

Phosphatase An enzyme that catalyses the hydrolytic removal of a phosphoryl group.

Phosphorylase An enzyme that catalyses the cleavage of its substrate via nucleophilic attack by inorganic phosphate.

Phosphorylation A reaction involving the addition of a phosphoryl group to a molecule.

P:O ratio The ratio of molecules of ADP phosphorylated to atoms of oxygen reduced during oxidative phosphorylation.

Polypeptide A polymer of many amino acid residues linked by peptide bonds.

Polysaccharide A polymer of many monosaccharide residues linked by glycosidic bonds.

Protease An enzyme that catalyses hydrolysis of peptide bonds.

Protein A biopolymer consisting of one or more polypeptide chains.

Protein glycosylation The covalent addition of carbohydrate to proteins.

Proteoglycans A special class of glycoproteins that are heavily glycosylated. They consist of a core protein with one or more covalently attached glycosaminoglycan chains.

Purine A nitrogenous base with a two-ring structure in which a pyrimidine is fused to imidazole (e.g. adenine, guanine).

Pyrimidine A nitrogenous base having a heterocyclic ring that consists of four carbon atoms and two nitrogen atoms (e.g. thymine, cytosine).

Reducing agent A substance that provides (as it itself loses) electrons in an oxidation–reduction reaction thereby becoming oxidized.

Reduction The gain of electrons by a molecule, atom or ion. Loss of oxygen or gain of hydrogen by a molecule.

RNA A polymer consisting of ribonucleotide residues joined by $3'-5'$ phosphodiester bonds. The sugar moiety is ribose.

Ribose A five-carbon monosaccharide that is the carbohydrate component of RNA.

Salvage pathway A pathway in which a major metabolite, such as purine or pyrimidine nucleotide, can be synthesized from a preformed molecular entity, such as a purine or pyrimidine, rather than synthesized de novo.

Saturated fatty acid A fatty acid that does not contain a carbon–carbon double bond.

Standard redox potential (E_o) A measure of the tendency of a particular redox pair (e.g. nicotinamide adenine dinucleotide (NAD^+) and NADH) to lose electrons.

Steroid A lipid characterized by a carbon skeleton with four fused rings. All steroids are derived from the acetyl-CoA.

Sterol A steroid containing a hydroxyl group.

Substrate-level phosphorylation Formation of ATP by direct phosphorylation of ADP, without requiring mitochondrial respiratory chain.

Transaminase An enzyme that catalyses the transfer of an α-amino group (NH_3^+) from an amino acid to an α-keto acid.

Triacylglycerol (triglyceride) A lipid containing three fatty acyl residues esterified to a glycerol backbone.

Tricarboxylic acid cycle (TCA) A cyclical sequence of eight reactions that completely oxidize one molecule of acetyl-CoA to two molecules of CO_2, generating energy either directly as ATP or in the form of reducing equivalents (NADH or $FADH_2$).

Ubiquitin A small basic protein that binds to a protein and targets it for degradation.

Unsaturated fatty acid A fatty acid with at least one carbon–carbon double bond.

Urea cycle A metabolic cycle consisting of five reactions that synthesize the organic compound urea from two inorganic compounds: CO_2 and NH_4^+.

Very-low-density lipoprotein (VLDL) A type of plasma lipoprotein that transports mostly endogenous triacylglycerols, and also cholesterol and cholesteryl esters from the liver to the tissues.

Vitamin An organic micronutrient that cannot be synthesized by the body and must be obtained from the diet.

Water-soluble vitamin An organic micronutrient that is soluble in water.

Note: Page numbers followed by *f* indicate figures, *t* indicate tables, and *b* indicate boxes.

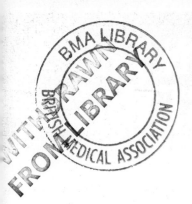